BREAKTHROUGH

BREAKTHROUGH

Elizabeth Hughes,

the Discovery of Insulin, and

the Making of a Medical Miracle

THEA COOPER and ARTHUR AINSBERG

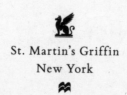

St. Martin's Griffin
New York

www.stmartins.com

Text design by Meryl Sussman Levavi

The Library of Congress has cataloged the hardcover edition as follows:

Cooper, Thea.
   Breakthrough : Elizabeth Hughes, the discovery of insulin, and the making
of a medical miracle / Thea Cooper and Arthur Ainsberg. —1st ed.
       p. cm.
   ISBN 978-0-312-64870-1
   1. Insulin—History.   2. Gossett, Elizabeth Hughes, 1908–1981—Health.
3. Diabetes—Treatment—History.   I. Ainsberg, Arthur.   II. Title.
   QP572.15.C66 2010
   612.3'4—dc22   2010021662

ISBN 978-0-312-61174-3 (trade paperback)

10   9   8   7   6   5   4   3

To my parents, who instilled in me a deep appreciation of stories; and to my husband, Craig, and my children, Jane and Ian, who continue to inspire me.

—T.C.

To the dedicated doctors, nurses, and staff at Mount Sinai Hospital in New York City, the Cleveland Clinic of Cleveland, Ohio, and the Mayo Clinic of Rochester, Minnesota, who have been my inspiration for the past thirty-five years.

—A.A.

CONTENTS

PREFACE

BREAKTHROUGH BEGAN AS A CASUAL GLANCE AT AN ARTICLE IN *The New York Times Magazine* in March 2003. It led to a consuming research project that would take us to medical centers, universities, libraries, archives, and other sites of significance located in twenty-five cities and towns in eight states and four countries over the course of nearly five years.

Initially, our research focused on Elizabeth Hughes, but we soon discovered that she was the nucleus of a constellation of characters, each of whom was as fascinating and enigmatic as Elizabeth herself. The discovery of these new characters led inexorably to more research and more discoveries. At a certain point our biggest challenge became choosing which of the many engaging characters and stories to focus on.

Eventually we decided to focus on four primary characters: Elizabeth Hughes Gossett, Frederick Grant Banting, Frederick Madison Allen, and George Henry Alexander Clowes. It was particularly difficult to relegate the captivating personality of Charles Evans Hughes to secondary importance. The remarkable J. K. Lilly Sr., along with his sons Eli Lilly Jr. and J. K. Lilly Jr., also introduced tangential story lines that were hard to resist.

This book is based on a true story, and relies heavily on primary historical sources and documents. With one exception, detailed in the section *Notes and Sources,* all characters are historical figures. Most dialogue and incidents have been drawn from contemporaneous sources, but in some cases have been invented or augmented for narrative purposes.

To the glory of God with thanksgiving for the wonder of life.

—Inscription on the grave of Eli Lilly,
Crown Hill Cemetery, Indianapolis

BREAKTHROUGH

PROLOGUE

I N 1918 AN ELEVEN-YEAR-OLD GIRL STANDS IN THE KITCHEN OF HER family's elegant townhouse gulping water from a glass with such ferocity that it runs down the sides of her face. It is her sixth glass. Elizabeth Hughes is the daughter of Charles Evans Hughes, one of New York City's most highly respected and familiar citizens. In a few months her diagnosis will be confirmed, and what had been a happy, active childhood will be devoured by the mounting symptoms of ravenous hunger and insatiable thirst. She has diabetes mellitus, also known as type 1 or juvenile diabetes.* It carries a prognosis of eleven months of suffering followed by death.

Most of the food a person eats is turned into glucose, or sugar, for his or her body to use for energy. A healthy pancreas makes the hormone insulin, which helps glucose get into the body's cells. A diabetic either doesn't make enough insulin or can't use it well.

Symptoms of diabetes were described on Egyptian papyrus as early as 1550 B.C. The recommended Egyptian treatment was to eat a boiled assortment of bones, wheat, grain, and earth for four days, a diet perhaps no more satisfying than that prescribed for the disease in 1918. Progress toward understanding and treating diabetes has been slow and halting. It wouldn't be given its current name until the second century A.D.—thousands

---

* There are two major types of diabetes: Type 1 diabetes is defined by the body's failure to produce insulin; type 2 diabetes is defined by the body's resistance to or insufficient production of insulin. Type 1 diabetes is also called insulin-dependent diabetes, or juvenile diabetes, because it affects mostly children, teenagers, and young adults.

of years after its appearance on papyrus. Aretaeus of Cappadocia, a celebrated Greek physician, coined the term "diabetes" after the Greek word for "sieve" because the symptomatic incessant thirst and urination made the body act as a sieve. Three centuries later, Indian physicians noted that the urine of their diabetic patients tasted sweet, like honey, but they did not know why. For the next thirteen centuries, little more was learned.

In the eighteenth century an Englishman named Matthew Dobson determined that the sweet, sticky substance found in diabetic urine was sugar. His important contribution ushered in a series of advances during the nineteenth century. In 1856, Claude Bernard, the French physician known as "the Father of Physiology," postulated that the pancreas was the probable source of the disease. In 1889, Germany's Oskar Minkowski and Josef von Mering definitively confirmed the central role of the pancreas. After removing the organ from a dog, the animal exhibited all the classic symptoms of diabetes. This monumental discovery launched a decades-long search for a mysterious substance in the pancreas. Germany's Paul Langerhans described a cluster of cells that he separated from the pancreas in 1869, but he did not investigate its purpose. In 1889, France's Edouard Laguesse named these cells the islets of Langerhans after their discoverer and suggested these cells lower blood glucose levels. As the twentieth century dawned, Belgium's Jean de Meyer named the mysterious pancreatic substance "insulin"—from the Latin word for island—yet its existence was only a scientific speculation.

Around the world, the search for insulin continued. Germany's Georg Zuelzer claimed to have isolated the pancreatic substance in 1906, going as far as obtaining a patent in 1912. Unfortunately, he was unable to produce enough consistently effective extract to prove it. America's Ernest L. Scott made similar claims and met similar failure in 1912. And so medical science continued to struggle with how to use insulin to alleviate diabetes. For type 1 diabetics, this struggle was a matter of life and death, Elizabeth Hughes included.

In 1918, despite thousands of years of medical scrutiny, physicians could only watch helplessly as diabetic children like Elizabeth died. They yearned for a cure or at least a treatment that would prolong their patients' lives until the cure that had eluded medicine for centuries could be found. That was exactly what Dr. Frederick M. Allen accomplished with his "starvation treatment," a drastic diet that usually succeeded in keeping diabetics alive, albeit as living skeletons, for months beyond their prognoses. To be sure, some patients starved to death under his care, but Allen reasoned that they would have died anyway. In 1918 this desperate course was the only hope that diabetics had. The years 1914 to 1922 were known as the Allen era of diabetes research. Elizabeth Hughes would become one of Allen's most tragic and successful patients.

Ironically, a cure for diabetes couldn't have been farther from the mind of the man who would be at the very center of its discovery. In 1918 Frederick Banting was too busy tending to wounded soldiers in the fetid trenches of Cambrai, France, to think about medicine's next marvel. When the war allowed him a rare quiet moment, he likely thought about his fiancée, Edith, walking to church on the dirt roads of Alliston, Canada, or the family farm where he had grown up. His aspirations were to marry and find a job as an orthopedic surgeon. In these goals he would be thwarted. Instead, he would find himself bound for a destiny of international fame and fortune that he was ill equipped to manage. This trajectory would be launched, in no small measure, by Elizabeth Hughes.

Elizabeth Hughes could not have foreseen how these very different men would figure prominently in her life. In 1918, she was a healthy, adventurous American girl, destined for all the promise and privilege that her famous parentage afforded her. Everything would change in 1919.

ONE

Christ Church Cranbrook, Bloomfield Hills, Michigan, 1981

ON TUESDAY, APRIL 28, 1981, MOURNERS BEGAN TO CONVERGE ON the wet streets around Christ Church Cranbrook in Bloomfield Hills, Michigan. Emerging from their late model cars, they tucked under umbrellas and made their way through the raw spring air toward the carillon bells ringing from the tower. Inside the sanctuary, organ music soared from the south wall of the nave, drawing the eye upward to the intricately carved wood, stone, and brilliant stained glass. As the mourners were ushered into pews, they nodded solemnly to one another; most everyone knew each other. They were gathered to acknowledge the passing of and pay tribute to the remarkable life of a seventy-three-year-old woman who had died three days before. Her name was Elizabeth Hughes Gossett.

Although most of the mourners would likely claim to have known Elizabeth well, only a few people in the church knew just how remarkable her life really was. Dr. Lowell Eklund, dean of continuing education at Oakland University in Rochester, Michigan, rose to the pulpit to deliver the eulogy. He mentioned Elizabeth's "intellect, wisdom, quiet yet irresistible leadership." He mentioned her distinguished service as a trustee of her alma mater, Barnard College, in New York City. He said that she, like her father, America's most famous lawyer, jurist, and politician, had been a lifelong advocate of self-directed scholarship and perpetual inquiry. It was this spirit, he said, that had led her to play an important role in the founding of Oakland University in 1957.

Did Eklund know that the circumstances of her early life had *forced* her to pursue her education as a self-directed and largely solitary endeavor? If he knew, he didn't say.

As heiress to the legacy of a great American statesman, she carried forth her father's ideals with "modesty, dignity and grace," he said. Dr. Eklund described her as "a champion of civil rights in speech, in document and in action." He went on to say that she had cofounded, with her friend Chief Justice Warren Burger, the Supreme Court Historical Society in 1974. But did Eklund know why this daughter was especially compelled to protect her father's legacy, of how the great man had risked everything for her sake?

Sitting in the front pew with his smooth, clean hands folded in his lap was William T. Gossett, to whom Elizabeth had been married for fifty years, a former member of the church vestry. Around him were seated their three children, Antoinette, William, and Elizabeth, and next to them were their spouses, Basil, Mary, and Fred, respectively. Also seated in front were the eight grandchildren, the eldest of whom was David Wemyss Denning, son of Antoinette and Basil. In 1981 he was a twenty-four-year-old medical student. Dappled light, steeped in the rich jewel tones of the towering east window, played over the heads of the family like the lightest touch from an invisible hand.

David knew that Eklund would not mention what to his mind was one of the most important and remarkable facts of his grandmother's life. This fact had also been omitted from his grandmother's obituaries in *The New York Times*, *The Washington Post*, *The Los Angeles Times*, and the leading Michigan papers. In 1922, Elizabeth Hughes was among the first children to receive an experimental pancreatic extract called insulin. By the time of her death, she had received some 42,000 insulin injections over fifty-eight years, probably more than anyone on earth at that time. And yet, through Elizabeth Gossett's own steadfast efforts only a few people knew this, and those few were sworn to secrecy.

How ironic to hear Eklund describe Elizabeth as a lover of history; it was a perfect alibi for someone who had made a lifework of obfuscating her own history. This effort had been so successful that Dr. Eklund had no knowledge of the brave, bright spirit whose childhood had been tempered in the crucible of death's daily and intimate companionship.

The last will and testament of Elizabeth Hughes Gossett arranged for the disposition of her jewelry, personal effects, and works of art. After the will was executed, there remained in her estate an odd collection of cryptic relics, like a muddle of jigsaw puzzle pieces from different puzzles:

+ Thirty or so letters tied with a satin ribbon. The letters had been written by Elizabeth during 1921 and 1922, mostly to her mother ("Mumsey"), when Elizabeth was fourteen and fifteen years old. The letters had been written from New York State, Bermuda, and Toronto, marking points on her peripatetic attempt to evade the death that pursued her relentlessly.

+ A small, hand-knitted sweater of fine, faded blue wool, which looked to be made for a child eight or nine years old.

+ An old photograph of a modest house in Glens Falls, New York, showing a rocking chair on the front porch. On the back of the image were the words, *Save one life and save the world*, written in indigo ink in an elegant hand.

+ A square of canvas removed from its frame, bearing a rough oil painting of a farmhouse rendered in pigments of burnt umber and cobalt.

+ A small brown glass medicinal vial with an age-yellowed label on which the words had faded to illegibility.

These mute artifacts were all that remained of Elizabeth Hughes's life before her miraculous transformation into an entirely different girl. What follows is the improbable story of *that* Elizabeth—*the Elizabeth that Elizabeth erased*. This is the story of Elizabeth Hughes, who "vanished" in December of 1922 without a memorial service or a funeral, without anyone ever really even noticing.

TWO

Fifth Avenue, New York City, April 1919

Dr. Frederick M. Allen gazed around his meticulously tidy office at 5 East Fifty-first Street in Manhattan and prepared to make the trip, thirteen blocks uptown, to 32 East Sixty-fourth Street: the home of Gotham's distinguished citizen, Charles Evans Hughes. Allen was a brilliant medical investigator, the author of *Glycosuria and Diabetes,* the most extensive history of the search for a cure for diabetes. Known as "Dr. Diabetes," he had held research positions at both Harvard Medical School and the Rockefeller Institute. This notoriety was a mixed blessing, rather like being a very good and experienced executioner. If you must have one, you want a good one, but you hope to never need one.

Allen was self-conscious in the presence of men of great importance and wealth. He had no way of knowing that Hughes had come from a background even more humble than his own. Born in Iowa in 1879, Allen moved to California when he was eleven, where his father grew oranges. He attended the University of California as an undergraduate and continued through medical school, graduating just a year after the 1906 San Francisco earthquake. He then volunteered at an animal lab at Harvard, where he was eventually hired and earned a small stipend of $47.50 per month.

After three years and four hundred dogs at the Harvard animal lab he borrowed five thousand dollars from his father—fully one-fifth of his father's entire worth—to publish *Glycosuria and Diabetes* in 1913. At the time he had not published a single journal article, but he had a guileless faith that his book, written in painstaking longhand, would open the doors to a scientific career. Shortly after the book was published, the Rockefeller Institute of Medical Research offered him a position as chief physician of an investigative ward of its hospital at York Avenue and Sixty-sixth Street in Manhattan. Allen accepted the offer and relocated to New York.

In his new role, he succeeded in applying the knowledge gained at the Harvard animal lab to humans in a hospital setting. Unfortunately, he found that not only was working with human patients more frustrating than working with dogs, it also produced inferior results. Humans were unreliable subjects, difficult to control. They promised to comply with instructions and then failed to do so. They forgot. They cheated. They misunderstood. They succumbed to temptation with infuriating regularity. No amount of chiding seemed sufficient to persuade them of the importance of *complete* cooperation, and their repeated deviations and indiscretions jeopardized the integrity of his findings.

At Rockefeller Allen soon became known as an intensely dedicated worker. He was also impatient and thin-skinned. He did not mix well with his well-born colleagues and he was unpopular with the diabetic patients under his care. He was let go, and his position was turned over to another doctor, a political favorite whose background as a chemist, although vaunted, was not especially relevant to the work in which Allen had invested so much. It was a scalding professional rebuke.

By this time the United States had entered the Great War in Europe and Allen was sent to serve as an army doctor at General Hospital No. 9 in Lakewood, New Jersey. He published a second book, *Total Dietary Regulation in the Treatment of Diabetes,* which cited exhaustive case records of 76 of the 100 diabetes patients he had observed during his five years at Rockefeller. After his military discharge he struggled to launch a private practice in New York City. Only the most hopeless patients sought him out, and always as a last resort. He treated primarily children who were dying. One four-year-old boy, admitted to his care in the spring of 1917, had won a contest for being the most perfect baby a year or so before. As these patients survived weeks and occasionally months beyond their prognoses, more doctors referred their patients to him and he recovered from the humiliation of his Rockefeller years.

By the end of the first decade of the twentieth century, Dr. Frederick Allen and Dr. Elliott Joslin had become the two most widely recognized diabetologists in the nation. The small-boned and well-mannered Joslin had inherited significant wealth, attended Yale University, and graduated as valedictorian of his Harvard Medical School class. At Harvard, Allen and Joslin forged an unlikely friendship that would endure for decades. They contributed in different but complementary ways to the study of diabetes. Allen's expertise was in the alchemical combination of fasting, undernutrition, and exercise to stem the progression of diabetes. He was the first to see that it wasn't just carbohydrates that stressed the metabolism, but protein and fat as well. Therefore, the best approach was to find, for each patient, the minimum amount of food required to live. This proved to be a highly exacting calculus that varied from patient to patient and, for each patient, from day to day and from hour to hour. The expression "The cure is worse than the disease" may not have been coined for the Allen treatment, but it fit.

Joslin focused on improving the medical chronicle of diabetes. At the time, there was no standardized protocol for medical documentation. Joslin believed that improving the way patient data was recorded could improve the diagnostic process. He began a diabetic registry, the first such system for recording diabetic patient data outside of Europe. Throughout their careers Allen and Joslin regularly conferred with each other about patients. Both experimented with a new model of working with diabetic patients that involved educating them about diabetes and enlisting them as participants in their own treatment. This was a significant departure from the typical doctor-patient relationship at that time. Not all patients were open to such modernity and to assuming some responsibility for their own care.

On this day in April, Allen was to tell Charles and Antoinette Hughes that Elizabeth would not likely survive through the summer. Her only hope was to completely surrender to his extremely onerous therapy. While errands such as the one that occupied him on that April morning in 1919 were not unknown to Allen, clinical care could hardly be called his strong suit. Allen preferred the study of disease to the care of those unhappy individuals beset with it. He was a portly, balding, forty-year-old bachelor with thin lips and a gaze both exacting and remote; he looked like a man whose job it was to deliver bad news.

He was nervous. It was imperative that this meeting go well, which was no mean feat considering the meeting's purpose. He was building a private practice for the first time in his life. The admission of such a high profile patient as Elizabeth Hughes would be invaluable in establishing his new venture. The patient's father, Charles Evans Hughes, knew everyone. For someone as challenged in salesmanship as Allen was, the advocacy of such a highly regarded public figure would be a huge coup.

The doctor's scalp began to perspire where the smooth leather hatband fit against the thinning hair of his head. He stopped to pull a handkerchief from his jacket, his too-large hand fumbling in the narrow inside pocket. Although Allen had now established himself as a prolific author he had not written the slender, red book he was carrying, intended as a gift for the Hugheses. *Starvation (Allen) Treatment of Diabetes,* by Lewis Webb Hill, M.D., and Rena Eckman was a mere 134 pages and written in language that a lay practitioner or a patient could understand. It plainly stated the singular revelation, for which Dr. Allen was credited: Diabetes was a problem not just with carbohydrate metabolism, but with protein and fat as well. Instead of detailing case histories, it contained instructions for food measurement and preparation. It even contained dozens of recipes. It was this book that Allen gave to his new patients and their families. First published in August 1915, the book was now in its third printing. Unlike Allen himself, the book was a popular success.

When he reached Fifth Avenue, Allen turned right and set off at a plodding pace uptown. He came to the window of an opulent haberdashery. Behind the glass was an artful composition of fine wool, polished leather, sterling silver, and starched, white linen. But Allen did not see any of this. He was scrutinizing his own reflection in the glass. He studied his girth, the length of his arms proportionate to his torso, the exact slope of his shoulder, and, most of all, his facial features, which gave the impression of stern disapproval even when he felt none. He raised his eyebrows in an attempt to soften his features and create a more sympathetic appearance, but this only made him look alarmed. His brows settled back into place and his face resumed a look of grim resolve, but this time it was authentic. He sighed. It was bad enough contending with the complications of human patients, but to have to contend with the parents of the human patients was a whole new dimension. Still gazing into the glass, he imagined himself sitting in the home of Charles Evans Hughes, facing the great man. Then he rehearsed the words he would soon have to say in earnest.

Elizabeth is suffering from severe juvenile diabetes mellitus—the inability of the body to make use of glucose. The human body needs glucose to function, much like an automobile needs gasoline. In diabetics, the pancreas does not function correctly, and the body becomes unable to metabolize glucose. There is no way to restore the pancreas. There is no cure. I'm afraid Elizabeth will be dead within a year.

Allen's daydream was abruptly interrupted as he became aware of a salesman standing inside the window, watching him. The man smiled a lubricious smile and beckoned him in. Allen turned suddenly from the window, his cheeks flushed in embarrassment.

A brand new Cadillac brougham livery cab rolled past him to the corner, its backseat empty. He did not enjoy walking but he had made a commitment to take more exercise. It was, after all, a central element of his treatment. Although he often rationalized to himself that there was no reason that a nondiabetic such as himself should adopt the treatment prescribed for diabetics, he had come to appreciate that there was something unseemly about his corpulence given that his name had become synonymous with starvation. He didn't want Mr. and Mrs. Hughes to see him arrive in a car. He checked his pocket watch and plodded on, allowing the shiny black sedan to continue its journey.

At the corner of Fifth Avenue and Sixty-fourth Street he paused. Looking south, he could see forty blocks of towering concrete, steel, and glass, all the way down to that architectural curiosity, the Flatiron Building. He had come a long way from his father's California orange grove. He turned to the northwest to the lush green heart of Manhattan— Central Park. Directly ahead he could see the Arsenal and the Menagerie in what was called the Children's District of the park. Beyond that he could imagine the Dairy and, to the left, the Pond with its swans and graceful stone bridges. It was all so serene. He winced at the unhappy conversation that was before him, the misery he would soon be delivering to the inhabitants of 32 East Sixty-fourth Street. They would ask him for a solution, a way out. But once they learned what the solution was, they would wish they'd never asked. Between the disease and the treatment there was no lesser evil. He knew that even then, they were awaiting his arrival. With a heavy sigh he proceeded down Sixty-fourth Street, fixing his attention resolutely on the stone steps that led to the home of Charles Evans Hughes.

THREE

The Breakfast Room of the Home of Charles Evans Hughes,
New York City, April 1919

THAT SAME HOUR, ANTOINETTE AND CHARLES EVANS HUGHES SAT in the breakfast room grimly awaiting Dr. Allen's arrival. At the age of fifty-seven, Hughes was a former Republican Party presidential candidate, former Supreme Court justice, and former governor of New York. Although he held no public office at that time (he would be named secretary of state in 1921), he continued to command such a dominant public profile that the name Charles Evans Hughes had appeared in the headlines of *The New York Times* well over a hundred times in the previous twelve months. "Work Done by Legal Aid; Society Headed by Charles E. Hughes Helped Many Inducted Men"; "Hughes Won't Act With W. R. Hearst, Refuses Membership on Mayor's Committee"; "End War Policies Now, Says Hughes; 'In Saving the World Have We Lost Our Republic?' "; and "Hughes Points to Flaw in Covenant; Suggests Seven Amendments, Including Specific Recognition of the Monroe Doctrine."

Antoinette was his constant companion, his soulmate, confidant, and the mother of his four children—Charles Jr. (called Charlie), twenty-nine, Helen, twenty-seven, Catherine, twenty, and Elizabeth, twelve. They had been married for nearly thirty-one years. As she gazed across the table on this morning, she did not see the fearless and formidable figure whom Teddy Roosevelt described as "a bearded iceberg," but a helpless father, head bowed in grief and frustration at his utter inability to protect his own child from a premature death, a diagnosis that would be almost certainly confirmed within the hour. She reached across the table and clasped his hand. He held on with a genuine urgency. Although the world would soon be forever changed by a series of medical breakthroughs and a more open attitude toward illness and medical therapy, in 1919 the Victorian attitude toward illness prevailed. It was governed by secretiveness, superstition, and patent medicines and their fallow promises.

They had much to be grateful for, and Antoinette forced herself to think of these things now. Topping the list of blessings, certainly, were the safe return of Charlie from the War to End All Wars and the recovery of Helen who, it seemed safe to say, was finally free of the terrifying pneumonia that had followed her bout with the Spanish flu. Yes, there was much to be grateful for, and it seemed there had been just as much to endure. She and Charles had soldiered through it with characteristic aplomb, but it had depleted their emotional and spiritual reserves. So this morning they were nearly undone to find themselves again facing the prospect of losing a child. Even the family pet, a canary named Perfect, which normally filled the house with song in the morning hours, sat silently on his perch. The entire house seemed to be waiting, listening together to the percussive pendulum of the grandfather clock that stood like a stoic sentry on the first landing.

Their youngest child, Elizabeth, had persuaded her mother that she felt well enough to go on a Girl Scouts field trip, Catherine was in her final year at Wellesley, Charlie was at work downtown at his father's law firm, and Helen was in her sickbed on the floor above. Antoinette was reminded of another time, ten years before, when they sat across the same kitchen table, then in the governor's mansion in Albany. On that morning they were trying to discern if and how to respond to an anonymous threat to kidnap their baby Elizabeth, the much-heralded first child born in the gracious brick Queen Anne style mansion on Eagle Street.

As a reformer, Charles had introduced many initiatives, including new banking laws, a simplified ballot, and a direct-primaries act. When he turned his reform efforts to bookmaking at the horse races, Charles received an anonymous threat to kidnap Elizabeth, and his own life was threatened. He had faced threats to his own life before and had always refused to be swayed by them. But a threat to his child was different.

How could he weigh his responsibility to his baby daughter against his sworn oath to serve the people of New York? Together he and Antoinette had decided to stand firm. The danger passed without incident. Now they again faced an unseen foe that threatened to take Elizabeth from them, but this time it was no hollow threat. If Elizabeth's diagnosis was to be as dire as diabetes, then her parents would once more be forced to make hard choices.

And who better to make hard choices than the illustrious Charles Evans Hughes? After two two-year terms as governor of New York he was appointed associate justice of the Supreme Court of the United States, and he and Antoinette moved to Washington. Six years later Hughes was nominated by the Republican Party to run as their candidate in the 1916 presidential election.

Indivisible as they were, Antoinette had accompanied Charles on the campaign trail, the first wife ever to do so. They spent the better part of 1916 traveling the country by trains, boats, and the then relatively new automobile. Throughout the meandering 20,000 mile expedition, Antoinette remained fixed at her husband's side, taking in the soaring glory of Yellowstone, the modern engineering of a copper mine in Butte, Montana, and many other sights along the way. She made a temporary home for them in the railroad coach and, from coast to coast, invited newspaper correspondents into the car for loganberry juice and chocolate cookies. According to one observant journalist,

> She watches Mr. Hughes, mothers him, makes him take care of his voice, admitting, however, that at times she finds him a "very willful child." When he has talked as long as the schedule calls for, or the occasion seems to demand, she pulls his coat tails or gets someone else to do it. . . . "She is my confidential adviser," Mr. Hughes recently admitted.

During the entire campaign, she missed only one of his speeches, and that was because a well-meaning ladies group in Missouri had planned a reception for her during Charles's speech. After politely disabusing them of the idea that she was tired of hearing his speeches, she was driven to the hall where she was refused entry until he was finished.

In November 1916, Hughes lost to the Democratic incumbent Woodrow Wilson by a slim margin, and the Hughes family left the beloved four-story brick Georgian they had built in Washington, D.C., in 1911. By 1917 he had resettled his family in New York City and reestablished himself at Hughes, Rounds, Schurman & Dwight, where he was a founding partner. Charles and Antoinette were relieved to think that most of life's wrenching drama was behind them. They could not have been more wrong.

As was his habit when stressed or anxious, Charles Evans Hughes hurled himself all the harder into his work, both paid and unpaid. By his own estimate, he devoted "fully one-third of [his] time . . . to matters of more or less public interest, outside of [his] professional work." Perhaps the most personally significant work he took up during this period was the Draft Appeals Board. A month after America entered the war in April 1917, Congress passed the Draft Act, and at the end of July, Charles Evans Hughes was tapped to be chairman of the District Draft Appeals Board for New York City. It was a formidable task requiring the processing of a thousand cases each day, each of which decided the fate of a young man. The Board comprised thirty eminent members organized into six subcommittees that met in the old Post Office building. To aid them in managing the huge volume of paper, a massive clerical staff was drawn from the city's leading banks and the New York Telephone Company. As they began the task, the cavernous corridors were already crowded with boxes of mail and lines of people waiting to make their appeal. Four thousand pieces of mail arrived each day. Hughes was responsible for personally signing—in quadruplicate—the papers of every man who went into the military and every man who was exempted from service. He refused to have a stamp made, because each signature might represent the death of a man. He served as chairman of the Draft Appeals Board until May 1918.

The war ended officially at eleven o'clock on November 11, 1918—the eleventh hour of the eleventh day of the eleventh month. Before memorials could be erected to the dead, the most virulent and deadly influenza virus in history had begun to make victims of the war's survivors: the returning soldiers, the nurses, the siblings, the parents, and the widows. In the churning, bloody wake of the war, the great influenza epidemic of 1918—"the Spanish Flu"—swept over the earth. It was called the Spanish flu primarily because it received the most press coverage in Spain, where journalists were not hampered by the imposition of wartime censorship as were journalists in countries participating in the war. The postwar movements of so many people all around the world and the cramped quarters of hospitals, troopships, and barracks ensured transmission and accelerated the virus's broad and rapid geographic dispersion from the Arctic circle to the Fiji Islands. Ironically, many of the families fortunate enough to welcome a soldier home were the very ones who fell ill first, little realizing that in welcoming back their soldiers, they were also embracing their own deaths. Surviving soldiers carried on the shoulders of their neighbors in hometown victory parades were soon carried on the same shoulders, in coffins. For many, peacetime was worse than war.

By the time it was over, the Spanish flu would claim fifty million lives worldwide, more than three times the number killed in World War I; in the United States it afflicted over 25 percent of the population. In one year, the average life expectancy in the nation dropped by twelve years. Unlike other outbreaks, this flu targeted not only the young and the old, but also adults between twenty and forty years old.

But even the flu had a more optimistic prognosis than juvenile diabetes. While the mortality rate for the influenza of 1918 was between 2 and 20 percent, the mortality rate for juvenile diabetes was very nearly 100 percent.

Helen Hughes fell ill in the autumn of 1918, and by that winter she was too sick to work. That winter, Elizabeth also took sick with the flu. And so the youngest and oldest Hughes girls kept each other company convalescing at the family home. Although there was a fifteen-year difference in their ages, Helen's deep interest in girls made her an excellent companion for Elizabeth, and Elizabeth's ebullience buoyed Helen through the cold, dark months of January and February. If Helen was the child who most resembled her mother, Elizabeth was the child who most resembled her father. Helen's round face always bore a gentle, contemplative expression, and she wore her hair pinned atop her head in a knot, just as Antoinette did. At twelve and a half, Elizabeth's fiercely curious mind seemed to boil with questions, propelling her into constant investigative action. Her dark hair was smartly bobbed and she frequently sported skinned knees, the result of her tireless explorations in her beloved back yard—Central Park. If Helen seemed to hold a quiet stillness within her, Elizabeth was perpetually in motion.

Of the four Hughes children, Elizabeth was the only one who inherited her father's peculiar mental talent—a photographic memory. While Elizabeth was too sick to venture outside the house, she and Helen made flash cards with the silhouettes of familiar tree leaves on them. Helen marveled at Elizabeth's ability to memorize the flash cards after seeing them only once. Soon Elizabeth could even recite the names of the trees in alphabetical order—backward and forward: ash, aspen, beech, birch, buckeye, cedar, chestnut, elm, fir, holly, juniper, maple, oak, pine, spruce, sweet gum, sycamore, tulip, willow. To pass the long hours they listened to the Victrola. Helen taught her how to knit. Sitting together listening to Al Jolson's "Hello Central, Give Me No-Man's Land" and Irving Berlin's "Oh! How I Hate to Get Up in the Morning," they knitted scarves to send overseas for the war reparation effort.

Elizabeth's and Helen's bedrooms were purposefully positioned at opposite ends of a long hallway, so that hushed conversations about Helen's illness held away from the older sister's door were often within earshot of Elizabeth's door and vice versa. They made a pact that they would spy, eavesdrop, and use any means possible to glean whatever information they could about the other's illness and share it.

By March 1919, Elizabeth seemed to have recovered, except for her unusually ravenous appetite and unslakable thirst. Helen's condition developed into pneumonia. So it was that while Helen remained confined, most of the espionage fell to Elizabeth. Spying was somewhat of an avocation for Elizabeth, an avid birdwatcher. Further, the Hughes household was frequented by many famous visitors, not the least of whom was close family friend, former president William Howard Taft. Antoinette and Charles often entertained guests in their home. During parties Helen typically joined the adults and Catherine flirted with the Secret Service men in the kitchen while Elizabeth peered between the balusters of the second-floor landing, often equipped with her father's birding binoculars.

Elizabeth sometimes sat at Helen's bedside and read the newspaper to her. Of particular interest to them were the issues of women's suffrage and spiritual direction that were polarizing public opinion at that time. Religious leaders of varying stripes speculated about whether the influ-

enza epidemic might be divine retribution for applying the ingenuity of
the human mind to war. Had America lost its way? Faltered in her great
experimental mission of freedom and equality? A third great awaken-
ing of religious fervor seized the American people.

Helen was absolutely passionate about preparing the next generation
of women to be active and influential participants in their government.
She felt certain that women would soon have the vote. This generation
of girls would vote, yes, and so much more. Helen was desperate to get
on with her life. She had only just begun a promising career with the
Young Women's Christian Association, where she pioneered the founding of high school girls clubs and served as a member of the national board
of the YWCA and as field student secretary in the Middle Atlantic States
and New England. And she simply *had* to be well enough to attend her
fifth class reunion at her beloved Vassar in Poughkeepsie in June. After
that she hoped to return to the beautiful 700-acre YMCA-YWCA campus on the western shores of Lake George in Silver Bay, New York,
where she had spent so many happy days in previous summers.

But for now Helen lay upstairs, helplessly listening to the inexorable
cadence of the clock on the landing. When her lungs felt particularly
leaden, she would count out sets of ten tocks until her fear of suffocation
subsided. On that April morning it seemed the whole house was counting
with her.

Just when she expected the familiar Westminster chime to sound the
hour, another sound echoed through the silent house. Dr. Allen knocked
at the door.

FOUR

The Library of the Home of Charles Evans Hughes,
New York City, April 1919

In early April, Antoinette had taken Elizabeth to Dr. Allen's office on Fifty-first Street to be examined. Now Allen sat in the library of the Hughes home to discuss his findings. Charles and Antoinette both knew that Dr. Allen's verdict carried a special gravity and no recourse; it was highly unlikely that his opinion would be refuted by anyone. And so it was with a sense of profound dread that Antoinette and Charles heard the words *she will likely be dead in six months.*

"How can you say that with such certainty?" Antoinette asked, forcibly modulating her voice to sound calmer than she was.

Allen was not insensitive to the harshness of the news, but he was not one to mince words, particularly when consideration for the parents' emotional well-being was purchased at the expense of the child's physical well-being.

"Without treatment, the life expectancy of a juvenile diabetic is less than a year from the onset of symptoms."

"Yes, but surely there are miracles. Not every single child who—," Antoinette continued pleadingly.

"I'm afraid so," Allen countered.

"Come now, Doctor. There are exceptions," Charles weighed in.

"I have yet to see one. I could refer you to Dr. Elliott Joslin's work for statistical confirmation, but I'm afraid you really don't have time for research." Allen was thinking, at that moment, of Joslin's sad testament, the diabetic ledger. The ledger recorded the names, ages, and addresses of the diabetics he had treated since 1893; it was like the passenger manifest of a doomed ship. While his ledger represented a uniquely useful record of diabetes for medical research, it also documented the lack of progress in the clinical treatment of diabetes. All of the patients listed in the ledger died prematurely of diabetes or its underhanded complications such as coma and gangrene. For a moment the three sat in silence.

"The decision you have before you is a critical one," Allen resumed after a time. "Unfortunately, it's a decision you will have to make quickly. I am here to provide you with the facts."

"We appreciate that, Doctor." Charles spoke now. The deep authoritative tone of his voice comforted Antoinette. "But isn't there something we can do? Some measure that can be taken?"

"There is no cure. But there is a way to buy time."

"Go on," said Hughes.

"We must starve her."

"But she's so thin!" Antoinette blinked uncomprehendingly.

"A normal girl Elizabeth's age consumes 2,200 calories daily," Allen explained. "I propose that we begin Elizabeth with a fast followed by a diet of 400 calories, almost none of which will include carbohydrates."

"And this will help her to gain back the weight she has lost?" Charles asked the doctor.

"Certainly not. But it will keep her alive."

"For how long?" Antoinette asked.

"It's hard to say," Allen replied. "If she survives the diet she might live with her diabetes for up to eighteen months. Elizabeth's symptoms began in . . . November? December?"

Antoinette nodded grimly.

"How long would Elizabeth have to remain on this diet before she could eat normally again?" Charles asked.

"She will never be able to eat normally again," Allen said. "Every gram of food that she eats will be weighed and measured and the preparation supervised for the remainder of her life."

"Four hundred calories . . . What *can* she eat?" Antoinette asked.

"Eggs, cream, bran rusks, all in extremely limited quantities," Allen said. "Vegetables boiled three times to purge them of carbohydrates. No desserts or bread ever."

Antoinette's mind raced with the implications: no corn or potatoes, no birthday cake, no Sunday morning flapjacks, no roast goose with stuffing at Thanksgiving. Antoinette considered the practicalities of caring for Elizabeth at home. Would she eat at the table with the rest of the family, watching everyone else consuming what she could not? Would it be worse for her to take all of her meals alone in her room? She tried to imagine Elizabeth, gaunt and silent, spooning up tiny bites of bran rusks and boiled cabbage in the kitchen while the sound of laughter and lively conversation floated in from the dining room. And how could they possibly ensure that the maids, who adored Elizabeth, would not sneak food to her, particularly if it looked like she would die if she didn't get it?

"It would be easiest for all," Allen continued, "if you could begin to reconcile yourselves with the idea that food, previously seen as the staff of life, is now a deadly poison."

"Easiest?" Antoinette sputtered. "But she's hungry all the time."

"It's hard to believe that starvation could be the answer to hunger," Charles explained.

"The less food, the more life." Allen leveled his clinical gaze at Antoinette. "To starve is to survive."

Antoinette pressed her lips together as if she was afraid of the vitriol that might escape them. Having met Americans from coast to coast during the 1916 presidential campaign, she got along with people of all ages and walks of life. She was known as a gracious hostess and a charming dinner companion, providing measured and thoughtful contributions to conversations on a variety of subjects. But when she met Dr. Allen, she was seized with a palpable dislike of him, which was only reinforced in this, their second encounter.

"I assure you, Mrs. Hughes," Allen continued, "it will get far worse. Some of my patients weigh as little as thirty pounds—which is why I insist on inpatient treatment."

"Elizabeth would not live at home?" Charles asked.

"The sanitarium is the safest place for Elizabeth."

"But we have so little time left with her!" Antoinette protested. "Can't we keep her at home?"

"I can extend that time, if you consent to commit her to my care," Allen asserted.

"At what cost to Elizabeth?" she countered.

Hughes noted his wife's ears turning a vivid pink.

"How do you keep from going too far?" Hughes interjected. Allen looked back blankly. Hughes continued. "Have you ever lost a patient to starvation?"

"Most certainly," Allen replied. "The treatment is very difficult. The dietary restrictions are severe, and even a slight deviation can cause the onset of coma. Once that has occurred there is nothing I or anyone else can do."

At that exact moment the sanitarium did not yet exist, except in Frederick Allen's mind. As he sat in the parlor of the Hughes home, Allen was finalizing plans for a private sanitarium on Fifty-first Street for the treatment and study of diabetes. Having been thoroughly disgusted with the politics and favoritism at the institutions where he'd worked, Allen had determined to open his own facility, never to have his work subject to the vicissitudes of personal popularity again. Within the walls of his own facility he would have complete control. He could monitor every aspect of his patients' existence, every morsel of food and drop of liquid consumed, every minute of exercise undertaken, and blood and excreta could be reliably analyzed at useful intervals. He could prolong the lives of diabetics by bringing their stressed metabolisms into something approximating a balanced state. Once that delicate state was achieved, patients would receive the vigilant care and scrutiny required to maintain it. With proper funding—and clearly Charles Evans Hughes represented a means to that end—he hoped his sanitarium might be fully operational in time to admit Elizabeth as one of his first patients.

The sanitarium would be housed in the mansion where his current office was located. Allen had arranged to rent the entire building furnished. The nurses would be trained dieticians, all graduates of the Domestic Science School in Framingham, Massachusetts. His three assistants, Drs. James W. Sherrill, J. West Mitchell, and Henry J. John, were all competent doctors from reputable medical schools. The linchpin of the whole operation would be Miss Mary Belle Wishart, that wonder of efficiency and professionalism. Allen had first encountered her at the

Rockefeller Institute, where she was assigned as his technical research assistant. Ever his devoted acolyte, she had followed him into the Army Service, serving with him at Lakewood, New Jersey, and now she would supervise the operations of his private sanitarium, which would allow him to focus on his real interest, research. The house contained three reception rooms, one dining room, one general kitchen, one diet kitchen, seventeen patient rooms, and accommodations for five nurses, three doctors, and Miss Wishart and her mother. An outside apartment would accommodate the six additional nurses to be permanently employed by the sanitarium. The house capacity, when full, would be twenty patients.

"Couldn't we hire a nurse," Hughes offered, "who could manage Elizabeth's diet while she lived at home?"

"A nurse trained as a dietician?" Allen asked dismissively. "A nurse experienced with diabetes?"

"Perhaps you could recommend one," Antoinette posited. "Someone trained at your own sanitarium."

"It is an extremely difficult regimen to maintain outside of a clinical setting," Allen replied. "There is the food preparation, the weighing and measuring, monitoring of blood glucose levels, urine testing, the schedule of meals and exercise, all of which must be followed to the letter and carefully recorded."

Antoinette felt her face flush with anger. *At best, Allen could delay the progress of the disease—delay, not even stop it. At worst, he would ensure that Elizabeth's next few months (and possibly her last few months) would be excruciatingly painful. And even if his treatment does extend the postdiagnosis time, is time the same as life? Is a year of agony better than two happy months?*

"Is committing Elizabeth to in-patient care really for her benefit? Or is it to spare us the pain of managing her diet?" she asked.

"Both."

"It sounds like it will get worse no matter what we do," Charles said.

"That is true," Allen replied. "But here she will worsen and die. With me she will worsen and live—for a while anyway." He sat back.

"We want to make her life as happy and comfortable as possible in whatever time remains," Antoinette said.

"I cannot make her happy or comfortable. I can only keep her alive."

For a moment Antoinette allowed herself to imagine a macabre farewell party where all of Elizabeth's favorite foods would be prepared in abundance and she would be allowed to eat as much as she wanted— perhaps the feast would even last an entire weekend. There was a contingent of respectable medical experts who believed that it was more humane to allow patients with severe diabetes to eat themselves to death than to subject them to the torment of the Allen treatment.

"Surely there is someone somewhere who is working on a cure," Hughes said.

"There are *many* people who are working on a cure. In fact, many of the leading experts believe that we are very close to discovering a cure. That is precisely why I urge you to do all that you can to keep your daughter alive. A cure could come at any time. What a tragedy if Elizabeth were to miss it by a matter of weeks."

"Who are they? Who is working on a cure?"

"Who isn't? Harvard, Johns Hopkins, the Mayo brothers—"

"But which *individuals?*" Hughes pressed him.

"A German scientist named Zuelzer used a pancreatic extract to relieve glycosuria—sugar in the urine. A Romanian named Paulesco used pancreatic extract to normalize blood sugar levels. Right here in New York City, Israel Kleiner and S. J. Meltzer are working on a pancreatic extract. A Scot named Macleod at Western Reserve University in Ohio. But these men are not clinicians; their work is strictly experimental. They are working with *dogs*."

Charles's face fell.

"We are close to the solution. We just haven't refined it sufficiently for practical use. We *know* the answer but we can't *use* it—yet. " In fact, Allen was well aware that medical science had known about the disease since antiquity and, worse, that it had teetered on a cure—a real cure— for nearly fifty years. It was as if the profession had run twenty-six miles of a marathon and then sat down as a group some one thousand feet from the finish line to discuss the race thus far.

The effort to study diabetes mellitus had improved the clinical ability to diagnose the disease, and because more children were diagnosed with diabetes, more premature-death certificates listed the disease as the cause of death. By 1920, the death rate from diabetes would be double what it was twenty years before, and the number of diagnoses was rising. It appeared that medical research was losing ground.

The rise in diagnoses fertilized a burgeoning business of fad diets, patent medicines, and hope cures hawked by unscrupulous opportunists, hucksters, and self-described healers. The oat cure, the legume cure, potato therapy, lime water, sweet wine, rancid meat, high carbohydrates, low carbohydrates, high-fat diets, low-fat diets, horseback riding, abstinence from plant products, even opium—each had been heralded as a miracle cure for juvenile diabetes.

By these therapies, and the soft-voiced, moist-eyed charlatans who proffered them, so many children had been hoped into death, and their families drained of precious savings in the process. Here was a kindness that actually killed.

"We will need some time to think about it," Hughes said.

"Of course." Allen could not hide his disappointment. "Of course you need some time," he repeated. "But I am primarily interested in what Elizabeth needs."

Antoinette bristled.

"We all want what is best for Elizabeth," Hughes said.

"Then you understand, Mr. Hughes, that for someone with Elizabeth's diagnosis, time is a very scarce commodity. If you wait too long, the decision will be made for you."

Hughes rose from his seat to show Dr. Allen to the door before Antoinette could speak. Without so much as a glance in her direction, he knew that the rims of her ears would be red as licorice laces.

"Thank you, Dr. Allen." Charles interrupted him.

"I cannot impress upon you strongly enough that—"

Again Hughes cut him off. "You may rely on our making every effort to come to a decision promptly."

"You may find this book helpful." Allen thrust the book he was holding at Hughes.

In less than a minute, Allen stood on the sidewalk outside the Hughes residence, squinting against the sun and hoping that he had not burned the bridge to beneficence. *Selling snake oil must certainly be an easier profession than this,* he thought.

For an instant he imagined himself leaving a very different kind of meeting—a meeting from which both parties would emerge happy. His pockets would be bulging with bills, and Antoinette would be clutching a bottle of magic elixir, distilled from frog's teeth, shark's tears, and the spittle of the Mexican gila monster. Hughes would be clapping his shoulder and chuckling as he stood with Allen at the door.

Allen started off on foot, but once he was out of sight of the Hughes residence, he hailed a cab. Moments later, settled into the back of the car, he clenched his jaw repeatedly as if chewing on the one question that always bedeviled him after meetings such as the one he had just left: *How could a mother even consider declining a treatment that would save her child from certain death?*

FIVE

New York City, April 1919, Later That Afternoon

AFTER DR. ALLEN LEFT, CHARLES IMMEDIATELY WENT TO WORK AT his office at 96 Broadway in Lower Manhattan. Charles walked the nearly five miles in his dark worsted suit, spring topcoat, fedora, and black bluchers. The journey was prolonged by the frequency with which he was compelled to stop to allow himself to be greeted by someone. He rarely passed through a street or avenue without a hat being doffed to him or a nod of approving recognition.

By the time he spotted the distinctive Gothic steeple of Trinity Church, he would be glad for the privacy of the cool, dark recesses of the narthex. He entered, breathing in the sweet smoky tang of incense. It was a familiar smell. Trinity was located directly across the street from the building in which his offices were located and, although he was not Episcopalian, he came here occasionally during the workday to think about a particularly vexing problem of law. Usually the tomblike atmosphere cheered him, reminding him of his own mortality and unimportance and putting the niggling problem into proper perspective. He turned into a pew and sat down. The cool air lay upon his neck like the palms of an alabaster saint. He closed his eyes.

Later he would cross the street and enter his building, where the guards and elevator operators would all greet him by name. They would let him off at his floor, and he would go into his son's office and tell him of the meeting with Allen. But for now he would sit in the hushed darkness and allow Charlie to work happily unaware of the grim prediction delivered by Dr. Allen. He imagined Elizabeth tramping through the woods of Westchester, calling out the names of trees as she passed happily beneath their boughs. Of all his children, she seemed the most engaged with the natural world. Charlie was intellectual, Helen was spiritual, Catherine was social, and Elizabeth was fascinated by all things earthly: beetles and birds, shells and stones, the seasons and tides.

Elizabeth had been something of a natural phenomenon from the very start, having been born nine years after Catherine, her next oldest sibling. Both Charles and Antoinette had always quietly believed that Elizabeth was destined for some great and special purpose, and it seemed to him not just tragic but wrong that she should be prematurely taken from the world. His eyes stung with the thought of it.

Abruptly, he roused himself from the hard pew and crossed the street. He threw himself into work as if he could outpace, through his professional activity, his utter powerlessness to help his two doomed daughters. "I believe in work, hard work, and long hours of work," he often said. "Men do not break down from overwork, but from worry and dissipation." Hughes never stopped working at the highest level. Between November 1918 and February 1921 Hughes made twenty-five arguments (including three rearguments) before the U.S. Supreme Court.

Back at home that evening, he and Antoinette would try to reach a decision as they had reached so many decisions: They would come to an answer by asking questions, and not just asking them but asking them relentlessly, until both questions and questioners were exhausted and a direction became clear.

Reason had always been his religion. He pursued law over the objections of his parents, who had hoped he would enter the ministry. And yet today he found himself wondering if such a question as Dr. Allen had posed earlier could be answered by reason. Could he honestly claim even a modicum of objectivity in such circumstances? If he could not rely on reason, what could he rely on?

Charles and Antoinette could and did and would always rely on each other.

Antoinette thought of Elizabeth's ruddy, mud-flecked face when she had returned from the Westchester woods. The pockets of her jacket were full of stones and cones and samaras. Exuberant but trembling with exhaustion, she had gone directly to bed.

"Let's give Dr. Allen the benefit of the doubt," she began. "We would be keeping Elizabeth alive to wait for a cure. Is it foolish to think that it would come now? For us? When it has eluded so many for so long? And even if it does, isn't there an inherent conflict of interest? Dr. Allen's livelihood depends on the patient being sick enough to need his treatment."

"But my dear, do you really believe that if a cure were to become available he would hesitate to provide it to his patients?"

"I suppose he is bound by the Hippocratic Oath, but . . . a sanitarium is no place for our Elizabeth."

Charles thought of his father, Reverend David Charles Hughes, who had died ten years before. He was an impoverished Methodist minister of Welsh descent, who doted on his only child's mental, physical, and spiritual development. The elder Hughes's letters to his son at college covered the gamut, from the importance of wearing warm socks to the perils of card games. Charles wondered what his father would say about this situation. *Does Christianity require that a believer submit to the will of heaven and allow nature to take its course? Was it right to subject a child to a living hell if it was the only kind of living she could do?* It seemed to Charles that his father never deliberated or doubted a moment in his life.

Charles heard his father's stentorian voice intoning *Prayer changes everything.* So Charles and Antoinette sank to their knees in Charles's study and they prayed. They prayed for Elizabeth's recovery. They gave thanks for Helen's recovery. They prayed for more faith. They prayed for the strength to accept whatever happened. They gave thanks for the privilege of making choices. They prayed for God to direct their thinking in all things. And then they sat together, waiting and listening.

By the age of five Charles was reading the Bible and his mother was teaching him French, German, and arithmetic. His parents enrolled him in school, but after only a few weeks he was bored. On his own initiative he prepared a document entitled "The Charles E. Hughes Plan of Study," which he presented to his parents. The plan sought to prove to his parents that he could better educate himself at home than his teachers could at school. The plan described in detail a daily schedule and curriculum, involving his rising early in the morning to complete his studies so that he could spend his afternoons playing baseball and Red Lion with the neighborhood boys. His parents agreed. By the age of eight he had read *Pilgrim's Progress, Robinson Crusoe,* and nearly all of Shakespeare's plays, his favorites being *The Tempest, Twelfth Night,* and *The Merry Wives of Windsor.*

It was nearly dawn. Outside, in the early light, the delicate blush of cherry blossoms breathed a gentle mood up and down Fifth Avenue, and the riotous red and yellow of Dutch tulips proclaimed spring's arrival from the Park Avenue window boxes. Although in many ways it represented the most difficult of all possible choices, Charles and Antoinette decided to hire a nurse and keep Elizabeth at home for as long as possible, adhering to the Allen treatment on an outpatient basis. In order to secure Elizabeth's dedicated cooperation, they would have to tell Elizabeth about her diagnosis and, worse, the prognosis. They would also have to inform the help in the house, insisting on both their compliance and discretion. And they would have to withdraw her from school. In this, Elizabeth would follow her father's example.

By the time Charles and Antoinette trudged the steps to the second floor the inveterate urban sparrows and pigeons and starlings had begun their morning conversation. What they didn't know as they reached the top of the stairs was that the landing had been occupied until moments before by Elizabeth. She had overheard the entire discussion, stifling her horror with a fistful of balled-up nightgown.

SIX

Toronto, Canada, and Cambrai, France, 1917–1918

THE CASUALTIES OF WORLD WAR I WERE OF A SORT AND A SCALE never before seen. For the first time, dogfights screamed through the skies, filling them with fire and smoke, and on the seas German U-boats quite literally undermined the superlative British fleet. The war introduced tanks and dirigibles, machine guns, blinding chemical gas, and long-range guns, including the biggest in the world, a howitzer named Big Bertha. And it killed profligately. Great Britain and its empire lost over 1 million soldiers; France, 1.3 million; Russia, 1.7 million; Germany and its allies, 3.5 million. During the fighting, the loss of life per day exceeded five thousand souls. To replenish its devastating losses, Britain passed five versions of the conscription act, each one broader than the previous one until the last, when they were calling up all men, married or unmarried, of any profession, from the ages of seventeen to fifty-one. For nearly three devastating years America claimed political neutrality, watching the carnage from across the Atlantic (while manufacturing weapons and selling them to the Allies).

Advances in military technology had far outstripped the advances in medical technology. Injuries were of a type that doctors had never seen: bones pulverized into unrecoverable shards, a profusion of disfiguring facial injuries, and a mysterious new condition called shell shock. The terrible destructiveness of the new weaponry, coupled with the revoltingly unhygienic environment of the trenches, made for an acute need for medics and more medics on the battlefield.

England had sent out the call and Canada responded. The University of Toronto's Medical School reorganized and condensed the curriculum of the fifth and final years of training of the class of 1917 so that its members would be graduated a year early and sooner sent overseas. Upon graduation, the entire class of 1917 enlisted in the Canadian Army Medical Corps (CAMC). Practically speaking, their final credits were to be earned in the trenches. In 1917 the population of Toronto was nearly 90 percent Anglo-Celtic. "God Save the King" was the Canadian national anthem. The Union Jack figured prominently on the Canadian Red Ensign national flag. A half million Canadian soldiers fought in Europe, and more than sixty thousand of them died.

Frederick Banting, a mediocre student in the class of 1917, was among the first to volunteer. It was the third time he had tried to enlist. He first appeared at the army recruitment center on August 5, 1914, the day after Canada entered the war, but his poor eyesight prevented his enlistment. He tried again in October and was again rejected. By December 1916, his medical training, coupled with the desperation born of the terrible loss of life, made possible what had not been possible before. It would be one of many experiences in Banting's life where he succeeded by persistence through repeated failures and against compelling evidence and poor odds.

Banting was of Scottish and English descent. His family had come to Canada in the middle part of the nineteenth century. Banting was born to Margaret and William Banting in 1891 on a farm in Alliston, Ontario; he was the youngest of four. He had one sister and three brothers (a fourth brother died as an infant); the sibling nearest in age to him was his sister, four years his senior. Fred was especially close to his mother, Maggie.

As each of the Banting sons turned twenty-one, his father gave him a horse, a harness, a buggy, and $1,500, which he could spend any way he chose. All three of the older Banting boys used their money to establish farms. Fred spent his money on education.

When he entered Victoria College at the University of Toronto, he had no definite objective in mind. Like the parents of Charles Evans

Hughes, Banting's parents hoped he would pursue the ministry. Although he maintained the habit of attending church every Sunday through his college years, it was largely to please his mother. He was interested in art and had a fine baritone singing voice. He was athletic and played football and baseball. Although Banting enjoyed college life, his grades were not especially good. He had to repeat English composition and struggled with spelling throughout his life, but he persevered, spurred by the understanding that if he failed he would have to return to cleaning out henhouses, threshing wheat, and mending fences.

According to one story, Banting's interest in medicine came about as the result of his witnessing an accident one day in which two workmen fell from a scaffold and appeared to be seriously injured. Fred ran for the doctor. He was impressed by the effect the doctor's arrival had on the crowd that gathered around the men. They were immediately relieved and stood at a respectful distance to watch as the doctor set to work with steady and sure hands.

Edith Roach was part of Banting's plan to improve himself. They met in the summer of 1911 when Edith's father, a Methodist minister, moved his family to Alliston. She was also a student at Victoria (with a scholastic record considerably better than Fred's). The last thing Lieutenant Banting did before leaving Toronto in late February 1917 was to give Edith Roach a ring and ask her to wait for him.

Banting's ship crossed the Atlantic, landing in the CAMC depot at Westenhanger, in Kent, the southeasternmost county in England. From there he went to Granville Canadian Special Hospital at Ramsgate, where he worked with Dr. Clarence Starr, a highly respected orthopedic surgeon from Toronto who would play an important role in his future. Although such an arrangement was excellent training for a newly minted surgeon, Banting was anxious to get into the action. He would soon be afforded the chance.

The medical corps suffered more battle casualties than any other arm of the service. On the Western Front, stretcher bearers, ambulance drivers, and doctors fell beneath the same shells as the soldiers whose wounds they were charged with dressing. In the winter of 1917, Banting was sent to replace a doctor who was killed by shrapnel while looking out a window in a shattered home at Cambrai.

Cambrai is roughly a hundred miles north of Paris and a hundred miles southwest of Brussels. During the Great War, it was in enemy hands and deemed the key position on the German front line. Although the battlefields of Cambrai are today among the least visited of the Western Front battlefields of World War I, the fighting that began there in November 1917 is well remembered in the annals of military history. It was the first instance of a revolutionary method of attack—a mass assault using both tanks and aircraft. The routed Germans studied this method and later developed the blitzkrieg methods that the German army successfully employed in World War II.

As a medical officer of the 44th Battalion Banting served with the 13th Field Ambulance, stationed at a place called Lilac Farm, near Cambrai. The 13th Field Ambulance was commanded by Lieutenant Colonel W. H. K. Anderson. Banting's immediate superior was the second in command, Major L. C. Palmer, an able surgeon who, like Starr, would play an important role in Banting's future medical career. Fred was popular among his comrades, joining in soccer and volleyball games during the brief respites from duty. He was cool under pressure, and courageous, too. According to an oft-repeated apocryphal tale, he once walked into an enemy dugout, armed with nothing more deadly than a swagger stick, and emerged with three German prisoners whom he immediately put to work. The official history of the unit contains the following paragraph:

> Captain F. G. Banting, Medical Officer of the 44th, goes forward with the attack—and, with his medical detail, establishes the first dressing station in Drury Quarry. His work is beyond praise. Pressing into service a captured German medical detail he worked incessantly throughout the operations—clearing hundreds of wounded in addition to the men of his own unit.

Dressing stations were ad hoc operating theaters, which were set up in any available structure, such as a barn or farmhouse or even a primitive dugout. The wounded were evacuated from the battlefield by horse-drawn ambulances. Human stretcher bearers transferred wounded men from the ambulances to the operating tables in the dressing station and back to the ambulances for transport to the casualty clearing stations farther from the front.

At Lilac Farm the dressing station was a partly wrecked barn, not far behind the firing line, and Captain Banting often came under heavy German fire. Many of the wounds to combatants were catastrophic, and surgical decisions had to be made in seconds. Amputations were common. In this era, before the introduction of sulfa drugs, infection was a primary concern among wartime surgeons. When faced with a choice between dressing a potentially infected wounded limb and a sanitary amputation of that limb, the latter was often preferred. The soldier's chances of survival were better with amputation.

While everyone at the front could hear the distinctive long whistle of an incoming shell and know that it would end in an explosion, one man in Banting's unit, an Italian stretcher bearer, had trained his ear to discern the difference between an "overhead," in which one should remain standing, and a "ground burst," in which it was better to lie flat. At the first scream of an incoming shell, everyone in the unit would look to the Italian, who would signal whether the incoming round was "overhead" or "ground burst." Much to Major Palmer's amazement, Fred Banting had trained his ear to hear nothing at all. Occasionally Palmer would find Banting studying a pocket anatomy textbook with such concentration that he seemed oblivious to the shells screaming all around him.

On September 28, 1918, Banting was operating at his dressing station at Lilac Farm. As a result of several casualties, Palmer and Banting were the only officers at the station. That morning, the Germans were using "whizzbangs," which were shells that had no incoming scream and could be heard only seconds before landing and exploding. These confounded even the Italian stretcher bearer.

The Germans were in retreat, but firing furiously as they went. A Canadian artillery officer set up an eighteen-pounder in the barnyard and aimed it over the ridge at the Germans. The Germans were determined to put this gun out of action, and the whizzbangs pelted the farm with such intensity that both the Canadians and their German prisoners were taken aback. One of the prisoners, a German major, ventured out onto the steps of the farmhouse to admire the storm of shrapnel and was promptly decapitated where he stood.

A piece of shrapnel tore open Banting's sleeve and chewed into his right forearm. It was a deep wound, and the ragged metal severed the interosseous artery. Palmer took Banting by the shoulder and guided him to the shelter of a brick wall. There he quickly tied a tourniquet above the elbow, removed the fragment, and applied a dressing.

Palmer ordered Banting to the casualty clearing station and pointed to a waiting ambulance. Until this moment, Banting had accepted his superior officer's help without protest, but now he looked in the direction of the abandoned dressing station and begged to stay near the action, where he was clearly needed. The shells were crashing down around them. There was no time to argue. Just as Palmer was about to say so, a runner arrived with a note: Cambrai had been taken by the Allies and they needed a new dressing station there immediately. Palmer hesitated, considering whether to take Banting along. Then Palmer decided to go ahead to Cambrai, taking some sergeants with him to dress the wounded. He ordered Banting to the ambulance and left.

At Cambrai, the tanks had torn and churned the earth together with the rain so that it was nearly impossible to find a place to set up the dressing station. Then there was a sudden and fierce counterattack, and the Germans retook the town. As the German infantry flooded into the area, Palmer hid in a cellar, where he could hear the German boots on the floorboards overhead. It seemed that he crouched there for hours, barely breathing, hoping none of the soldiers would think to explore the cellar. Around midnight, the British again advanced and the Germans again retreated. Back at Lilac Farm, the wounded continued to arrive in a steady stream. Banting took care of them as quickly as he could, dressing them and dispatching them to be transported to the same casualty clearing station to which he himself had been ordered hours before. Each time a stretcher arrived, he told himself that this would be the last one, or that as soon as there was a break in the shelling, he would report to the casualty clearing station to get his arm checked. The shells continued to rain down, and the wounded continued to arrive. Hours passed. Whenever Banting decided that it was time to go, he would look down at the young man on the table before him and ask himself if this was the face he would walk away from. The answer was always no; the next would be the one. By the time Major Palmer made it back to Lilac Farm after his ordeal, it was four o'clock in the morning. He was stunned to see Banting standing at the table, just as he had left him seventeen hours before.

At the moment of Palmer's arrival Banting was trying to force his stiffened fingers to scissor open a blood-soaked pant leg. Palmer gazed beyond Banting to the far wall, where the bodies of those who would not be moving on to the casualty clearing station had been laid side by side under a drape of filthy cloth. Palmer grabbed Banting by the left shoulder and directed a hard glare at the surgeon's grimy, blood-spattered face. Banting met his gaze without malice or fear.

"Which one should I have left, sir?" he asked. Banting nodded to the soldier bleeding before him on the stretcher. Palmer looked down. It was the Italian stretcher bearer. The left side of his jaw was torn away, and the pulpy tissue of his face was spattered over his shirt like a bloody bib. The tissue was flecked with small white chips of bone. His left eye was swollen shut, but his right eye stared up at Palmer, wide with terror. Without another word, Palmer walked away.

When Banting had patched up the Italian and sent him on to the casualty clearing station, Palmer returned and put his hand on Banting's neck and walked him to the ambulance. Haggard with fatigue and weak from the loss of blood, Banting did not resist. Banting eased himself into the seat next to the driver, and within seconds his chin had dropped to his chest. Palmer tapped the roof of the vehicle and it hurtled off over the muddy, shell-pocked field with the sleeping officer.

At the casualty clearing station Banting was given morphine and told that he would be evacuated to England. The next thing he knew he was at the Number One General Hospital in Manchester, and his wound had been debrided.

Banting sent word to Dr. W. E. Gallie whom he knew from Toronto. Permissions were promptly secured, and Gallie was soon in Manchester, examining Banting's arm. He determined that the wound on the dorsum of the forearm was infected and there was a slight ulnar nerve lesion. Banting remained at the hospital in Manchester for two weeks, at the end of which he took a turn for the worse. He was transferred to Buxton, where there was discussion about amputating his arm. The surgeons told him he had a choice between losing his arm and losing his life if the infection persisted. It was an argument that Banting had made to others, but he had never been on the receiving end of it. He would have none of it, arguing with such force and irascibility that no one dared to cross him. Further, he insisted that he and only he should direct his care. Ultimately he prevailed. The resident surgeons left him alone to take his chances. No doubt some were surprised when the infection cleared up.

Banting's refusal to comply with military orders won him the Military Cross. His refusal to comply with medical advice won him the use of his right arm. With this arm he would save the lives of millions of diabetic children. His would be the medical breakthrough that Dr. Frederick Allen had so long believed was imminent.

SEVEN

War, Peace, and Politics, 1914–1918

THE DEMOCRATIC CANDIDATE FOR THE 1916 UNITED STATES PRES-idential election was the incumbent, Woodrow Wilson. The nation was consumed with one central question: Should the United States enter the war? For more than two excruciating years, America had stood by while Europe suffered appalling losses. At the time, the United States was a nation of recent immigrants, and many Americans had strong ties to Europe. A vast number of them were crying out for America to join. Pitted against Wilson was the only person ever to resign a seat on the Supreme Court to run for president of the United States, Charles Evans Hughes.

Woodrow Wilson's campaign slogan was "He kept us out of war." Charles Evans Hughes agreed that the United States should remain neutral. Many others believed that the nation's passivity was shameful.

One who held this opinion with special fervency was a forty-two-year-old Scot named John James Rickard Macleod. He was the chair of the physiology department of Case Reserve Medical School (now Case Western Reserve University School of Medicine) in Cleveland, Ohio, one of the preeminent medical schools in America. A discipline within biological science, physiology is the study of the normal mechanical, physical, and biochemical processes of the tissues and organs of animals and plants, including nutrition, movement, and reproduction. In Cleveland, Macleod distinguished himself as a medical authority and a favorite teacher. In 1913 he published the monograph *Diabetes: Its Pathological Physiology,* adding this title to a growing list of journal articles, book chapters, and lectures that bore his byline. But as his professional career was escalating, so were the tensions in Europe, where both his family and his wife's family lived. Since moving to Ohio, Macleod and his wife had spent every other summer with family in Aberdeen, Scotland, but when Britain went to war in 1914, their trips overseas stopped.

The son of a hardworking, popular reverend with the Free Church of Scotland (Presbyterian), John was the eldest of five, having two brothers and two sisters. His brother Clement had followed him into medicine, and in November of 1914 he enlisted and was sent immediately to France with the Royal Army Medical Corps (RAMC). America watched from across the Atlantic, and with increasing agitation, so did the eldest Macleod.

When the Germans sank the British luxury liner *Lusitania* in May 1915, causing the loss of 128 American civilian lives, Macleod was sure that America would enter the war at last. The tragedy drew a hue and cry from the American people and supported the rising tide of anti-German sentiment. Many Americans of German descent suffered for this. Wilson sent three formal messages to Germany, each more strongly worded than the previous one. Some Americans objected to Wilson's response for being too mild, others decried it for being too strong. Secretary of State William Jennings Bryan resigned in protest over Wilson's handling of the matter.

On July 1, 1916, as Wilson and Hughes traversed the country giving campaign speeches, the Battle of the Somme began. It was to be the bloodiest day in the history of the British army, resulting in 57,470 British casualties, including 19,240 dead. Macleod was nearly mad with anxiety. How could American leaders continue to defend a position of neutrality in the face of such a devastating toll? In April, the Germans used poison gas for the first time. Meanwhile Americans hummed to songs by Irving Berlin and W. C. Handy as Ford's one-millionth car rolled off the assembly line and D. W. Griffith's Civil War epic, *Birth of a Nation* was released.

Macleod's vitriolic despair began to poison his relationships. He became increasingly critical of the university president, dean, and trustees, several members of the faculty, and Americans in general. His wife was unwell. His brother Robert, who had gone to sea as an engineer, died mysteriously in the Malay Peninsula. Clement, who had been away at the war for nearly three years, developed tuberculosis. He was awarded the British Military Cross (MC) and eventually returned to Aberdeen to die.

Within months of Woodrow Wilson's election to a second term as president, he who had campaigned on the slogan "He kept us out of war" committed to sending American troops across the Atlantic. The American Expeditionary Force began training in the spring of 1917; it would be the largest force ever to leave American shores. But it was too late for Macleod.

After fifteen years at Western Reserve University School of Medicine, Macleod made up his mind to bring an end to what had been a largely successful career as a prolific researcher and teacher. As far as Macleod was concerned, America had abandoned the British Empire, and so he would abandon America. He resigned the professorship of physiology in 1918.

Macleod was a world authority on carbohydrates and metabolism. Any medical school in the United States would have been delighted to add him to its faculty roster. Had he chosen Harvard, he would be near to Joslin. Had he chosen Yale, he would be near to Allen. Macleod transferred to the University of Toronto, deliberately resituating himself within the dominions of the British Empire.

In June 1918, Jake and Mary Macleod moved into a lovely English country-style house, built by an English architect, in the Rosedale section of Toronto. Sir Robert Falconer, president of the University of Toronto, had been courting Macleod since 1916. He knew that he had scored a great victory in signing him to the medical school faculty. What he could not yet know was just how great a victory it was. In this single act, he had committed the university to the pages of history in indelible ink and would secure for Canada its first Nobel Prize.

EIGHT

Glens Falls, New York, April 1920

CHARLES EVANS HUGHES SAT AT HIS DESK HOLDING A LETTER IN-viting him to deliver the commencement speech at Wellesley College in June 1920. His middle daughter, Catherine, would be among the graduating class. When he agreed to deliver the commencement speech several months before, he had had only the dimmest idea that by June Catherine might be his only daughter. On this particular afternoon in April, he was struggling to think of anything hopeful to say to young women, or anything hopeful to say at all. It had been a punishing year since Allen delivered his diagnosis.

In the spring of 1919, Helen returned to work for a month or so before attending the long-anticipated reunion at Vassar College. But instead of the lively weekend with friends that she expected, she was suddenly taken ill again. This time the doctors did not deliver a good report. In July 1919, Mr. and Mrs. Hughes were stunned to learn that she was suffering from advanced tuberculosis.

The Hughes's penchant for privacy, dignity, and decorum meant that they preferred to address Helen's illness, like Elizabeth's, as discreetly as possible. Antoinette, Helen, Elizabeth, and Blanche moved to a rented house in Glens Falls, New York, where Charles had spent his early childhood in a small house on Maple Street. Glens Falls was conveniently near to the well-known therapeutic communities of Saratoga Springs and Ballston Spa, which competed with each other for the title the "Queen of Spas." In 1919, the therapies for the restoration of health and vigor included fresh air, sunshine, rest, and "taking the waters." Each summer, the visitors from New York City alone numbered in the tens of thousands.

Some of the water from the celebrated springs in Saratoga tasted like rotten eggs, some like wet dog fur, and some like steel submerged in seawater, but health-seeking tourists were nevertheless eager to stroll the beautifully designed Congress Park where elegant marble fountains were connected directly to individual underground springs such as Coesa, Hathorn, and Geyser. Each spring had its unique mineral composition, degree of carbonation, and particular medicinal properties. For example, the waters of Geyser Spring were prescribed for acid stomach, while the waters of Hathorn Spring were recommended for constipation.

All through the summer and fall Charles commuted the two hundred miles to Glens Falls from Manhattan every Saturday morning, returning to the city on Sunday. It was a grueling schedule. He drove himself at such a frightening pace and with such fervor that during one of his weekend visits Antoinette cautioned him that she could only manage one patient at a time and that if he insisted on having a nervous breakdown, he would have to wait until Helen had fully recovered her strength. Helen struggled to do just that. She desperately wanted to visit her beloved summer haven, the serene campus of Silver Bay, an insurmountable thirty-five miles north of Glens Falls. She was so weak that she could barely make it from her bed to the porch without being wracked by uncontrollable coughing that turned her face a frightening purple and exhausted her physically, spiritually, and emotionally.

By the summer of 1919, Elizabeth and her nurse, Blanche Burgess, had become inseparable. Blanche was a thirty-year-old war widow from New England. With no husband or children, Blanche devoted herself completely to Elizabeth. The pair had been living mostly at home, but there were periodic stays at Allen's sanitarium so that Elizabeth could be assessed and treated and Blanche could receive more training. Wherever she went, Blanche took a gram scale, a 100 cc graduated measuring cylinder, and the various equipment and solutions necessary for urinalysis. Elizabeth seemed to take to in-patient care quite well, a fact which Allen hoped Elizabeth was reporting in her near daily letters to her mother.

Week by week, the more dire Helen's situation became, the cheerier Elizabeth's letters were. She seemed determined to counterbalance the despair that she knew her mother was feeling. She had taken to addressing her long, chatty letters to "Dearest Mumsey." She was fascinated with photography and made good use of her new camera. The Physiatric Institute was among the first institutions of its kind to make radio available for the entertainment of patients. Each room featured a headset and the common rooms were equipped with speakers. She was an avid reader of newspapers and adventure stories. She signed her letters—"ME!" The signature was so emphatic that whenever Antoinette encountered it she imagined Elizabeth stomping her foot and hollering: *I am still here!*

All through July and August the oppressive heat bore down, and the evenings rang with the songs of cicadas, crickets, and peeper frogs. Antoinette and Charles doted on the increasingly frail Helen who was, quite literally, drowning in her bed. As her condition worsened, she slept more and more deeply. The weight and fabric of her dream life took on a vivid and realistic quality that she had never before experienced. In her dreams, she frequently found herself walking over the soft lawns of Silver Bay and all throughout the next day she could not fully dismiss the idea from her mind that she had actually been there and breathed the sweet easy air.

As Helen slipped away, Antoinette was nearly driven to insensibility by her utter helplessness in the situation. It didn't help that that year's hit song was, Bert Williams's "O Death Where Is Thy Sting?"

Charles described his Helen as "a ray of sunshine," and "just pure gold!" and "a rare and joyous spirit, radiating happiness not only in our home but in all her associations. Dedicating her life to good works, she realized my ideal of a beautiful character." On through the autumn and winter she struggled against the sodden dark that closed in around her like the reedy stream around *Hamlet*'s Ophelia. Each shallow inhalation filled her pale, sunken chest with a lacerating pain.

Christmas of 1919 was a bleak affair for the Hughes family. The only bright spot was when Charlie and his wife, Marjory, who had been a classmate of Helen's at Vassar, came with their two sons, four-year-old Charles Evans Hughes III and three-year-old Henry Stuart

Hughes. Elizabeth, weighing in at a mere 62½ pounds, watched her two nephews enjoy the newly popular Christmas treat—the candy cane. At Christmas Elizabeth was at the outside edge of the postdiagnosis survival range, having lived twelve months since the onset of symptoms. She was plagued by colds and tonsillitis that upset her metabolism, and Allen struggled to maintain the dietary inflection point that would balance her metabolism and keep her alive. That winter the elusive magic combination of carbohydrate, fat, and protein seemed to fluctuate from hour to hour. Elizabeth was consuming fewer than five hundred calories a day and losing weight and strength, but she was alive—for now. But within months, the unmistakable signs of the final starvation would begin: muscle wasting, dry, scaly skin, and hair loss.

Dr. Howk, Helen's doctor in Glens Falls, waited until after the holiday to tell Charles and Antoinette that there was no hope for their eldest daughter.

The Hugheses were not alone in beginning the New Year under a cloud of worry and fear. A stock market crash had begun on November 13, 1919. It followed the postwar boom and added to the many postwar problems that were destroying President Woodrow Wilson's health. Over the 660 days that the crash ultimately endured, the Dow Jones Industrial Average plummeted from 119.62 to 63.9, a total loss of just over 46 percent. But the nation would soon see that there *were* ways to make money, illegal ones.

In January 1920, the Eighteenth Amendment went into effect and the great experiment of prohibition began. The nation began sorting itself into two populations. The pietistic Protestants (largely Methodists, Northern Baptists, Southern Baptists, Presbyterians, Congregationalists, Quakers, and Lutherans), having won the legislative battle, grew in strength and number. After America's dark night of struggle and anguish, the country was returning to the spirit of its founding, and a bright new era was dawning. This was the movement in which Helen had so hoped to participate. But America could not recover its prewar innocence, and while the pious gathered in places like Silver Bay to teach youth a wholesome way of life, another population was gathering together in smoke-filled speakeasies. A culture of flappers and bootleggers began to flourish also; they met furtively to play cards, listen to jazz, and drink contraband whiskey and gin. Women bobbed their hair, hiked up their hemlines, and climbed into automobiles to sit behind the steering wheel as America roared into the 1920s.

The changing hairstyles and hemlines were emblematic of a major shift in the cultural identity of the American woman, and the decision of short or long was packed with political significance. Because hair and dress styles are such visible symbols, there was little room for the coy and the undecided, and by virtue of this, just stepping outside became a public declaration.

In the Hughes women, as in many families, the lines did not fall neatly along generational lines. Helen kept her hair long and continued to wear it in a conservative Victorian topknot like her mother. Although she worked for a women's organization, she supported rather than embodied the woman of the future. The beautiful, vivacious Catherine, on the other hand, bobbed her hair at Wellesley. Elizabeth followed suit.

Catherine, the tallest and prettiest of the three Hughes girls, had inherited the dark, flashing eyes of her paternal grandfather. Set in her smooth, perfectly oval face, they were completely bewitching. She loved fashion and looked wonderful in clothes; the styles of the 1920s suited her lean, athletic shape to perfection. She was popular and seemed always to be surrounded by a crowd of young people. All through her career at Wellesley, Catherine's spirited and playful manner belied the tragic burden of her family, for while she was playing tennis and attending dances, both her older and younger sisters lay dying.

Elizabeth's weight hovered in the low sixties; Allen continued to cut her calories in an effort to gain control over her metabolic slide into diabetic danger. On January 11, 1920, Helen turned twenty-eight years old. She was too weak to blow out her own birthday candles.

On February 10, 1920, Antoinette wrote a letter to Charles:

> *Oh the pathos of it! I have never struggled with myself more desperately than I have this week, with the result that I have kept up through the day, but the nights have been hideous. I thought after all that we went through last summer I was prepared for anything but I was not prepared for the definiteness of Dr. Howk's statements. My imagination ran riot and the many practical matters with their complications nearly drove me mad.*

Certainly one of the "complications" on her mind was the presidential election in November 1920, just seven months away. The Republican National Convention was to be held even sooner, in June. People were already predicting that Hughes would likely emerge from the convention as the Republican nominee. Charles would not campaign without her, but how could she manage to accompany her husband on a nationwide presidential campaign with two daughters racing each other to the cemetery?

Helen Hughes would never see Silver Bay again. She never left the house in Glens Falls. She died on April 18, 1920. She was buried in lot number 12673 on Elder Avenue at Woodlawn Cemetery in the Bronx, New York. There she joined her paternal grandparents, the Reverend David Hughes and Mary C. Hughes, also buried in the family plot.

Woodlawn's necropolis of three hundred thousand residents occupies four hundred acres of extraordinary history, architecture, and natural beauty. These were but small comfort to the Hughes family on the April morning they buried Helen.

From where Antoinette stood beside the coffin she could see two small stones memorializing children in adjacent plots. And there was the enormous monument of Theo Malmberry, a twenty-four-year-old Columbia graduate, which stood just across from the Hughes family plot. They saw it each time they had visited the graves of Charles's parents and the sad gray eyes of the tall stone angel seemed to greet them with particular kindness when they had filed past her this morning. Between the war and influenza, so many families had suffered so much grief in these last years.

That morning the sky was piercing blue, the air perfumed with the earthy pungency of the dark wet mound of earth beside the grave. The last stubborn drifts of snow had melted and the crocuses were blooming, dappling the lawns with touches of lavender, saffron, and white. The branches of the large gingko tree that grew at the edge of the plot were knobby with new buds. The world was stirring from its long dark dream, but Helen would never awake.

Just as Antoinette's body had been changed by Helen's arrival in the world—her pelvis splaying and her breasts filling with milk—so Helen's departure had expressed itself on her physically. Every inch of Antoinette's body ached—her teeth, her scalp, her eye sockets, and the quick of her fingernails—as a part of her life, as elemental as the rhythm of her heartbeat, was lowered into the dark wet ground. It was all she could do to keep herself from climbing in after the coffin.

Charles's posture lacked its former upright carriage; his spine was slightly pitched forward, as if he were carrying something heavy on his back. He would later say that Helen's death was the greatest sadness of his life. To the end of his days he never spoke of her without a quaver in his voice.

Hughes shook a shovelful of earth over the open pit. The sound of it dropping, clod by clod, onto Helen's coffin echoed among the sad stones of the cemetery. Even the hardened gravediggers, watching from a respectful distance, seemed gentled by it. *Man cometh forth like a flower and is cut down* (Job 14:2).

All the woe in the world seemed to press in upon this huddled family, swaddled in baleful black wool, damp with tears and anguish in the still stone city of aggrieved memory. How few and vulnerable they seemed now, this family of great stature and privilege and promise, how pathetic the flickering power of their personalities against the great dull darkness of uncomprehending sorrow. There were Charles and Antoinette and Charlie and Marjory and their two sons, Charles III and Henry, fidgeting at their tearful mother's knee. Catherine, who would be graduated from Wellesley in just two months, wore a mask of ashen stoicism. Elizabeth was too weak to attend the burial, but she was certainly not far from her mother's mind.

For Antoinette, it was not just Helen's interment that weighed on her, but the thought that this same group would almost certainly be gathered here in this spot within the year to bury Elizabeth, perhaps even before grass had taken root in the fresh earth over Helen's grave. Helen had been twenty-eight. Elizabeth would not likely see fourteen.

Antoinette was mistaken. It would be twenty-five years when the next Hughes would be laid to rest in the Woodlawn family plot, and this time it would be Antoinette herself. Elizabeth would never be buried in Woodlawn cemetery. In fact, Elizabeth would never be buried at all.

NINE

❧

The Idea of the Physiatric Institute, May 1920

O N THE MORNING OF HELEN'S FUNERAL, DR. FREDERICK ALLEN
squared himself at his desk at the sanitarium on Fifty-first Street.
Before him on the dark green blotter was a heavy brass paperweight
engraved with the words "The less food, the more life," a gift from Belle
Wishart, his loyal and capable superintendent, given to him at the opening of the sanitarium nearly one year before. Across the room stood a
tower of boxes: A shipment of the latest printing of *The Starvation (Allen) Treatment of Diabetes* had just arrived. The Allen treatment was
working. Although some patients died of starvation, many others lived
past their prognoses—albeit in agony. Each day these patients remained
alive was a day that a cure might be discovered. The sanitarium was
regularly occupied. Elizabeth's health had improved since Christmas, no
doubt due in part to her resilient spirit and flawless adherence to the
prescribed regimen.

Several unopened envelopes lay on the blotter. He opened the first
one. It contained an invoice from a pharmacy for basic supplies for urine
testing: copper sulphate, potassium hydroxide, sodium citrate, sodium
carbonate, distilled water. The second envelope, sent by registered mail,
held the news that the property in which both his practice and the sanitarium were housed had been sold. He was to vacate the premises by July
15, 1920.

His first reaction—fury—quickly dissipated. The sale of the building prompted him to make a change that he had been mulling over for a long time. Now, at last, he had a reason to make the leap. He envisioned creating an institute that would symbiotically bring/together clinical work and research under one roof. However, unlike the Rockefeller Institute, it would do so in a spa-like setting, which would encourage fresh air and daily exercise. This unique combination of features would attract both established scientists and postdoctoral students, the best scientific minds from around the world to seek a cure for diabetes and other diseases. The institute would welcome patients from all walks of life, supplying the most luxurious accommodations to those who could afford to pay and allowing charity patients to pay in kind with work-exchange arrangements. He had even dreamed up a name for his vision. The Physiatric Institute. Allen could hardly think of the words without grinning. The Physiatric Institute—from the Greek words *physikos* (physical) and *iatreia* (healing)—would be the nation's first institution dedicated solely to the care and study of metabolic disorders, particularly juvenile diabetes.

Time was short. Allen's mind raced with dozens of incremental tasks that would be needed to realize his vision. He sat down at his desk and started to make a list, his pen moving furiously over the tablet. In no time he had filled an entire page. The very first task on the list was a visit to Charles Evans Hughes.

It was now one year since Allen had walked from his office to deliver the grim news of Elizabeth's fatal diagnosis. Although the sanitarium was on the verge of being shut down (after which he would be technically unemployed), Allen had never felt as optimistic as he did that afternoon in early May 1920 as he walked up Fifth Avenue to the corner of Sixty-fourth Street to present his master plan for the Physiatric Institute to Charles Evans Hughes. He carried the proposal in a slim portfolio in anticipation of laying it before the man whose judicial demeanor was so aloof and austere that the press had dubbed him "the Baptist Pope." Allen could not possibly have known how keenly willing Hughes would be to help him, how precious the prospect of being able to do something, anything, to help ease the suffering of his desperately ill daughter Elizabeth.

This would be the fourth time Dr. Allen had given the presentation. The first he had confided in his most trusted colleague, Miss Wishart. Emboldened as he was by her enthusiastic support, he proceeded to share it with his fellow physicians at the sanitarium. Then he told the entire staff of the sanitarium, assembled for a compulsory meeting at which he also announced the imminent closure of the sanitarium.

Much to his amazement, and perhaps for the first time in his professional life, his idea met with unanimous support and the entire staff expressed an interest in following Dr. Allen to his new enterprise. In view of his history of difficult interpersonal relations, this response moved him deeply. He felt that he was being carried forward by a force of destiny.

A uniformed maid ushered Dr. Allen into Hughes's study, leading him gingerly through the hushed, dimly lit house. Hughes looked up from the draft of the Wellesley commencement speech. (He would speak of vigilant adherence to democratic ideals: *Unless we have in peace time, that dominant sentiment which prompts a continuous and self-sacrificing devotion to public ends, the sacrifices of patriotism in war will have been in vain.*) His face was gray and drawn. Clearly, the last few months had taken their toll. With little introductory small talk Allen explained the circumstances necessitating his relocation and placed the proposal in Hughes's hands. Hughes took the sheaf of paper and dealt four pages in the style of a croupier, laying them side by side before him on the desk. He turned his preternatural mind to the pages and, as if he were reading them simultaneously, he gathered them and replaced them with the next four pages. Allen watched in silence, pressing his damp palms together.

The proposal described the purchase of the "Cedar Court" estate owned by Mr. Otto H. Kahn, located one mile outside the city of Morristown, New Jersey, thirty-eight miles from New York City. The property sprawled over 176 lush, level acres, 136 of which had been tamed and trimmed into luxuriant gardens and grounds while the remaining 40 acres were farmland. To Hughes, it sounded like a promising location for bird-watching, in other words, an ideal environment for Elizabeth.

The main building was an Italianate mansion of magnificent proportions. The living space in the residence, including a wing connected to it by a glorious glass-enclosed pagoda, totaled forty rooms. These would comfortably accommodate the administrative force and thirty full-pay patients, with alterations to be made as necessary to accommodate fifty or more according to the extent of the need. The other structures on the property included a superintendent's cottage, caretaker's cottage, two farmhouses, several greenhouses, and, best of all, a dairy designed for pasteurization and storage that could be adapted easily into an animal research laboratory to house thirty dogs.

The estate had cost Kahn over a million dollars; he would sell it for $250,000. The contract called for $10,000 in cash up front and another $20,000 in two months. Allen would need investors both now and later, for even if he were to succeed in raising enough money to purchase the property, there was the cost of operation to consider. Mr. Kahn had employed between fifteen and twenty-two men year-round just to maintain the grounds; Dr. Allen's proposal called for five full-time groundskeepers. Because the property had been vacant and deteriorating for several years, there were repairs to consider, and the nine hot-air furnaces would have to be replaced with central steam heat before the first winter. It was an undertaking of enormous magnitude and complexity but it was worth the effort if it meant that Allen and his patients would never again be evicted.

The medical purposes of the Physiatric Institute would be progressive and educational, treating patients as partners in their therapy. Only those patients who would seriously commit themselves to their own improvement would be admitted, and they would be selected regardless of their ability to pay. Each case would be carefully studied to determine the proper diet to keep the disorder under control. Dietary prescriptions would be highly personalized and require dedicated and individual attention from staff members. Patients would be taught their diet so that they could continue their treatment at home, either alone or under the supervision of a local physician. Patients would keep their own detailed charts describing the preparation and circumstances of each morsel of food ingested, and the time of day and, for the first time, they would perform their own regular urine tests.

Allen had worked out the operating costs of the new enterprise in a general way, basing his figures on the per-person cost of room and board at the Fifty-first Street sanitarium. His plan was to charge thirty paying patients enough to support thirty charity patients. He was so committed to the ideal of the institute that he was prepared to forfeit any personal compensation for his work there. He did not include a personal salary in the budget. Allen believed he could depend entirely on his practice in New York City for personal income. He could not imagine how much it would cost to keep such an enormous property heated but he believed, naïvely, that grants and donations would materialize to make up for any operating deficit.

The first step toward the goal would involve the formation of a corporation to be run without profit to its stockholders. Allen would need the kind of investors who could attract more of the same. He thought the timing of his approach to Hughes was good. For an entire year he had overseen the care of Elizabeth, slowly earning her parents' trust. Elizabeth was four feet eleven inches tall and weighed seventy-five pounds when he first examined her. Although her weight plummeted soon after she came under his care, he had kept it relatively stable for most of the year, gradually increasing her diet to seven hundred calories or more. For the most part he had accommodated her parents' wish to keep her living at home. He had trained Blanche (well, really, he had Miss Wishart to thank for this) in dietetic food preparation and glucose testing. Blanche had proved to be surprisingly dedicated, keeping excellent records and developing an aptitude for timely and accurate urine testing. Elizabeth herself had proved to be perfectly reliable in honoring his dietary constraints, gram for gram, and taking regular exercise as directed. As a result, she was—quite literally—living proof of the success of the Allen treatment.

As Allen left the meeting with Hughes, he paused at the corner and looked south over the architectural marvels that crowded the narrow island of his adopted home. There was the soaring Singer Tower and the majestic Woolworth Building, the behemoth structures of Penn Station and Madison Square Garden, which somehow managed to be both graceful and gargantuan. Allen was confident that forces even more powerful than Charles Evans Hughes were working on his behalf in the universe. It seemed that new wonders were revealed daily, from aspirin to X-rays. Dirigibles transported people through the air, and subways transported them underground, and rotary dial telephones enabled them to speak directly to whomever they wished without going anywhere at all. Why wouldn't Hughes support the Physiatric Institute? Despite all the initial misgivings about undernutrition, Allen had saved Elizabeth from certain death, at least for the time being, which was really the only time there ever was. How could Hughes refuse him?

Hughes did not refuse him. After satisfying himself by privately commissioning an investigative report on the venture, Hughes agreed to serve as honorary chairman of the Physiatric Institute. The name "The Hon. Charles E. Hughes" would top the list of fifty honorary chairmen on the letterhead, including many of the most recognizable names in New York. As chairman of the Draft Appeals Board, Hughes had been responsible for thousands of life-and-death decisions. As honorary chairman of the Physiatric Institute, he would be responsible for many more lives— including Elizabeth's. But despite Hughes's support and the infusion of ten thousand dollars of Allen's own personal savings to launch the venture, the financial stability of the Physiatric Institute was tenuous. The campaign to raise money fell short and Allen was forced to invest an additional ten thousand dollars of his own money. But he remained wholly committed to the idea: The institute was to be the last resort and the best hope for diabetic children everywhere. Allen's future was set, or so he thought.

On October 30, 1920, just six months after the Hughes family gathered at Woodlawn Cemetery and Allen proposed his grand vision to Charles Evans Hughes, and one week before the United States presidential election, a twenty-eight-year-old unknown Canadian surgeon would be awakened suddenly from a fitful sleep. He had an idea.

Frederick Allen would keep Elizabeth alive long enough to benefit from that idea.

TEN

Banting's House in London, Ontario, October 30-31, 1920

ON SUNDAY, OCTOBER 30, 1920, JUST BEFORE MIDNIGHT, DR. FREDerick Grant Banting was scratching in the cold, hard earth outside a white brick house at 442 Adelaide Street North in London, Ontario. He had propped a small candle on the ground so that he could see what he was doing, but the flame kept flickering and sputtering out. The symbolism was not lost on him. On that day and at that hour, Banting felt as discouraged about his professional prospects as Frederick Allen felt hopeful about his own. Squatting there, clawing at the ground, his feelings of dejection were especially acute. As he sifted the frost-hardened dirt through his large, square hands, he catalogued the myriad missed opportunities and bad breaks that had cascaded upon him since his return from the war.

The next morning, Monday, October 31, he was to give a lecture on carbohydrate metabolism and the pancreas at the University of Western Ontario. Just a few weeks earlier, Professor Frederick Miller, head of the Department of Physiology, had offered Banting a lecturer position in the Department of Surgery and Physiology, which brought in an additional eight to ten dollars per week. Banting was barely qualified to teach the class, but he had assured Professor Miller that week by week he could keep ahead of the students. Some weeks he did so by the slenderest margin imaginable. He often had trouble sleeping the night before he was to give a lecture, and tonight was no exception. He had spent the day preparing his talk and brooding about his life.

He felt lost, not just in the curriculum of physiology but in the inscrutable geography of his life. He had gone from being a country farm boy to being a medical student to being a decorated officer in the Canadian army and now he found himself unemployed and in debt, casting about for direction, plagued by resentments about the past, and paralyzed with fear about the future.

Only four months before, on July 1, 1920, he had driven a wooden spike into the same ground in front of the big white brick house on the quiet, residential street. Atop the spike was a sign bearing the proud inscription DR. F. G. BANTING. He had purchased the house from a local shoe merchant, Rowland Hill, with the expectation of settling there and building a future with his intended, Edith Roach.

The total purchase price was $7,800. Fred borrowed some of the $2,000 down payment from his father, and the Hills took a mortgage for the balance. They agreed that the Hills would continue to occupy the house for up to a year while their new house was being built, and Fred would use a small bedroom on the second floor and the front parlor for an office. He wouldn't need the whole house until he and Edith moved in to begin their married life. With the purchase of the house he was finally making good on a proposal he had made four years, half a world, and a war ago. It was to be a symbol of his moving forward from a difficult period of transition back to civilian life.

In the four months between, nothing had happened and everything had gone wrong. He and Edith continued their tortured engagement, seeing each other nearly every Saturday, but each week was more painful than the last. Twice she had returned the engagement ring, and once he had asked for it back, yet neither Fred nor Edith seemed capable of ending it once and for all. The week before, he had buried the ring to prevent himself from offering it to her again. Now he was scraping away at the earth looking for it.

As he piled the stones beside the hole, forming an accidental cairn, he tried to recall the first event in the avalanche of his misfortune. Amidst the thundering horror and pitiless carnage of Cambrai, he had thought every day about returning to life in Toronto, but the Toronto that he imagined returning to bore scant resemblance to the city he found when he returned. During the war, women had stepped in to fill many of the traditionally male jobs that had been vacated by soldiers.

Consequently, the soldiers returned to an employment shortage that was exacerbated by high inflation and a sea change in gender roles. And the population continued to grow so rapidly—from 86,000 in 1885 to 521,000 in 1921—that the city government's main occupation was building up the infrastructure to sustain it.

Edith had changed as well. While Banting had been in the trenches, developing a colorful vocabulary and quite a few other bad habits, Edith had completed her studies at Victoria College, taking the gold medal in Modern Languages. She had also adopted some modern ideas and attitudes. For one thing, she had begun to earn her way in the world as a high school teacher in Ingersoll, some ninety-six miles southwest of Toronto. With Edith employed but relocated and Banting in Toronto but penniless, their long-awaited reunion got off to a bad start and deteriorated from there.

The city held annual veterans' parades to honor the half-million Canadian soldiers who fought in Europe, and built a war memorial in front of city hall, but it did not honor the veterans with what they wanted—jobs. Banting found temporary work at Toronto's Hospital for Sick Children, assisting surgeons C. L. Starr and W. E. Gallie, whom he knew from the CAMC, but he was not invited to stay on. As he reflected years later, "Surgeons were very plentiful in Toronto. It was my greatest ambition to obtain a place on the staff of the [Hospital for Sick Children], but this was not forthcoming."

While in Toronto, he had reconnected with Bill Tew, a classmate who had been class president in their final year of college. Tew was working at Burnside, the obstetrical unit of Toronto General Hospital. They discussed setting up private practices, and together decided to try the second largest city in Western Ontario, London, where there would be less competition. With some reluctance Banting left Toronto in June 1920.

Fred's attempts to persuade Edith that the move to London was a move toward their future together fell on deaf ears. Edith was now one month shy of her twenty-fifth birthday. She had waited for Fred for four years. Although she had offered to support them until Fred could get his feet under him professionally, he was adamant that they would not wed until he could support her. He held fast to traditional ideas about marriage and grand ambitions for work. He was interested in innovative orthopedic solutions and in new surgical techniques—he took pride in a prosthetic foot he had fashioned for a child—but he hadn't yet managed to settle into a secure arrangement. Apparently, Edith had been waiting for him only to wait for him. Still, she hoped he would surprise her with an invitation to move to London on her birthday. He did not.

Now Fred stared at the darkened windows of the big, brick house, as if he could will his happy future to materialize before his eyes. He tried to imagine Edith moving about in the kitchen or singing children to sleep in the nursery upstairs, or himself busily preparing prescriptions in the small apothecary that adjoined his office, readying for a full schedule of patients the next day.

Such scenes had certainly not materialized in his life. After he opened his practice, weeks passed without a single patient. Bill Tew had also opened a practice in London, but his office was located in town and was developing nicely. Banting's income for his first month in business had been four dollars. That had come from a sad and shaking alcoholic desperate for a prescription for alcohol—during prohibition this was the only legal way to procure spirits. In August his income rose to $37, in September to $48, and in October to $66, but his expenses still surpassed his income. He was restless during the long idle days that stretched interminably between patients and spent the numbingly quiet hours in the unfamiliar town reading war poetry and medical textbooks.

Just a few days after Banting knelt in the dirt to look for the ring, a poem entitled "The Second Coming" was published, written by Irish poet William Butler Yeats. It wrenchingly captured Banting's disillusionment and despair:

> *Things fall apart; the centre cannot hold;*
> *Mere anarchy is loosed upon the world,*
> *The blood-dimmed tide is loosed, and everywhere*
> *The ceremony of innocence is drowned;*
> *The best lack all conviction, while the worst*
> *Are full of passionate intensity.*
> *Surely some revelation is at hand . . .*

About this time Ken Banting came to London, sent by the family on the unhappy errand of trying to straighten out the wayward youngest brother. Ken demanded to know what efforts Fred had taken to get his practice off the ground. Had he advertised? Had he gone door-to-door to introduce himself to families in the area? Had he made the rounds at the local hospital? The truth was he had done little more than sit in the parlor waiting for patients to arrive, and he had the results to prove it. Of course, he had also devoted a good deal of every day to brooding on why he hadn't followed his friend Bill Tew's lead and opened a practice in town. And then there was always the daily agonizing over his feelings about Edith.

"If it doesn't take off, what will you do? How will you pay your mortgage?"

"All right. All right!" Fred snapped. "I've secured a job as a medical demonstrator at the University of Western Ontario. Did you know that?"

"Medical demonstrator? How much does that pay?"

Fred hesitated before admitting that it was only two dollars per hour.

"I've been thinking of joining up with an oil expedition," Fred said suddenly. He had only just heard about this from Bill Tew the previous afternoon. Bill wasn't interested in the opportunity for himself, and he had mentioned it almost as a joke. In fact, Fred had hardly given it another thought until just that moment. "They're considering taking along a doctor. It could be quite an adventure, wouldn't you say?" Fred added gamely.

Ken did not smile.

"So you'll marry Edith, park her in the house, and leave for the Northwest Territory?"

"Well . . . I'm not so sure what's to become of Edith and me."

"So it's over between you and Edith and you're selling the house?" Ken, ever the practical farmer, flew into a rage. "Then sell the ring and use the money to start paying off Pa, who, if you care to know, sacrificed quite a bit to lend you that money!"

Fred was shamefaced. He sat silently and took the tongue-lashing that his brother delivered. It seemed to go on and on.

As Fred's cold-cramped fingers continued to claw in the dirt, Ken's reproach rang in his head. How *would* he tell his father that he was selling the house so soon after borrowing the money to buy it? Banting would try to put a respectable gloss on it, concoct some story about putting his affection in cold storage in order to better devote himself to the demands of scientific research. He would make the case with conviction. His father would accept it. They would both know it was a lie, but his father would be too kind to deny his son this fragile pretense of dignity.

And then, suddenly, it was between his fingers—a white gold band with a small stone caked with dirt. He laid it on the palm of his hand and looked at it as if it were an exotic moth: perfectly formed, delicate, moribund. His back and legs ached from squatting. Exhaling, he rose slowly to his full height of six feet and squeezed the small, dirty ring in his right fist. A mean smirk twisted across his face as he considered hurling the ring at the house. The windows stared back, reflecting the starlit clouds skating across their unblinking surfaces.

It was after midnight—October 31, 1920.

Banting went inside and plugged the sink, then scrubbed the earth from his hands and the ring. At one o'clock in the morning he sat down and thumbed through the November issue of *Surgery, Gynecology and Obstetrics,* which had arrived in the mail the previous afternoon. Professor C. L. Starr of the Hospital for Sick Children had mentioned that there was an article in this issue that might interest him. It was a twelve-pager entitled "The Relation of the Islets of Langerhans to Diabetes with Special Reference to Cases of Pancreatic Lithiasis." The article began:

> Any reference to the pancreas as secreting a hormone necessary for the utilization of sugar by the tissues of the body is misleading as that function is, accurately speaking, exercised by only a very small portion of the organ, the so-called "islets" of Langerhans, so that what is generally understood as the relation of the pancreas to diabetes is rather the relation of the islets to that disease.

It was written by an American pathologist named Moses Barron, who was working at the University of Minnesota. Barron wrote about a rare case of pancreatic lithiasis (a pancreatic stone) that he had encountered during a routine autopsy. He noticed that while all of the acinar cells (that produced digestive enzymes) had atrophied, most of the islet cells (that produced hormones) were intact. This observation prompted him to research the literature related to the pancreas. He discovered that his finding was consistent with experimentation in which the pancreatic ducts were purposely blocked by ligation, or being tied off.

Bored, Banting cleaned traces of dirt from beneath his fingernails, then slumped in the chair and drifted into a restless sleep. He awoke twenty minutes later and tried again to concentrate on the article. He found the subject numbingly dull. Endocrinology—pity the poor bastards in that field! Imagine spending your life scrutinizing the murky ooze secreted by some obscure, oddly shaped gland. Orthopedic surgery—now that's where the action is. Any discipline that involves bringing a saw into an operating room is bound to be exciting. At least it had seemed that way when he was performing amputations in the trenches.

He was compelled to press on. The lecture loomed before him, just a few hours away. He imagined himself standing in the lecture hall before the expectant faces of the students. It would be just his luck that there would be some smart aleck among them who would try to humiliate Banting by asking questions he couldn't understand, never mind answer, revealing him for the incompetent instructor he feared he was.

After several tries, Banting got through all twelve tedious pages and again slipped into sleep. But at two o'clock in the morning he found himself awake, still clothed, still sitting in the chair by the bed, the journal still open in his lap. What had awakened him? A noise outside? A dream? No. He was awakened by the force of an idea.

He took the small black notebook from the bedside table and scribbled twenty-five words in a barely legible, sometimes misspelled, loopy, half-awake hand. These twenty-five words scrawled at two o'clock in the morning on October 31, 1920, would eventually lead to the solution of a medical mystery that had persisted for thousands of years. The notation was:

> *Diabetus [sic] Ligate pancreatic ducts of dog. Keep dogs alive till acini degenerate leave Islets. Try to isolate the internal secretion of these to relieve glycosurea [sic].*

The idea was essentially this: By ligating the pancreatic duct and allowing the acinar tissue of the pancreas to degenerate over six weeks, he could eliminate the destructive interference of the digestive enzyme and isolate the islet tissue and its elusive secretion. This secretion, sufficiently purified, had been shown to allay the symptoms of diabetes in animals.

It was not a new idea, but Banting was so unfamiliar with the literature that he wasn't aware that Lydia de Witt had described the same idea as early as 1906. He didn't know that in 1911–1912, a graduate student, Ernest Lyman Scott, had also come to the conclusion that the previous attempts to isolate the elusive internal secretion had failed because of the interference of the digestive enzyme, which destroyed the effective principle of the islet secretion before it could be identified. Scott even tested his theory by injecting depancreatized dogs with the isolated pancreatic extract and obtained results that confirmed his hypothesis in three out of four cases. Banting was not aware that, as recently as 1916, a Romanian physiologist named Nicolas Paulesco also injected dogs with a pancreatic extract that normalized their blood sugar levels. Paulesco had even named the magical extract "pancreine." (But Paulesco's work had not yet been published in English.) Unfortunately, these early researchers were unable to consistently reproduce their results. The process was exasperatingly complicated and delicate. In other words, not only was it difficult to extract and isolate insulin, but even if you did it was hard to prove it.

Banting's initial idea was neither original nor successful, but he persisted in it, and his persistence led to a solution that was *both* original *and* successful. He would later say that if he had been more familiar with the literature on the subject and had known about the previous attempts, he would not have pursued his idea at all. Fortunately for Elizabeth Hughes and millions of other children, he knew next to nothing.

ELEVEN

Toronto or Bust, October 1920 to April 1921

Banting resolved to approach Dr. Miller later that same morning, immediately after delivering his lecture, to explain his insight. He could hardly bring himself to wait that long. He would ask Miller for the resources to test his theory: a laboratory, an operating room, several dogs, and a salary sufficient to allow him to devote himself entirely to the work.

After the lecture, Banting met with Miller and explained his idea and the way it had come to him. He was so excited that twice Miller was forced to ask him to slow down. Although the details of the experiment were not entirely worked out, Miller understood that Banting believed he had arrived at a way to isolate a pancreatic extract. Miller also understood that Banting was absolutely convinced his idea would work and that he was determined to convince Miller of the same. Miller tried to sound encouraging, but biochemistry and the problems of the metabolism were not his area of expertise, so he was not in a position to assess the idea scientifically. In any case, he could not grant Banting's request because there were no laboratories available. The science department at Western was then in the midst of a comprehensive capital campaign and the new building was under construction. Miller and Banting sat silent for a moment, and then Miller's expression suddenly brightened.

"You might be the luckiest man in history," Miller said, his eyes twinkling.

"Why do you say that?"

"Because one of the greatest authorities on metabolism is in Toronto. I don't know why I didn't think of him immediately."

"Who is it? Who?"

"Does the name J. J. R. Macleod mean anything to you?"

"No."

"Well, it should. He wrote a textbook on diabetes—and now he's at the university!"

"He is? I don't remember a Macleod."

"He wasn't there when you were. He came a few years ago from one of the big medical schools in the United States. It was quite a coup for Toronto. If I remember right, he's an associate dean of the medical school and head of the physiology department. He'll have more labs than he knows what to do with! And your timing couldn't be better because Toronto's physiology department got a one million dollar grant not too long ago, so their laboratory facilities are top-notch."

"Will he talk to me?"

"Why not? You're an alumnus, and the subject will likely appeal to him since it's in his research field. You can tell him I suggested that you call on him. There's probably no better person on earth to advise you than Professor Macleod."

Banting left the meeting with Miller with one thought: If his brainstorm resulted in a medical breakthrough, it would vindicate him. It would prove his worth to Ken, Edith, and all the people who declined to hire him in Toronto. It would prove that the unhappy chapter in London had not been a waste of his time and his father's money. Whenever doubt crept in, he asked himself, "Why not me?" Hadn't Einstein been a lowly patent clerk when he had his epiphany about relativity? Hadn't he struggled to find a job after graduation, just as Banting had? Hadn't he claimed that imagination was more important than knowledge? Science failed when it neglected to ask the bold questions and when it dared not challenge the historical record. In November 1919 *The New York Times* headlines proclaimed "Lights All Askew in the Heavens. Men of Science More or Less Agog Over Results of Eclipse Observations. Einstein Theory Triumphs." The *Times* of London carried the headline "Revolution in Science. New Theory of the Universe. Newtonian Ideas Overthrown." The stories reported on the confirmation that the solar eclipse of May 29, 1919, had borne out Einstein's predictions, and Einstein, Banting told himself, had begun with a hunch just like his own. It was the age of big ideas. The heroes of the day were Edison, Tesla, von Zeppelin, Einstein, Curie. Would the name Banting be added to the list? He made plans to travel to Toronto.

Banting's confidence grew with each mile of the one-hundred-twenty-five-mile trip from London to Toronto to meet the great Professor Macleod. By the time he entered Macleod's office in early November 1920, he was filled with such zeal that his hypothesis seemed unassailable. Banting's first impression was that Macleod was a small man in a big office. Fifteen years older than Banting, Macleod was distinguished looking, dressed in a Harris tweed suit. His manner was formal and reserved. He had pale, freckled skin, a slightly receding hairline of fine sandy hair, and a brushy mustache.

Macleod was predisposed to feel warm toward Banting, not just because he was an alumnus but because he was a veteran of the CAMC, which had risen with courage and alacrity to fight in Europe. Macleod had been back in Toronto only a few months after having spent the summer in Scotland, the first trip home since the war. There he had reunited with his parents and sisters and spent what were to be his last days with his brother Clement, a veteran of the RAMC and, like Banting, a recipient of the military cross. (Clement would die less than two weeks after Macleod met with Banting.)

Banting was not at all as Macleod had expected him to be. He was self-conscious and inarticulate. Nervous, he refused to take a seat. Instead he paced the length of the office, cracking his knuckles and speaking in rapid, blustering bursts and then halting in midsentence, scowling and starting again on a different tack. Banting spoke with a surgeon's urgency rather than a researcher's deliberate calm. The proposal he set forth—if you could call it that—was hardly well considered. Essentially, Banting swaggered into the office, chattered about the rudiments of a research project, and demanded the means to carry it out. Watching him pace in front of his desk was like watching a wild animal: fascinating but you don't want to get too close.

"You operate on several dogs, locating the ducts connecting the pancreas to the duodenum. You tie off those ducts, closing them off completely, and close the incision. After seven weeks or so, the dog is recovered from the surgery and the acinar tissue that produces the digestive enzyme is atrophied. Then you open up the dog again and harvest the islets of Langerhans, which should contain only the secretion from the islets. Meanwhile, you've depancreatized another dog, rendering it diabetic. You take the harvested secretion and introduce it to the depancreatized dog, measuring the sugar in the urine and blood before and after. If the diabetic condition is relieved, then I'd say we've succeeded. If the dog dies, we failed."

"I see. And how exactly do you propose to introduce the harvested secretion to the depancreatized dog?"

"You could inject it intramuscularly or intravenously. You could even transplant the ligated pancreas into the depancreatized dog, grafting it into the abdomen somehow. I haven't worked out the particulars yet. The point is to see how long you can keep the diabetic dog alive."

"Very interesting," Macleod said. "You realize that it's not entirely unprecedented."

"What do you mean?"

"I mean to say that work like it has been done. Perhaps you could explain to me how your idea is different than previous efforts."

"Why?"

"Why? To show how your effort would be original and worthy of support."

"I'm not trying to be original. I'm trying to find something that works!"

"Well, yes, but let's start with what has been done. A review of the literature might be a good way to begin."

"Why?"

"Why? To learn from it, of course. The study of diabetes is a rapidly advancing area of research. Some of the greatest scientific minds of our time have been applied to the problem. Aren't you interested in their findings?"

"I'm more interested in finding a cure for diabetes than in reading about how others have tried and failed."

Macleod almost guffawed.

"I admire your zeal, Dr. Banting, and your idea is interesting, but there is a long history of failure to prepare an extract of pancreas that contains the effective property and I think you'd do well to familiarize yourself with it."

"But no one was using pancreases with ligated ducts!"

"That's not precisely accurate, as you would know if you had read the history. Are you sure you won't have a seat?"

"No, thanks."

"You're aware that no one has as yet shown conclusive evidence that this internal secretion actually exists. There's a group within the research community who believe that it doesn't."

"So?"

"You do realize you are standing on the campus of a research university, don't you, Dr. Banting?"

"Look, I get you. You are a researcher. An academician. I am a sawbones. Most of what I know I learned on the battlefield. One thing I learned is that I'd rather save lives than win arguments."

"Nevertheless, you have come to an office at the University of Toronto to ask for research funding."

"Yes, but I'm only in it for the clinical application. Lives could be lost while I'm wasting time in the medical library."

"Dr. Banting— Won't you please sit down?"

"I said no, thank you!"

Macleod, flummoxed and beginning to wonder if Banting had wandered over from the psychiatric ward of the Christie Street Veterans Hospital, simply watched in silence as Banting paced in front of his desk.

"I know what you're thinking. Why should you give someone with no research background money and a lab."

Macleod said nothing.

"Well, you just should! See here, I'm not a talker. You know it and I know it. I could stand here for another forty-five minutes and try to persuade you—not very eloquently—or you could just say yes now and save us both some time."

For the first time, it dawned on Macleod that Banting might have anticipated starting immediately. He might even have a suitcase outside the office door and a bag of surgical instruments.

"Surely you don't expect me to give you an answer on the basis of this brief conversation. There are procedures, Dr. Banting. You must submit a written proposal."

Banting stopped pacing and glowered at the word "proposal."

"How can I say yes if I don't even know what you're asking for? How much money? What kind of lab? How long will you need it? How many dogs? Will you require an assistant?"

"Just let me get started. You won't regret it. I'm telling you this idea is going to work."

Macleod suppressed a grin. If Banting wasn't so menacing, he would be amusing. His appearance was a bit clownish—the lumbering posture, the overly large hands, the horsey facial features. Macleod found himself alternately moved to compassion and apprehension.

However Macleod felt about Banting as a man, he couldn't help but feel a bit sorry for him as a scientist. It was commonly understood among researchers that if there were a way to prove once and for all the existence or nonexistence of this elusive substance, it would be through isolating it. Despite the ex-soldier's blustering confidence about ligating pancreatic ducts, Macleod knew it was an extremely tricky procedure.

Macleod himself was pursuing a theory that the best solution could be found in the sea. Teleostei comprise a class of ray-finned fish including trout, bass, salmon, and tuna, and game fish such as Atlantic sailfish, swordfish, and marlin. In these fishes islet tissue is contained within one or more easily recognizable nodules. Since the islet tissue is anatomically discrete from the acinar tissue, it would be easy to harvest and there would be no danger of contaminating the islet secretion with the acinar secretion. If Macleod's idea were proved, it would allay the most daunting impediment to developing a practicable extract for clinical use.

Macleod had begun to make plans to pursue his fish pancreas research at St. Andrews in New Brunswick during the summer of 1922. He had gone so far as to contact the captain of a commercial fishing boat, the *Venosta,* to procure a supply of the bony fishes all through the summer. Macleod hoped to complete a paper by the following autumn, and for that purpose the negative findings that Banting's effort would certainly produce could be useful in adding support for the fish pancreas direction.

"I'll tell you what," said Macleod. "Go to the medical library, do a bit of looking around in the literature, and then write me a letter telling me what you'll need for your research."

"And you'll grant me the funding?"

"I will absolutely take it under consideration."

"You mean you'll think about it."

"The university has entrusted me to allocate its resources judiciously and as long as it is all right with you, I intend to do so."

"When can I expect your answer?"

"When will I receive your letter?"

Banting left in a huff, vowing never to waste another moment with J. J. R. Macleod or any of his highfalutin, tweed-wearing, backward-looking ilk.

As the weeks wore on, Banting's high resolve was softened by financial imperative and a growing restlessness. Five months after he unearthed Edith's engagement ring, he once again found himself seeking to reclaim something he had discarded. On March 8, 1921, he wrote to Macleod expressing his wish to work at Macleod's lab in late May, June, and July—"if your offer . . . still holds good." He proposed to begin work on May 15, 1921.

Despite having written the letter, Banting remained ambivalent about what to do: apply to accompany the oil expedition in the far North Country or spend the summer operating on dogs in Toronto. He learned that the expedition was to go to the Mackenzie River Valley, a pristine region populated with moose, caribou, lynx, and grizzly bear. The Northwest Territory was roughly twice the size of Ontario, covering nearly one-fifth of Canada. Of the two options, he was leaning toward the call of the wild. He was burning for adventure, and the idea of a group of men in the wilderness promised the camaraderie he had so enjoyed during the war. He decided to interview for the oil expedition, but since he'd already written a letter to Macleod, he dropped it in the post anyway. Banting decided that he would accept whichever offer came to him first.

Macleod considered Banting's letter. He and Mary would be in Scotland for much of the period of Banting's research effort, so granting Banting the lab would not pose much of an inconvenience to him personally. On the other hand, Macleod wondered whether it was irresponsible to allow such an unknown and apparently volatile character to have unsupervised access to the facilities.

Three days later, Macleod replied to Banting agreeing that he could begin his research on May 15 at the University of Toronto. When

Macleod's letter reached Banting, he was leaning so heavily toward the oil expedition that he did not reply for a month. However, when the news came that the oil expedition would not take a doctor along after all, Macleod's offer became considerably more attractive. On April 18, 1921, Banting wrote to Macleod accepting the offer.

TWELVE

Presidential Politics, 1916 and 1920

EVER SINCE THE WAR ENDED, AMERICANS HAD BEEN ARGUING ABOUT peace. As Wilson's term neared its end, his strength and health were in decline. For nearly two years he had fervently and tirelessly promoted the Fourteen Points and his vision of a cooperative international body whose mission was to promote peace—the League of Nations. Charles Evans Hughes spoke out against the United States joining the League. He believed the United States should reserve the right to decide such a serious matter as whether to go to war on a case-by-case basis, taking each situation as it arose, rather than arrange its alliances in advance. On September 25, 1919, Wilson collapsed after a speech urging the ratification of the covenant of the League of Nations. On October 2, he suffered a serious stroke that left him paralyzed on his left side and blind in his left eye.

In 1920 the U.S. Senate rejected the covenant and the United States refused to join the 44 member states in the League of Nations. Political isolationism gained popularity among Americans, and politicians discussed placing limits on immigration. While Wilson was incapacitated, he was sequestered from even his vice president and cabinet members. Edith Galt Wilson, Wilson's second wife, spoke for the president during the remainder of his term, thus earning her the title "American's first woman president." Although the seriousness of Wilson's condition was withheld from the public, one thing was evident—he would not run again.

Looking toward the presidential election in November, the Republican Party felt that it was their year, and the leaders cast about for a candidate. Hughes, now fifty-eight years old, was once again being considered for the Republican nomination. Since he was first elected Governor of New York in 1906 his name had been bandied in conversations of consequence by men who mattered, often in smoke-clouded back rooms and private clubs. Until now he had adhered to Benjamin Franklin's credo that one should never seek out a public office and never refuse one when asked.

Yet in 1920 Charles and Antoinette were nearly ruined by grief. The idea of a second presidential nomination weighed heavily on them; they spent many an evening in quiet discernment, trying to come to terms with how to respond to the call if it came. Could they possibly summon the strength to endure the campaign, never mind the actual presidency were they to win? And what of Elizabeth, and the miserably practical matter of the timing of her death? Were Charles to run, he would rely on Antoinette to accompany him on the campaign trail as she had in 1916. But how could she leave Elizabeth when she was so desperately ill? Could they bear to commit her to the Physiatric Institute full time? Could they afford it financially?

Hughes had not aspired to be president. He viewed public office as "a burden of incessant toil at times almost intolerable, which under honorable conditions and at the command of the people [it] may be a duty, and even a pleasure to assume, but it is far from being an object of ambition." He was a very private, deeply thoughtful man of frugal tastes. He walked to his office, usually came home to eat a spartan lunch with his wife, dressed conservatively, and trimmed his own beard. One colleague on the Court recalled that later, when he was chief justice dining in the justices' dining room, he ate the same meal every day: two boiled eggs, a demitasse of coffee, and a bowl of soup. Although friendly to all, Hughes had few close friends. His closest relationships were with his wife and children.

"What would we do if she were to pass away in six months?" Antoinette asked.

"We would have to cancel campaign appearances and come home," Charles replied softly.

"And what if she didn't die right away but lay in a coma for weeks? Would we then withdraw from the race?"

It was a ghastly business to consider such practicalities, but to ignore the reality of Elizabeth's condition and proceed without considering its impact would be a disservice to the party and to the American people. In any case, *who would vote for a man who could leave his fatally ill daughter to run around the country kissing other people's babies?* Ironically, a decision not to run would disappoint no one more than Elizabeth.

In 1920 Elizabeth was enthralled with illustrious people, and the idea of living in the White House sent her into excited fantasy. She imagined a daily parade of prominent visitors from royalty to movie stars and countless parties and receptions. Besides, Helen had impressed upon her how important it was to be where things really got done, especially now and especially for women. The 19th Amendment would be ratified in August 1920. Elizabeth could not abide the thought that her condition might cost her father the chance to be president—and the nation the presidency of Charles Evans Hughes!

One of her earliest memories was being held in her father's arms on the balcony of their suite at the Waldorf Astoria Hotel on election night in 1916. Hughes had seized the lead early and he was favored to win the election. He had even won New Jersey, which had been predicted for Wilson. It all came down to California. Waiting for the final results, father and daughter breathed in the night air and looked northwest from their aerie above Fifth Avenue (where the hotel was then located), to the very center of the narrow island of Manhattan, to Times Square. There, huge celebratory bonfires surged and spat sparks at the stars that seemed to wheel above their heads. Like everyone else, they kept a close watch on the 357-feet tall Times Building at the corner of Forty-third Street and Broadway where, according to tradition, the searchlight would signal the election results. The signal light was visible for thirty miles, and voters from Paterson, New Jersey, to Tarrytown, New York, to Staten Island could read the message from the Times Tower.

At midnight, the signal flashed from the tower: "Hughes Elected!" The chant of the throng of two hundred thousand people gathered in Times Square rang like a temple bell—"Hughes! Hughes! Hughes!" It was pure magic. Then came the confirmation over the radio: Hughes had won. A breathless bellboy appeared on the balcony with an early edition of *The New York Times* bearing the front-page headline "The President-

Elect—Charles Evans Hughes." The boy's face was bright with the thought that he could forever after tell people that he had delivered a paper to the nation's president.

Bonfires burned in cities all across the nation on election night 1916. One such fire burned in Chickasha, Oklahoma, on the corner of Chickasha Avenue and Third Street in front of the First National Bank Building. Watching it was a twelve-year-old named William T. Gossett, who could not have imagined that a boy from Oklahoma would one day work for the eminent Charles Evans Hughes. Even more unimaginable was the idea that he would fall in love with his daughter.

While the bonfires still burned, and although the final results from California had not yet been tallied, Charles Evans Hughes went to bed.

The next morning the count was official. The popular vote was 8,538,221 votes for Hughes to 9,129,606 votes for Wilson. Hughes had lost by 3 percent of the popular vote. Women had voted for Hughes two to one, but their votes were counted only at the state level. The electoral vote was one of the closest in American history. With 266 votes needed to win, Wilson took thirty states and 277 electoral votes, while Hughes won eighteen states and 254 electoral votes. If Hughes had carried California and its 13 electoral votes, he would have won the election. Describing the episode nine years later, *The New York Times Magazine* remarked, "He went to bed the next president of the United States, and woke up a mere man."

Of all of the positions Hughes held, he found the work of the court the most satisfying. He had even said so in his letter accepting the 1916 nomination: "I have not desired the nomination. I have wished to remain on the bench. But in this critical period in our national history I recognize that it is your right to summon and that it is my paramount duty to respond. . . . Therefore, I accept the nomination." The letter, dated June 1916, was addressed to the chairman of the Republican National Convention, Warren G. Harding.

Hughes's six years as an associate justice of the Supreme Court had been a very happy time for the Hughes family. So confident were Antoinette and Charles in projecting a long and stable life in Washington that they used what was left of their savings to buy a quiet lot on the southwest corner of Sixteenth and V Streets, and build a gracious brick Georgian at 2100 Sixteenth Street NW in the Sheridan-Kalorama neighborhood. It was their ideal home in every detail. In November 1911 they moved in, fully expecting to live there for the rest of their days. Antoinette, Catherine, and Elizabeth tooled around town in an electric car. Charlie had just been graduated from Harvard Law School and was beginning his practice in New York City. Helen was at Vassar. Catherine and Elizabeth were attending National Cathedral School, a girls' school on the grounds of the National Cathedral in Washington, D.C., an institution also attended by Roosevelts, Rockefellers, and Firestones. Grandmother Hughes occupied the top floor of the house, which she shared with Elizabeth—the youngest and oldest members of the household.

It was during this time that Elizabeth first began to appreciate the privileges and responsibilities of being born the daughter of Charles Evans Hughes. He set an inhumanly high standard for himself and others and was not shy in expressing his disapproval. There was an unspoken feeling, shared by all the Hughes children and by Antoinette, that one must never disappoint him.

Shortly before the Republican National Convention of 1920, which met in Chicago, Illinois, from June 8 to June 12, 1920, Senators Henry Cabot Lodge, James W. Wadsworth, and William M. Calder met in Washington to discuss who should be nominated as the Republican presidential candidate. The senators each had their favorite candidates, on whom they did not agree, but they could all settle on Hughes as an acceptable alternative for the nomination. And so the senators approached Meier Steinbrink to present the idea to Hughes to see what his response might be to being nominated.

Steinbrink, a leader in the Republican Party, had a good relationship with Hughes, forged through assisting him in two major undertakings: the Draft Appeals Board and an aviation inquiry. Hughes and Steinbrink met for lunch at the Lawyers Club. Steinbrink was alarmed at the change in his friend's appearance. He seemed to have aged ten years. He anticipated that Hughes might not even hear him out, and so he asked him to refrain from comment until he had finished his proposal. Hughes agreed. Then Steinbrink told Hughes that the senators wanted to be able to vote for him for president and why.

As promised, Hughes listened to Steinbrink to the end. Then, struggling to maintain his composure, he beseeched Steinbrink to understand that he and Mrs. Hughes were dispirited and bereft after the nearly yearlong vigil that had preceded Helen's death. In a most uncharacteristic decision, he asked to be relieved of the duty to run for president of the United States and asked that his name not be mentioned as a possible choice. He doubted that he had the strength and stamina to meet the national and international challenges that the next president would inherit, the same ones that had most certainly caused Wilson's physical collapse. He never mentioned Elizabeth's condition.

Like most people, Hughes believed that whoever was nominated at the Republican Convention would be elected. He predicted to Steinbrink that the man who assumed the office at this most unhappy time of international unrest would likely not live to finish his term. Hughes did not want to be that man. His ominous prediction would prove to be accurate, but ironically the bulk of the international peacemaking responsibilities would soon fall to him anyway.

In the late summer and autumn, the 1920 presidential election swung into high gear. Leading the Republican ticket was the same man who had officially proffered the 1916 nomination to Hughes—Warren G. Harding. He was a junior senator and newspaper publisher from Ohio. His running mate was to be the stoic governor of Massachusetts, Calvin Coolidge. Harding was a great admirer of William McKinley, and it was during McKinley's presidency that Harding began his political career as senator. He had a winning personality and a strong, handsome, face. With these assets he had transformed a struggling local newspaper, *The Daily Star* of Marion, Ohio, into one of the most successful in the nation.

The Democratic presidential candidate was James M. Cox, governor of Ohio and his vice presidential candidate Franklin D. Roosevelt. On October 30, 1920, the day Banting had his epiphany in London, Ontario, *The New York Times* published an article entitled, "Roosevelt Makes 12 Speeches in Day; 'Things Look Awfully Good,' He Says at Ossining, 'and We're Going to Win.'" It was his eighty-first day on the road; he had been in thirty-one states.

In October 1920, having forfeited the opportunity to run for president himself, Charles Evans Hughes announced his support for his party's choice. Although Harding was in the journalism business, he could bloviate with the best of them and played fast and loose with language besides. Harding is responsible for the introduction of at least one new word to the English lexicon, a word minted on the campaign stump. The word was "normalcy," and it drew Americans to it like the peal of a dinner bell.

"America's present need is not heroics, but healing," Harding declared. "Not nostrums, but normalcy; not revolution, but restoration; not agitation, but adjustment; not surgery, but serenity; not the dramatic, but the dispassionate; not experiment, but equipoise; not submergence in internationality, but sustainment in triumphant nationality."

William Gibbs McAdoo, a Democrat, called Harding's speeches "an army of pompous phrases moving across the landscape in search of an idea."

For the first time the American women's vote for president would be counted. On August 18, 1920, one day before Elizabeth's thirteenth birthday, the Nineteenth Amendment was ratified by Congress. All through the day, Elizabeth fought the impulse to weep as she thought of Helen, who had so dearly longed to see this momentous event and missed it by four months to the day. Now that it had arrived, it came with such bitter irony for the Hughes family. Not only had Helen not lived to cast a vote, but it was certain that Elizabeth would not live to do so either.

By election time in November 1920 the colds and tonsillitis that had so weakened Elizabeth's system throughout the spring had temporarily abated. To stabilize her metabolism Dr. Allen had decreased her diet to five hundred calories per day. In October she weighed sixty-five pounds; the following March her weight fell to fifty-four pounds.

The Harding-Cox presidential election returns were the first to be broadcast by a commercially licensed radio station—Westinghouse-owned KDKA. When the news was official that Warren Harding had been elected twenty-ninth president of the United States, Elizabeth sobbed in Blanche's lap.

In fact, the diminutive Harding's first act in office was to reach up and appoint a giant as his first cabinet member. Charles Evans Hughes accepted the position of secretary of state. For the first time in five years, Americans felt safe knowing that international affairs would be guided by such a capable mind.

When her parents told Elizabeth the news, she was so elated that she announced that she would bathe in the White House fountain. Catherine's response was just the opposite: She had fallen in love with Chauncey Waddell, an attorney just beginning his career in New York City. She persuaded her parents to allow her to live in the Bronx with her brother and sister-in-law, Charlie and Marjory, where she could more easily continue her courtship. And so Charles, Antoinette, and Elizabeth were moving back to Washington after all.

Hughes was to take office in March 1921. Antoinette prepared to leave the home in which both Elizabeth and Helen took sick. What were they to do with Elizabeth while they looked for a house in Washington? The Physiatric Institute seemed like the best option, at least as a temporary measure until they were settled. The only ones who would be pleased at this prospect were Dr. Allen; a diabetic named Eddie, whom Elizabeth would help to secure a pet canary; and a little boy named Teddy Ryder, who weighed only twenty-seven pounds and who, in July of 1921, would celebrate his fifth and almost certainly final birthday inside the institute.

THIRTEEN

The Physiatric Institute, Morristown, New Jersey, 1921

ALTHOUGH IT HAD BEEN QUIETLY ACCEPTING PATIENTS FOR MONTHS, the Physiatric Institute officially opened with much fanfare on April 25, 1921. Several hundred physicians and surgeons attended the ceremony. Speeches were made by Dr. Henry Pritchett, president of the Carnegie Foundation as well as by Dr. Frederick Allen himself, who made sure that *The New York Times* reported that "patients in all degrees of financial circumstances" could find help there. It was quickly filled to overflowing.

As Antoinette struggled to begin a new chapter in Washington, she was pelted with letters from Morristown. Elizabeth's letters to "Mumsey" provided detailed descriptions of the exacting regimen that dominated her existence. A typical breakfast might be one egg, two-and-a-quarter heaping tablespoons (125 grams) of thrice-boiled string beans, and one tablespoon of cream and coffee. At ten o'clock she might have half of a small orange (50 grams). For dinner (at noon) she could have two and a half heaping tablespoons of cod, two heaping tablespoons of thrice-boiled Brussels sprouts, five small olives, a half pat of butter, and tea. Her supper would be one egg and one egg white, two heaping tablespoons of thrice-boiled spinach with a half pat of butter and tea. She fasted one day a week.

The advanced kitchen at the Physiatric Institute experimented with a number of creative recipes. The great quest was always to produce a palatable bread substitute, and various bran cakes and bran muffins, made with washed bran, soya, and casoid or Lyster's flour, were forever being plied on the patients. Because of the paucity of food and the unpalatable nature of what food there was, great care was taken to prepare and arrange the patients' meals. Cucumber cups and egg tulips were popular features. Eggs occupied a starring role in the caloric cast list, and the indefatigable dieticians worked magic with them, inventing dozens of ways to prepare them, such as: steamed egg, baked egg in tomato, dropped egg with parsley, egg farci I, egg farci II, egg à la Suisse, eggs au beurre noir, and chicken broth with egg balls.

Everyone at the Physiatric Institute, both patients and staff, were preoccupied with food and the lack thereof in some way. When he had the strength, the small, skeletal Teddy Ryder liked to work on his scrapbook. This was a favorite pastime of several patients at the institute. Teddy spent hours flipping through colorful, glossy magazines and cutting out photographs of food, which he lovingly pasted into a book under the watchful gaze of the nurses (who were commanded to do so by Allen himself to ensure that he didn't eat the paste). The scrapbooks of healthy children are emblematic of their lives, comprising report cards, homemade valentines, pressed flowers, and photographs, but the scrapbooks assembled by the children at the Physiatric Institute were emblematic of the lives they could not lead, the childhood they were not having. The game *What would you eat if you could eat anything?* took the place of the usual children's game *What do you want to be when you grow up?* By necessity, ambitions of these children were more short-term.

Teddy had been diagnosed with diabetes mellitus the previous year, at the age of four. His desperate mother, Mildred, took him to doctor after doctor, but the prognosis was always the same, and always grim. One doctor tried to deter her from seeking treatment and allow the doomed child to eat as he liked and enjoy the little time he had left. Dr. Allen made an incredible claim to Earle and Mildred Ryder—that he might be able to keep their son alive for up to two years.

The Ryders had heard about Dr. Allen's methods while making the rounds with Teddy. Many of the doctors they'd seen disapproved of Allen's methods as being too cruel to be practical. Nevertheless, on November 19, 1920, they committed Teddy to the Physiatric Institute. At Morristown his caloric intake was steadily reduced until, at some stages, he received only 224 calories a day (as compared with a normal child of his age's intake of 1,500 calories a day). He ate mostly jellies, thrice-cooked cabbage, and washed bran cookies. When he went home to Keyport, New Jersey, for visits, the neighbors would shake their heads and make disparaging remarks about the quack doctor who had duped the Ryders into starving their poor son to death. How could they place their trust in such a man when the prescribed treatment was so clearly harmful to Teddy? When he went home for Christmas in 1921, there was no Christmas tree. Mr. and Mrs. Ryder hadn't expected their son to survive until Christmas Day. Somehow he persevered, listlessly compiling his scrapbooks.

Blanche apprenticed in the sanitarium kitchen under the cold scrutiny of Miss Mary Belle Wishart, who was a strong advocate of education. She had studied at the University of Missouri and Cornell Medical College. Every dietician on the staff had completed dedicated training in domestic science. Wishart shared Dr. Allen's belief that Elizabeth could be better treated as an inpatient, and she was, at first, skeptical of Blanche's ability to manage Elizabeth's diet at home.

Elizabeth and Blanche set themselves to proving the skeptics wrong. Together they read two books by Dr. Joslin, two by Dr. Allen and of course, the little red book. They transcribed what they learned onto flash cards and drilled each other on the equivalencies of carbohydrates, proteins, and fats. Instead of being a *victim* of diabetes, Elizabeth became a *student* of diabetes. Elizabeth embraced the study of diabetes as if her life depended on it, which it did. *One gram of fat equals 9.3 calories. One gram of protein equals 4.1 calories. One gram of carbohydrate equals 4.1 calories. One calorie equals the amount of heat necessary to raise the temperature of one kilogram of water by one degree centigrade. One kilogram equals 2.2 pounds.*

Elizabeth took a particular liking to a sullen boy named Eddie, who was a year older than she. Both Elizabeth and Eddie were fond of birds. They talked about whether European starlings were crowding out the American robin population and whether passenger pigeons were truly extinct. They kept a list of migratory warblers, orioles, tanagers, vireos, and woodpeckers that they had spotted on the institute grounds. Thinking of the cheerful presence of the Hughes's pet canary Perfect, Elizabeth suggested that Eddie keep a pet canary at the Institute. She raised the idea with Dr. Allen, who frowned on it. He was not an animal lover to begin with, and he was concerned about the effect of the animal presence on so many weakened immune systems. Elizabeth argued that each time the patients took their mandatory daily exercise they were exposed to hundreds of germs and that in general, person-to-person contagion was more likely than animal-to-person contagion. Besides, she reasoned, having something to care for would help lift Eddie's spirits and give him a reason to get out of bed. And did he know, she asked, that the canary was named for the Canary Islands off the coast of Spain and didn't it make sense to have a bird named after islands since the islets of Langerhans was the reason he'd opened the institute to begin with? When Elizabeth set her mind to accomplish something she was hard to resist, even for a man like Allen, and he agreed to the bird on a trial basis.

Like most boys in that day, Eddie was interested in the war. He became especially interested in messenger pigeons, because an uncle had served with the U.S. Army Signal Corps in France, which had made extensive use of the birds. The most famous war pigeon of all was Cher Ami, who saved the lives of two hundred men in October 1918 when a U.S. Army battalion of the 77th Infantry Division became trapped behind enemy lines. They were surrounded and outnumbered by the Germans. To make matters worse, the American artillery started firing hundreds of rounds into the ravine where Major Charles Whittlesey and his men were trapped. Each pigeon that Whittlesey had sent out to tell the Americans to stop had been shot out of the sky. Cher Ami was his last one.

The major scribbled a note: "We are along the road parallel to 276.4. Our own artillery is dropping a barrage directly on us. For heaven's sake, stop it." He rolled up the note and inserted it into a tiny canister attached to Cher Ami's left leg. Then he released the bird. The flutter of wings prompted a torrent of German fire, but somehow Cher Ami rose above the bullets and flew twenty-five miles in twenty-five minutes. The American shelling stopped abruptly. The men were saved but the bird was mortally wounded.

Initially, Eddie threatened to name his canary "Drumstick" but finally settled on "Ami" to honor the martyred bird. Elizabeth often found Eddie out of his bed, doting on his pet canary, and touted her canary experiment as a great success.

★   ★   ★

Antoinette believed that "normalcy" was what Elizabeth needed. She did not approve of Elizabeth befriending Eddie, Teddy, or any of the other doomed children at the institute. On this one point, she and Dr. Allen were in full agreement. Increasingly Elizabeth depended on Blanche, not just for her dietary needs but also for companionship, entertainment, emotional support, and ultimately, her very life.

FOURTEEN

The University of Toronto, Summer 1921

On Saturday, May 14, 1921, Banting locked the house in London, Ontario, and left for Toronto. He had made plans to stay with his cousin Fred Hipwell and his wife, Lillian, until he found a place of his own.

Macleod asked two student research assistants, Charles Best and Clark Noble, to come to his office. He explained to them the opportunity to assist a surgeon in a research project for part of the summer. Both young men were biochemistry majors and so, he reasoned, some exposure to surgery would be good experience. Further, if they decided to pursue a career in medical research, they would almost certainly find themselves working in an animal lab; it would be good for them to know whether this environment appealed to them. Macleod suggested that they each take a turn under Banting and that they work out the details about how to do it between them. Noble and Best decided to split the summer into two four-week periods so that each would have part of the summer to spend with family and friends. They flipped a coin to see who would go first.

Shortly after his arrival in Toronto, Banting met Macleod in his office, and was introduced to a handsome, blond, twenty-two-year-old student named Charley Best. Macleod ushered them to the second floor of the Physiology building to the animal laboratory where Banting could pursue his idea over the summer months. It was hardly the gleaming vision that Banting had imagined. In fact, it looked more like the laboratory in Mary Shelley's *Frankenstein*. The counters, racks, and apparatus were shrouded with veils of dust and cobwebs. But the equipment looked new. A dedicated animal operating room was an idea ahead of its time; the scientific researchers on campus had not quite caught on to availing themselves of the facility. The three men stood in the doorway, speechless. Macleod broke the silence.

"I guess you'll want to begin with a thorough cleaning. I'll see to it that the janitor sends over some supplies," Macleod chirped, dropping two keys into Banting's hand.

"Here's a key for each of you. Any questions?"

Banting ventured into the center of the room, swiping his hand over the slate bench, furry with dust, then turned back to face Macleod. He opened his mouth to speak but didn't.

"Very well, then. I'll let you two get to it."

And then he was gone down the hallway. Banting turned to Best.

"Well, Charley. This is what you get for winning the coin toss with Noble."

"What makes you think I won?"

There was a long tense moment, after which Best broke into a broad grin. Banting laughed loud and long.

Just then they heard the janitor turn the corner of the corridor, bringing cleaning equipment.

"This looks more like archeology than physiology," Banting said. "Somewhere underneath all this I'm told there's an operating table. Shall we attempt to find it?"

"Now?"

Neither man was dressed for manual labor. Banting had observed Charley's pale soft hands, small and clean; they looked like they'd never held anything more demanding than a croquet mallet. Charley had grown up in West Pembroke, Maine, where his father was a respected doctor. He enjoyed a youth of culture and privilege, varsity sports, a sterling academic record, and a paid assistantship to the head of the physiology department. By contrast, Banting's mother had been the first white child born in a newly settled area of Ontario. Most of the boys in Alliston grew up in bare feet and overalls and left school before completing the eighth grade, just before they would have to take the entrance examinations for high school. All three of Fred's brothers pursued the farming life, but Fred remained in school, sometimes riding to high school on their horse, Old Betsy. Tramps and hobos wandered the countryside, sometimes stopping by the house to beg a meal or permission to spend the night in the barn. Arrowheads and spearheads frequently turned up in the field of the farm to the north of the Banting property, where there was a spring. Banting thought he would find out what his young assistant was made of. Banting threaded his arms through his suspenders and let them hang, then he unbuttoned his shirt and hung it on the doorknob.

"There's no time like the present," Banting said.

Somewhat reluctantly, Best did the same. And so one of the greatest advances in medical science began with bleach, a bucket, sponges, and mops.

As they scrubbed, Banting learned that Best was engaged to be married to a beautiful young woman, Margaret Mahon. Their courtship sounded like an endless string of parties and dances. Banting could not help but think of his tortured experience with Edith. Their courtship had taken place largely through the mail and in church, listening to Edith's father preach. But all that was behind him now: Edith, his practice, his friend Bill, and the big white brick house. Before him were eight weeks, ten dogs, and an idea.

Banting learned that Best's favorite aunt had died of diabetes. Banting's good friend Joe Gilchrist, a fellow member of the University of Toronto's class of 1917, had diabetes. For most CAMC veterans the war was over, but having fought for his country poor Joe now had to fight for his life.

In a few hours the animal operating theater was ready to receive its first patient and Banting and Best looked like coal miners. Macleod had estimated that over the course of the summer, Banting might use ten to twelve dogs. Each experiment would require two dogs—a donor dog and a recipient dog. The donor dog would be ligated and sacrificed to supply the pancreatic extract for the second, depancreatized dog.

Although Banting had never operated on a dog, it had not occurred to him that this might prove an obstacle to his success. It had, however, occurred to Macleod. On May 17 Macleod performed the first pancreatectomy with Banting and Best observing. Macleod demonstrated the correct procedure for depancreatizing and thus preparing the recipient dog for experimental treatment. In the Hédon procedure, which was the accepted practice of the time, the pancreas was removed in two phases. First, after cutting into the abdomen, Macleod cut away most of the pancreas, but left a small piece intact. He pulled this piece up and sewed it into place just under the skin. Then he closed the abdominal wound layer by layer with catgut. The small functioning piece of the pancreas would prevent the dog from becoming diabetic while it recovered from the surgery. Several days after the surgery, this piece would be snipped away and the process of depancreatization would be complete. The dog would become diabetic and die in about a week unless it could be kept alive by the administration of the pancreatic extract. Banting was surprised at the delicacy of the procedure, at how small and close the cavity was compared with a human being's.

Still, he reasoned, there was no way to learn but to do. Banting had performed his first operation in 1916, during his final year in school while working at the soldiers' convalescent hospital. A soldier with a large abscess on his throat needed it opened and drained so he could go overseas with his battalion. Seeing no other medical personnel, the orderly officer asked Banting to do it, assuming he was experienced. Banting thought he was as qualified as anyone, and so he did not object. The operation was a success and the soldier rejoined his battalion within forty-eight hours.

Banting and Best began with a literature review. They discussed Moses Barron's article of course, as well as work by Murlin, Kleiner, Hédon, Opie, Knowlton and Starling, and Mering and Minkowski. They read Macleod and Pearce's textbook, *Physiology and Biochemistry in Modern Medicine*. One of the most useful books they read was Dr. Frederick M. Allen's *Glycosuria and Diabetes*. (This was the book for which Allen had borrowed five thousand dollars from his father.) Best said he and Banting used it almost as a bible in the development of the work on insulin.

When Charley wasn't in the lab, he was often playing tennis or golf or enjoying the company of his perfect mate, Margaret. Banting's extracurricular activity ranged from the grim to the glum and often involved extended analyses of what went wrong with him and Edith. Occasionally, Charley encouraged Fred to go out with him and Margaret, and sometimes Fred would, gamely escorting one of the secretaries from the medical building, but the experience rarely rated higher than "pleasant, if awkward" for all involved.

At last Banting and Best began the work in earnest. Best would perform all the blood and urine testing and Banting would perform the surgeries. The first dog was accidentally killed by too much anesthesia. The second died from loss of blood. The third died from infection. By the time Macleod left for Scotland on June 14, 1921, Banting and Best had lost three dogs to surgical problems and ligated six dogs successfully, or so they thought. From Macleod's perspective, this was a bit of a bumpy start, but duct ligation was a difficult procedure, and the losses were not wholly surprising. If the ducts were tied too tight there could be infection, if they were tied too loose the acinar tissue would not atrophy. The experiment could also fail if the ducts were tied incompletely or incorrectly. Each dog's anatomy was different; what worked on one dog might not work on the next, and it was easy to overlook a duct altogether.

The conditions in which they worked were not optimal. The floor of the operating room could not be properly scrubbed because the wash water would seep down through the floor to the ceiling below. The operating table was wood and so could not be effectively sterilized, and the operating linen was stained and tattered. And then there was the heat—1921 was one of the hottest summers on record. The heat and the stench in the laboratory and the kennels were nearly intolerable.

Roaming the sweltering, abandoned campus fueled Banting's misery. He was practically penniless. Having already borrowed money from his parents to buy the house in London, he could not ask them to borrow more. In May and June he had made a little money performing tonsillectomies, and he had sold some surgical instruments for twenty-five dollars. At night, he often cooked his modest meals on a Bunsen burner at the lab, and he sometimes fished for an invitation to join the Hipwells. On Sundays, he frequented the free suppers at the Philathea Bible Class of St. James Square Presbyterian Church, which he had attended as a student.

In mid-June, Best left for ten days of militia training in Niagara. This left Banting alone in the lab to feed the dogs and clean their cages. He was living in a boardinghouse on Grenville Street, the same one he had lived in as a student, paying two dollars a week for a seven-by-nine-foot room. He blamed Macleod for this sad state of affairs and could not help but resent his comment that even negative results would be useful.

When Best returned in late June, he went to visit Margaret first, re-uniting with her and reporting his experience with the militia. Later he decided to swing by the lab for a quick look around. He arrived about 11:00 P.M. and much to his surprise found Banting there. More to his surprise Banting was boiling with rage. He launched into a tirade about the state of the lab, furiously pointing out example after example of smeared glassware, detritus encrusted on metal instruments, and dubious stains on countertops. Charley was astonished. As the assistant, he had only been following Banting's lead, allowing his superior to set the standard. Until this moment, he had thought Banting was pleased. If there had been disappointments, they had been surgical. Banting went on and on about the potential importance of this work, about what he had sacrificed, and about his soldierly expectations of loyalty, dedication, and honest effort. When Banting was finished, Best was shaking. For an instant Best looked like he might throw a punch, and Banting prepared for a fight. After a long hot moment, Best turned and in stony silence began to scour the lab. Banting left without a word. Best worked well into the early morning hours, cleaning every square inch of equipment. When Banting arrived the next morning, the lab was spotless. Not a word was said then or later about the night before. From that day on, Banting and Best were a team.

When the time came for Clark Noble to take over for Charley Best, everyone agreed that it was best for Charley to remain now that he and Banting had worked out the kinks in their relationship. The effort continued. Banting and Best depancreatized two recipient dogs in preparation for the harvesting of the atrophied tissue from the previously ligated donor dogs. On July 5, Banting opened up one of the donor dogs. He was shocked to find that the pancreas, which should have degenerated, was normal. The duct ligation had failed utterly. Now Banting opened all of the donor dogs, one after another. The mercury rose to 97 degrees Fahrenheit. Banting cut the sleeves off of his lab coat and tied a towel to his head. During the operation Best wiped runnels of perspiration from Banting's face and arms but still, sweat dripped into the open cavities. Banting discovered that in five of the seven dogs the duct ligation had failed. It was a crushing blow, but he swallowed hard and set himself to the task of re-ligating the five dogs. This time he used silk ligatures. Two of the dogs died within a day of the surgery. Then the two depancreatized recipient dogs died for lack of extract.

They were now seven weeks into their research and had nothing to show for it but carcasses.

After Banting and Best ran through the original allotment of dogs, they found their own supply on the streets of Toronto, either paying between one and three dollars each for them, no questions asked, or resorting to prowling around and capturing stray dogs themselves. Banting was quite fond of dogs and handled them as gently as possible, but the truth was that it was not always possible. He would later say that it was as if the dogs knew of the importance of the work and willingly participated. He said that one dog in particular got used to the routine of having its blood drawn and jumped onto the table when it was time.

On July 11 Banting and Best depancreatized Dog 410, a white terrier. They took the rest of the week off while they waited for it to heal. Charley told Margaret that he was tired of the work and the miserable conditions. On July 18, they removed the pedicle, or pancreatic remnant, from Dog 410. The dog became only moderately diabetic. Banting speculated that part of the pancreatic tissue remained in the dog or possibly the diabetic condition was slow to develop in it. They determined to wait and watch. In the meantime, they depancreatized Dog 406, a collie. Around this time they abandoned the two-step Hédon procedure, and began removing the pancreas all at once so that the dogs became diabetic immediately.

On Saturday, July 30 they chloroformed donor Dog 391 and removed its pancreas. The tissues had degenerated as expected. Adhering to Macleod's instructions for preparing the extract, Best sliced up the pancreas and put the pieces in a chilled mortar with Ringer's solution. The mortar was partially submerged in freezing brine until the pancreatic mixture partially froze. Then he macerated the contents with a chilled pestle and strained the mixture. The result was a pinkish-brown liquid, which was warmed to body temperature just prior to injection.

At 10:15 in the morning they injected four cubic centimeters (4cc) of the extract into recipient Dog 410. A normal dog's blood sugar should measure between .08 and .13. Before the injection Dog 410's blood sugar measured .20. One hour after the injection Dog 410's blood sugar had fallen to .12—a forty percent decrease. An hour later they administered a second injection and the blood sugar fell again, but just slightly, to .11. They were encouraged. At 2:15 Dog 410's blood sugar had risen to .14, despite another injection. That afternoon they tried feeding sugar water to the dog, in the hopes of testing whether the extract would allow the dog to metabolize it. They accidentally inserted the feeding tube into a lung and the dog nearly drowned. After fifteen minutes it seemed recovered and they tried again. This time they succeeded, but Dog 410's blood sugar began to rise into the .18 to .21 range, despite hourly injections of the extract.

After so many weeks they were finally in a position to record results in a viable patient. Despite this they left the lab at 6:15 P.M. and did not return until the following morning. When they arrived they found Dog 410 in a coma. They were able to take one blood sugar reading before it died. It measured .15. Inexplicably, they did not perform an autopsy. In a paper published in the *Journal of Laboratory and Clinical Medicine* in February 1922, they speculated that Dog 410 was likely dying from infection at the time they ran the final blood test.

On Monday, August 1, the collie, Dog 406, lay unconscious and close to death, either from infection or from diabetes. Banting and Best injected 8 cc of extract into a vein. The collie's blood sugar started to fall. At once the dog awoke, rose to its feet, and walked around the lab. Banting and Best cheered. Then, just as suddenly, the collie lapsed into a coma and died, despite repeated injections.

On Wednesday, August 3, they began an experiment on Dog 408, another collie. Injections of pancreatic extract on Dog 408 were definitively positive. They injected extracts of the liver and the spleen and showed that these injections did not produce the same effect. They tried boiling the pancreatic extract and injecting that and showed that that didn't work either. Over the next four days they injected the dog with the extract and each time the extract reduced the dog's blood sugar. On the fourth day, they conducted an all-night experiment, after which the dog died. An autopsy indicated infection. At last they had results good enough to report to Macleod. For the first time, Banting and Best gave their extract a name: isletin.

On August 9, Banting wrote to Macleod, "I have so much to tell you that I scarcely know where to begin." In addition to reporting the experimental results to Macleod, Banting also made five requests: (1) he asked to stay on and continue the work, (2) he asked for a salary, (3) he wanted a better room to work in, (4) he asked for a boy to take care of the dogs and clean the operating room, and (5) he asked that the floor of the operating room be repaired. On the issue of employing a boy to feed the dogs and clean their cages Banting was particularly insistent.

In the same letter, Banting listed sixteen questions related to their central question of whether they could cause a reduction in blood sugar by introduction of a pancreatic extract. These were questions concerning the chemical composition of the extract, the method of preparing the most potent form of it, the method of delivery, whether trypsin really did destroy the active principle of the pancreatic extract, and, of course, the clinical application. He wrote, "I am very anxious that I be allowed to [continue to] work in your laboratory."

Banting and Best realized that it would likely take three weeks to receive Macleod's reply, and he was due back in four weeks, so rather than wait for Macleod's return post, Banting and Best decided to assume that his answer to the first request would be yes and they would negotiate the other points once Macleod returned to Toronto. Ideally, this would provide them with more persuasive results to report to Macleod on his arrival.

Next they depancreatized two dogs, number 92 and number 409. Their plan was to give isletin to Dog 92. Dog 409 would serve as a control, meaning that they would allow it to recover from the surgery but not provide any isletin. As they worked, sweat dripped onto the operating table, the clamps and scalpels, and the linens that they used to wipe them. That infection continued to be a problem was hardly a surprise.

The results of the comparative experiment with Dog 92 and Dog 409 were unmistakable. On August 13, Dog 409 was barely able to walk while Dog 92, a yellow collie, was prancing around the lab, following Banting like a house pet. On August 14, they gave Dog 92 an overdose of extract to see if it would reduce its blood sugar to below normal. It did. They continued to experiment with different concentrations of the extract as Dog 409's condition worsened. On August 15, Dog 409 died. The extract seemed to be keeping Dog 92 in perfect health. She was an especially cooperative patient and Banting grew very fond of her.

On August 17 Banting and Best made extract using a dog's fresh whole pancreas and injected this into Dog 92 to see if the preparation would have the same sugar-lowering effect on the blood as degenerated pancreas. It did. In fact, using the fresh whole gland seemed to be even more effective than using the ligated gland. Yet they did not recognize this very important finding. Best continued to believe that it was necessary to eliminate the acinar secretion prior to preparing isletin. Their beloved Dog 92 began to weaken. There were no duct-tied donor dogs on hand to supply the wondrous extract.

On August 19, desperate to keep his favorite patient alive, Banting conceived of a way to procure the internal secretion. It was well known that the hormone secretin, which was produced by the duodenum, stimulated the pancreas to produce the digestive enzyme trypsin. Banting's idea was to open up a dog and use secretin to milk all of the digestive secretion from the acinar tissue. Then he could chloroform the dog and remove the pancreas, which would contain only isletin. From this, Best could prepare the extract. Time was running out for Dog 92; she could no longer rise to her feet. They hurriedly prepared for this procedure. The surgery was extremely complicated, requiring a resection of the bowel to procure the secretin. It took nearly four hours for the pancreas to be exhausted of trypsin.

On the evening of August 20, Dog 92 received the extract that was procured in this way. She responded marvelously. By the following morning their yellow collie was wagging her tail and following Banting around the lab again, resting her head in his lap when he sat down to make notes. That very afternoon he recorded that Dog 92 jumped down from her cage to the lab floor, a distance of some two and a half feet, and landed without falling. Banting would later describe the event as one of the greatest experiences of his life. But despite his elation, Banting realized that this could be only a temporary reprieve. Dog 92 would soon need more isletin to stay alive.

Over the next few days, Banting and Best carried out several experiments, mixing sugar and extract in a test tube, and injecting Dog 92 with a mixture of extract and trypsin to see if it would lower the blood sugar. It didn't. By August 22 they were again out of extract. They decided to use the opportunity to answer the question of whether the extract would work across species. After all, clinical application and not medical research had always been his goal. That day they repeated the procedure of stimulating the pancreas with secretin, operating on a cat this time. The cat died on the table but they decided to remove the pancreas and prepare the extract anyway. They injected the extract into Dog 92. She lapsed into shock. Dog 92 then began a long slow decline, her blood sugar gradually rising. For nine days she hung on, while becoming increasingly listless and weak. On August 31, the collie died. She had lived for a remarkable twenty days without a pancreas. Banting turned his face away from Best and wept. "I shall never forget that dog as long as I shall live," Banting wrote in 1940. "I have seen patients die and I have never shed a tear. But when that dog died I wanted to be alone for the tears would fall despite anything I could do."

Banting complained long and loud to anyone who would listen about the deplorable state of the lab and continued to blame Macleod for their difficulties and lack of progress. One of the people he persuaded to help him was Dr. C. L. Starr, who was making arrangements for Banting and Best to use the surgical research operating room from then on. Another sympathetic ear was Professor Velyien Henderson of Pharmacology, whose mannerisms had earned him the nickname of Vermin Henderson among the students of the class of 1917. Banting didn't think too much of him when he was a student, but he enjoyed getting to know him as an equal in the summer of 1921. Henderson agreed to let Banting know if a job became available in the pharmacology department. A salary would be a nice change; he was running out of things to sell. Henderson advised Banting to start thinking about writing a paper, so Banting and Best decided to make an effort to start taking better notes. As far as academia was concerned, making the discovery wasn't as important as publishing the discovery. Publication was a way to claim credit for the idea. And he wasn't about to let some beady-eyed Scot like Macleod keep him from it.

In late August Macleod said goodbye to his sisters and visited the graves of his brothers. He was now the only surviving son. His brother's children were fatherless. He and his wife were childless. Futility and grief weighed heavily on him. A recent letter from Banting, full of grandiose claims and indignant demands, had put him in a foul mood. Where was the sense in the world when a boor like Banting could make demands and a good, brave, talented doctor like Clement had been reduced to dry bones beneath the moss?

He and Mary steeled themselves for the two-week ocean journey, leaving their beloved Scotland behind, for how long they did not know. It was now apparent that it would be only a matter of time before violence once again shattered the hard-won peace in Europe.

According to the armistice that Woodrow Wilson negotiated in 1918, Allied hostilities would resume within forty-eight hours if the Germans deviated from the terms agreed upon. An Allied Reparations Commission toured Belgium, France, and parts of England to assess the damage. In April 1921 the amount was announced: 132 billion gold German marks (Reichsmarks), or £4,990,000,000, to be paid at the rate of 2.5 billion marks per year until 1961. France viewed the terms as too lenient. Germany viewed them as too punitive. Germany made its first payment in 1921, but as the year drew to a close the German economy was near collapse and would not be able to manage the 1922 payment. Britain agreed to a three-year hiatus, but Belgium and France began seizing German factories, commodities, and intellectual property, including the patent for aspirin—ironically, an anti-inflammatory compound.

Over the next four years one man would rise above all others as a dominant figure in world diplomacy, doing more to negotiate the seemingly intractable international relationships than anyone. This man was Charles Evans Hughes.

FIFTEEN

Washington, D.C., and Bolton, New York,
March to September 1921

WITH MUCH FANFARE, PRESIDENT HARDING TOOK OFFICE ON March 4, 1921, bringing with him an all-star cabinet. The appointment of Hughes as secretary of state enabled Harding to secure other prominent figures for his administration: Andrew Mellon became secretary of the treasury, Herbert Hoover became secretary of commerce, and Henry C. Wallace became secretary of agriculture. Harding also appointed former President Taft as chief justice. The Republicans set out to make good on their campaign promise: "Less government in business and more business in government." Florence Harding said that had she not been a political wife, she would have devoted herself to animal rights. Upon arrival in Washington, she promptly ordered the removal of all the animal heads—moose, deer, elk, bear, and bighorn sheep—that Theodore Roosevelt had hung as trophies in the State Dining Room.

In August 1919 the national debt had reached its highest point at $26 billion. In broad terms, the federal government's revenues from taxation in 1920 were nearly $6 billion—six times what they had been in 1917. While Harding worked closely with Mellon to achieve tax relief and introduce a federal budget system, he gave Hughes free rein to address international peace.

From the moment he first sat at the broad desk in the large office in the State, War, and Navy Building in Washington, Hughes had a perfect genius for directing the State Department. His typical routine was to arrive promptly at nine o'clock and leave at seven o'clock or later, often taking state papers with him for closer study after dinner. Twice each day, at eleven o'clock in the morning and at three-thirty in the afternoon, Hughes held a press conference.

Antoinette was also quickly drawn into active duty. She often hosted receptions and elaborate afternoon teas at their home on Eighteenth Street. Certain days of the week were designated for the wives of cabinet officers and other officials to be "at home," which signified an open-invitation reception. On Antoinette's first "at home" day, more than one thousand people visited with their calling cards. Traffic came to a stand-still for blocks. They ran out of food. And still people continued to arrive.

Barely a month after Charles and Antoinette moved to Washington, leaving Catherine in the care of her older brother, they had received a letter—*a letter!*—from Catherine informing her parents of her engagement to Chauncey Waddell. Antoinette was so stunned that she drove immediately to the State, War, and Navy Building and, mouth agape and letter in hand, marched into Charles's office in the middle of the day. Charles rose from his desk, alarmed. Antoinette handed him the letter without a word. She watched in amazement as his eyes scanned the familiar handwriting and then crinkled with mirth as his mustache spread over his smiling lips.

"That's our CaCa," he chuckled, referring to her by the nickname bestowed upon her by baby Elizabeth. "Independent to the end."

"But why has he not come to you to ask your permission?" Antoinette sputtered.

"The world has changed," Charles said, crossing to place a tender kiss on Antoinette's cheek. "We must trust her judgment." He placed the letter in the hands of his wife of more than thirty years. "After all, it's wonderful news! We're going to have a wedding!" Antoinette worried that the news might send Elizabeth into a depression at the thought that she, like Helen, would never live to marry.

The heat in Washington in the summer of 1921 was so oppressive that Antoinette arranged for Elizabeth and Blanche to spend August with longtime family friends in Bolton, New York, near Lake George, just twenty-two miles north of Glens Falls. This might well be Elizabeth's final summer, and Antoinette wanted to shield her from the prying attentions that her failing health would attract in Washington or Morristown. Elizabeth and Blanche would stay on through mid-September 1921.

At Stillwater Cottage, Elizabeth was attended to by maids and cooks who were wonderfully accommodating. She was reunited with family friends, the Hoopeses and the Hydes, with a longstanding tradition of summering in the area. As Elizabeth put it, "The clan has gathered." The natural environment seemed to restore her strength, and her letters were soon full of enthusiastic reports of her lively existence. Tellingly, they were almost completely devoid of the details of her daily diet.

The mornings were cold—the temperature only reached the midfifties in her bedroom—and Elizabeth often ate her breakfast in bed, beginning with hot cocoa. She was an avid reader of adventure stories, particularly stories of cowboys, scouts, and frontier life. She loved being outdoors and leapt at every chance to grab a fishing pole and climb into a row boat with Blanche, who would row them out to an island and serve a picnic lunch. Blanche would scramble Elizabeth's single egg in a Girl Scouts campfire cooking set while the other picnickers feasted on fresh-caught fish or chops and roasted corn on the cob. Every afternoon Blanche, or "Mrs. B." as Elizabeth had taken to calling her, enforced a nap of at least one hour.

> *There are 4 hydroairplanes [sic] here now, one of which is enormous, carrying 13 passengers beside the two pilots and having two liberty motors in it . . . it is all sort of camouflaged and painted like a fish. About everybody on the lake has been up sometime or other in one of them and they'll take you up to the narrows from Lake George for $10.00, a ride for 15 or so minutes. . . . Every time I see it up I heave a sigh, for I would so love to go, but I suppose it's foolish, nevertheless, among countless other things I'll do on August 19th, 1928 [her twenty-first birthday], I'll do that, and read* Wuthering Heights *as I go along!*

Elizabeth's letters included breathless descriptions of her fishing successes (black bass and perch) and bird-watching (bald eagles, great blue heron, wild duck) and the thrilling arrival on the lake of a fast new motorboat called the *Snark*. She joined the clan at country fairs and vocal concerts and tennis tournaments. On Sundays she attended the Baptist Church in Bolton Landing.

. . . last night really was the night of all nights and I shall never forget it. Evangeline Booth, Commander of the Salvation Army and her secretary came to dinner . . . It seems she comes up here almost every summer for her vacation and camps, but no one is supposed to know about it and she remains almost in seclusion . . . Oh, she is the most wonderful and remarkable person I've ever met and talked with . . . It was quite a dinner party too, my first real one, there being fourteen of us altogether and we didn't leave the table until quarter of nine!

Upstate New York was like a second home to Elizabeth, and she and Blanche were having a great summer. But Elizabeth worried about her mother back in Washington, who was still recovering from the loss of Helen just over a year before:

I want you to be very frank with me Mother, and promise absolutely to let me know if you get lonely and want me to really come home for some reason or other, for all the heat of Washington and the tropics put together wouldn't keep me back if I thought that. You'll promise, won't you?

On her fourteenth birthday the group celebrated with a lovely picnic lunch. Elizabeth ate her small portion of egg custard and cocoa while the others had coffee, sandwiches, salad, and watermelon. After lunch, Mrs. Hyde presented Elizabeth with a huge hatbox covered with pink paper to resemble a birthday cake, complete with fourteen blazing candles. Elizabeth wrote that according to the number of blows it took her to extinguish the candles, she would not be married for eleven years. Inside the hatbox were presents—books and RCA Victor recordings and a pincushion from her childhood friend Polly Hoopes.

Elizabeth began to collect bird nests and eggs, and even suggested that, when the time came, she might have the family canary, Perfect, sent to a taxidermist to add to the collection.

I don't know what's the matter with me when it comes to birds, but the more I study and watch the dear little things the more I become deeply fascinated, and it has a hold upon me that I simply can't explain. I'd rather hunt or read or talk birds than do almost anything else . . .

That summer she submitted a story about fishing to a popular children's journal—and it was published.

> *If my* St. Nicholas *has come (as it most doubtless has) please open it and look in the back for the "League," where you will find a familiar story about a fish called "A Proud Moment" by Elizabeth Evans Hughes, and also don't fail to notice that said story won a silver badge the next to highest distinction you can receive! Did you ever? When I saw my name and story actually in there I nearly fell over, but when I saw that I had won a silver badge on it, I was an absolute wreck, as you can well imagine . . . it inspired me with such "fresh veal and zigor . . ." Tell Father it's the first step toward his "life," that I'm bound I'm going to write one day!*

At night, as Elizabeth drifted off to sleep to the sound of crickets and peepers and the occasional hoot of an owl, she recited the names of the things she loved. She breathed each word as if it were a prayer: trees, songbirds, dogs, the first frost, thunderstorms, the smell of pine needles, the feel of pine needles underfoot on the forest floor, the wink of mica in sunlight, reading, writing, words in general, travel by train, travel by ship, the shape of leaves, the feeling of spray on her face as she raced across Lake George in a motorboat, picnics, ladybugs, pussy willows, the sound of rain, the smell of the earth in springtime, the crackle of campfires . . .

It was part devotional, part literary exercise, and part survival strategy. Conspicuously absent from the catalog was all manner of food. She and Teddy Ryder had adopted opposite approaches to achieve the same goal. Each was collecting reasons to stay the course, betting against the odds with the only capital they had—their willingness to endure the pain of living.

Without exception Elizabeth fell asleep before she finished her list.

SIXTEEN

The Washington Conference,
November 12, 1921, to February 6, 1922

A s Antoinette began to plan Catherine's wedding, Hughes set about planning what would be one of the most celebrated international peace conferences in the history of the world, the Washington Naval Disarmament Conference (the Washington Conference), over which he would preside. It would be his first major event as secretary of state. Europe was strewn with human wreckage and with Romanoffs, Hapsburgs, and Hohenzollerns dethroned and centuries-old social hierarchies dismantled. It was imperative to broker a new world peace. But how? In pursuit of a strategy to ensure the success of this momentous conference, Hughes maintained a weekday schedule seven days a week.

Occasionally he would emerge from one of his grueling intellectual workouts and announce to Antoinette, "It can't be done." And she would remind him that he had said that about many of the projects he had taken on. Then he would say, "This time is different. This time I've taken on more than I can handle." Then Antoinette would smile sweetly and remind him that he often said that, too. Her husband was literally trying to solve the problems of the world, and she was trying to keep him from destroying himself in the process.

In June, Antoinette traveled alone to Silver Bay to attend the ceremony of the laying of the cornerstone of Helen's chapel. The site selected was one where Helen often sat quietly during her time at Silver Bay. The architect was to be Mr. Collins of the Boston firm Allen and Collins. The structure would be built of locally quarried granite.

Antoinette led a procession of young and healthy YWCA women dressed in ankle-length, white cotton dresses across the wide summer lawn to the construction site. She was three months shy of her fifty-seventh birthday. Compared with the apple-cheeked women who followed her, she looked frail in her black dress and hat, as if her present form had been whittled from a larger, more robust person.

Appropriately, the Washington Conference began on the morning of November 12, one day after Armistice Day and the dedication of the Tomb of the Unknown Soldier. On November 11, 1921, at 8:30 in the morning, a military escort removed a coffin bearing the remains of an unidentifiable American soldier from the rotunda of the Capitol where it had lain in state under an honor guard for two days, resting upon the same catafalque that had supported the remains of presidents Lincoln, Garfield, and McKinley. The coffin was then committed to the sarcophagus, an event punctuated by three salvos of artillery, the sounding of taps and the national salute.

This solemn pageantry was a fitting prelude to the diplomatic salvo fired by the secretary of state on the following morning. The conference took place at Constitution Hall on Seventeenth Street, the home of the Daughters of the American Revolution. Several thousand people gathered in the cold on the streets outside in the hope of catching a glimpse of the notables as they arrived. Several hundred newspaper correspondents were in attendance to cover the event. Shortly after ten o'clock the attendees filed solemnly into the central hall where the tables were arranged in a large rectangle. The delegates settled into their seats in full anticipation of a bland and benign agenda consisting of the requisite welcoming speeches and mutual greetings, opening prayers, and logistical business of the conference. Instead, Hughes rose to the podium with a speech so volatile that it had been stored in a vault. Despite this precaution Hughes was so concerned about possible leaks and rumors that he asked Harding if he could deliver it right away instead of waiting until the second day of the conference. Harding agreed.

In a proposal that was bold beyond all expectations Hughes offered to scrap American warships and challenged Great Britain and Japan to do the same with their fleets, according to a 5:5:3 ratio. While those in attendance were turning to each other in disbelief, asking if they had heard Hughes correctly, the secretary of state continued. He next proposed a ten-year moratorium on capital ship construction. After a moment of stunned silence, a commotion swept through the dignitaries.

Tables were prepared and ideas were exchanged about how the ratio could be achieved. Reductions were assessed relative to existing strength, which was calculated to include both built ships and those under construction. It quickly became apparent that in order to achieve this goal all three powers would have to scrap part of their current fleet. Great Britain would have to make the greatest sacrifice in vessels already built. The United States would be called upon to make the greatest sacrifice of vessels both built and under construction. In all, the United States would scrap thirty battleships, or 845,740 tons; Great Britain would scrap nineteen battleships, or 583,375 tons; and Japan would scrap seventeen battleships, or 448,928 tons—all within ninety days of signing an agreement. The Hughes plan was both thrillingly idealistic and thoroughly concrete.

The admirals of the U.S. Navy were outraged. Hughes had violated diplomatic protocol by not consulting them first. They protested that such drastic reductions in naval power would jeopardize national security, particularly in the event of a war in the Pacific, where America would be exposed, especially in the Philippines. In fact, the policymakers of the Navy Department believed the U.S. Navy should be as large as Great Britain's and Japan's combined.

Japan preferred a ratio of 10:7 to the 10:6 ratio that Hughes proposed. Moreover, the Hughes plan called for the scrapping of the recently completed *Mutsu* battleship. The Japanese flatly refused to sacrifice *Mutsu* under any circumstances, claiming that the huge ship held special sentimental value for Japan because it was wholly the product of Japanese designers and engineers. The deliberations continued week after week through the winter holidays and into January. One *New York Times* headline blared: "End of Conference Still Not in Sight. Rainbow of Adjournment Again Fades from the View of Wearied Delegates." Day after day the fate of the world hung in the balance in these fragile deliberations, and the success of the deliberations rested squarely on the shoulders of Charles Evans Hughes. Returning to his office after the conference sessions, he paced the floors and worried about the outcome of his very high-risk, high-reward gamble to achieve world peace.

SEVENTEEN

*The Physiatric Institute, Morristown,
New Jersey, November 1921*

LATE ONE AFTERNOON IN THE MONTH OF THANKSGIVING, DR. ALLEN went into his study with the intention of writing a letter to Antoinette Hughes. It was a letter that he had avoided writing for quite some time, a letter he did not now want to write, but for Elizabeth's sake, he would.

Outside the window of Dr. Allen's office, Belle Wishart was crossing unseen through the early darkness to the groundskeeper's cottage, holding an empty birdcage before her like a lantern without a flame. The air was thick with the threat of a storm; she pulled her sweater more closely around her. There had been a sprinkling of rain that afternoon, and the grass was still wet. Miss Wishart moved slowly, lifting her feet high with each step like a wading shore bird.

Inside the cottage, the old man was sitting beside a woodstove, hunched over the seat of a chair that he was recaning with strong, knobby hands. Hearing Wishart approach, the old man unfolded himself, crossed to the Dutch door, swung open the top panel, and frowned.

He had been the groundskeeper for Mr. Kahn, and he hadn't had an easy time transitioning to the new regime. It wasn't that he minded the extra work or the restricted budget. It was that he could still see the place all lit up for a party on a summer night, with torchères blazing and jazz music floating through the portico and ladies in silk and gentlemen in spats strolling the topiary garden, smoking and laughing. It was hard to get used to the deathly quiet.

She came forward with the birdcage.

"Good evening," she said.

He nodded.

"Thank you," she said simply. The old man's hands remained in his pockets.

"Isn't that the cage the little girl borrowed?"

"Yes."

"Want me to get her another bird? I could catch one easy. A finch or a chickadee."

"It wasn't her bird. It belonged to another patient. A boy named Eddie."

"Does he want another bird?"

Miss Wishart shook her head. Reluctantly, the old man took the cage, lifted it over the lower part of the door and set it down on the floor.

"What'd he die of?"

"Diabetes."

The groundskeeper's eyebrows registered disbelief.

"Not the bird. The boy. Eddie died," Miss Wishart explained. "He ate the birdseed and it threw his meta— his system into shock."

The old man frowned, straining to understand.

"Thank you for the cage. For obvious reasons we will have no more birds as pets." Miss Wishart turned and began making her way with slow storklike steps back to the mansion house. He watched her for several steps and then, still frowning, called after her.

"Miss Wishart, ma'am. But what happened to the bird?"

Miss Wishart did not stop. She turned and called back over her shoulder.

"I opened the window and set it free."

The groundskeeper swung the top door shut, rubbed his grizzled face, and returned to the warmth of the woodstove, leaving the empty cage by the door. There it remained for weeks. He could not bring himself to look at it, unable to shake off the gruesome idea that Wishart had been lying, that the child might have eaten more than just the birdseed.

He had seen the small spectral faces that sometimes appeared at the windows of the great house. Even from a distance he could sense their desperation.

What could Allen do but use the tragic loss of Eddie as a cautionary tale for all the residents of the Physiatric Institute? If he did not do so, no good would come of his death, and that would add tragedy to tragedy. So Allen instructed Belle Wishart to tell the nurses to tell the patients the truth about what happened, providing facts and details as requested.

Although Allen hoped that Eddie's death would be a lesson to the patients, it was he who felt the most chastened by it. He was deeply ashamed of himself for the lapse in judgment, for allowing himself to be persuaded to permit the boy to keep a bird in the first place. There was a place for leniency to be sure, but it was in the accounts receivable department, not in the clinical treatment of patients.

In November 1921 Elizabeth's weight had dropped to fifty-two pounds and plateaued. She had been a semi-invalid for the better part of a year. Most of her hair had fallen out. Her skin was slack and parched. Allen took out the last letter he had received from Antoinette and smoothed the monarch page on his desk blotter. In it she informed the doctor that, because Elizabeth could not possibly sustain the stress of even a common cold, she intended for Elizabeth and Blanche to spend several months in Bermuda during that winter. He had never replied, being reluctant to disappoint her with his objections. But now Eddie's death quite literally forced his hand: He must never again allow a soft heart to jeopardize a patient.

He must speak up lest he lose the keel of his conscience. When a cure was found—as he knew it would be—they would thank him for keeping Elizabeth alive to see that great day dawn. But how to address this worrisome emotional intimacy? Blanche and Elizabeth traveled together to Lake George, Washington, New York, and—soon—Bermuda. They knitted sweaters together. They took daily walks on which they collected things to add to Elizabeth's prodigious collections of natural artifacts: shells, feathers, leaves, flowers, and seed pods. They were fond of reading aloud together, handing the book back and forth or huddling close with Elizabeth's head resting in the crook of her nurse's neck. Sometimes they read plays aloud, this way each taking on the roles of various characters. When hunger became unbearable, Blanche would gather Elizabeth into her lap and rock her.

Did Mrs. Hughes realize, he began, that the body's delicate metabolic balance can be upset by subtle emotional changes, climate changes, situational changes. He was concerned that Elizabeth's relationship with Blanche had become (how could he put it), emotionally exciting, and that this might prove detrimental to Elizabeth in the future. The Allen treatment was a comprehensive hormonal alchemy. For the good of the patients, he strove to maintain a constant and neutral atmosphere within the institute.

Indeed, it was easy to see the increasing intimacy between the two. Elizabeth had initially called her nurse Mrs. Burgess, then Mrs. B and then simply Blanche.

He stopped and began again. As she was no doubt aware, Elizabeth's treatment had been unorthodox in many ways. There was, for instance, the outpatient arrangement and the insistence on a private nurse. Indeed, it was this latter situation that placed him in the uncomfortable position about which he was compelled to write to her. Were Blanche employed by the institute, there would be no need to trouble Mrs. Hughes with his concern. In that case the course of action would be obvious, unpalatable, perhaps, but obvious. However, Blanche was employed by the secretary of state and her patient was the daughter of the secretary of state. Moreover, the secretary was among the major benefactors of the institute. It was his imprimatur on the letterhead, Dr. Allen knew, that had allowed Allen to raise the funds to launch the institute. And the future financial health of the institute, despite its good work and innovative business model, was far from secure.

He stopped again. This last effort piqued a particularly sore spot of indignation. He resented the need to split his time and energy between what he considered to be his real work and that greedy ancillary endeavor which was the work of supporting the work. Few were the days when he was free from the worry that, at any moment, this ancillary work would completely engulf his real work. On bad days he felt that, despite his medical degree and his reputation, his actual occupation was something between a professional sycophant and an emergency mason, constantly trying through all means of financial spackle, mortar, putty, grout, and crutches to shore up a structure that was forever on the verge of toppling. From the start the two roles had been at odds within him: He must do what was best for Elizabeth and he must be careful not to offend her parents. Hadn't he started his own institute in order to avoid politics?

He would try to adopt an avuncular rather than punitive tone. This thought brought an immediate smirk to his face. He thought about Otto Kahn, the dapper, well-loved, prominent New York financier and patron of the arts who had built the grand estate that now housed the Physiatric Institute. It occurred to Allen that Kahn was all of the things that he was not. Kahn made money for the rich. Allen denied food to the starving. Kahn's clients showered him with praise and invited him to tony social events. Allen's clients endured him because he was saving their lives. Allen was not warm. He was not suave. He was not dapper. Despite his being a successful doctor at the top of his career in a nation whose population of eligible men had been vastly depleted by the war, he had remained a bachelor until October, just weeks before, when, at the age of forty-two, he and Belle Wishart were married.

If Allen remained silent Elizabeth and Blanche would sail for Bermuda. They would be away for months. He could only imagine that their intimate connection would grow in such an idyllic setting. He imagined luxurious boat rides in sapphire water, picnics on the bluffs overlooking clusters of quaint whitewashed cottages, exotic birds, and the breeze infused with the scent of oleander. Weren't they to stay in a place called "Honeymoon Cottage"? Surely it was only a matter of time before pity would weaken Blanche's resolve to maintain the diet. And need he remind Mrs. Hughes that a cure was at hand?

He could not have known just how near.

As Allen struggled to write a letter in the stillness of the palatial Physiatric Institute, an unknown, impoverished surgeon sat in a laboratory in Toronto, smoking incessantly to mitigate the odor of dog feces as he struggled to write a paper that would document the summer's work.

In just a few weeks, and little more than a hundred miles from Allen's desk, Banting would deliver this paper to a group of eminent physicians, including Allen and Elliott Joslin. The paper, "The Beneficial Influences of Certain Pancreatic Extracts on Pancreatic Diabetes," would change the world dramatically, and within a decade Allen would be forgotten, his reputation eclipsed, and the Physiatric Institute abandoned forever.

EIGHTEEN

The University of Toronto, September to December 1921

Dᴜʀɪɴɢ ᴛʜᴇ ꜰɪʀꜱᴛ ᴡᴇᴇᴋ ᴏꜰ Sᴇᴘᴛᴇᴍʙᴇʀ 1921, Bᴀɴᴛɪɴɢ ᴅʀᴏᴠᴇ ᴛᴏ 442 Adelaide Street North. With grim determination he set about bringing the unhappy London chapter to a swift and final conclusion. In a single day, he sold the big white house and most of his furniture. What few belongings remained he loaded into his car. He could not get away from London and all that it represented fast enough.

When he returned to Toronto, Macleod's reply from Scotland was waiting.

Banting could remain at the university to continue his work, and Macleod assured him that he would do what he could to help him. He also agreed that Banting should use the operating room that Starr had arranged, at least until another solution could be worked out. There was a new anatomy building under construction, so there would be more operating facilities available. He advised them to be discreet in transporting dogs from one building to the other. The anti-vivisection movement had gained enough traction to make the University of Toronto administration nervous. This was yet another way that having someone like Banting on the campus was a potential liability. As far as presenting their research was concerned, his tone was generally encouraging but Macleod warned Banting that he had to ensure that there was no possibility of mistake. Macleod raised questions, no doubt intended to help Banting prepare to defend his work from the challenges that he would surely encounter in the scientific community. As was his wont, Macleod was cautious. He was known for telling his students, "One result is no result."

Banting's philosophy could not have been more different. To him, Macleod's letter indicated a vote of no confidence in the work that he and Best had done and a directive to suppress his imagination. Banting began to suspect that the great professor was not taking him seriously and perhaps never had.

On September 5 Banting and Best prepared two donor dogs by duct ligation. On September 7 they depancreatized two recipient dogs; these were identified as Dog 5 and Dog 9. These would be the last experiments of the summer. Macleod was due back very soon. The pressure was on to collect as much data as possible.

While they waited for the acinar tissue to degenerate in the two duct-ligated dogs, they tried to make some isletin by the secretin-stimulation method, but the dog died two hours into the surgery. They removed its pancreas anyway. They prepared an extract according to the prescribed procedure. That night they used the last 10 cc of the old extract on Dog 9, administering it by rectum this time. It had no effect.

Intravenous doses of the new extract, on the other hand, produced a dramatic reduction in Dog 9's blood sugar, lowering it from .30 at 6:30 P.M. to .07 by midnight. However, the injection itself appeared to cause pain to the dog. The following day's injections were much less effective on the blood sugar, and an attempt to administer the extract rectally had no effect.

On September 12 they tried to exhaust a cat's pancreas with secretin, but the cat died after ninety minutes of stimulation. They used its pancreas to produce an extract. They performed several experimental injections with this extract on Dog 9, including injecting the extract directly into the dog's heart. This produced a moderate decline in blood sugar, followed by shock and death. After performing an autopsy, Banting and Best determined that Dog 9 had died from emboli, or large particles of pancreas tissue, in the extract. Apparently, in their haste they had not macerated or strained the extract thoroughly enough. The control dog, Dog 5, was euthanized. The notebook suggests that its abdomen was infected.

On September 17 they again obtained extract from using the secretin-stimulation method and injected it into one last depancreatized dog. For the first time they tried the method of subcutaneous rather than intravenous injection. Best recorded the emergence of a hole the size of a quarter in the dog's skin at the site of the injection. Also, there was considerable bleeding from a superficial vein that had been partially degraded. The dog's blood sugar remained stable, neither rising nor falling. As these results were not definitive, they decided to suspend further experimentation until they had obtained trypsin-free extract. The summer's work was over.

In mid-September a junior member of the faculty in the pharmacology department left and Velyien Henderson wrote to President Falconer asking permission to hire Banting as his replacement. On September 21, the same day Henderson wrote to Falconer, Macleod arrived in Toronto. In late September or early October Banting and Best met with Macleod, who strongly encouraged Banting to repeat all of his experiments in order to confirm his findings. Banting reminded Macleod of his requirements: a salary, a boy to look after the dogs, a room to work in, and repairs to the floor of the operating room. Macleod was reluctant. Why fix up the old operating room when a new one would soon be available? He also pointed out that funds were limited; by directing further funds to Banting's project, some other researcher would suffer.

Eleven months later Banting wrote this account of the meeting:

> *I told him that if the University of Toronto did not think that the results obtained were of sufficient importance to warrant the provision of the aforementioned requirements I would have to go someplace where they would. His reply was, "As far as you're concerned, I am the University of Toronto." He told me that this research was "no more important than any other research in the department." I told him that I had given up everything I had in the world to do the research, and that I was going to do it, and that if he did not provide what I asked I would go someplace where they would. He said that I "had better go."*

Macleod relented. Banting suggested that Macleod could take an active role in satisfying some of his doubts about the work; he could participate in the experiments. Macleod demurred. Then Banting suggested that James Bertram "Bert" Collip might play a role on the team.

Collip was a brilliant associate professor of Biochemistry at the University of Alberta in Edmonton. In the spring of 1921 he happened to be in Toronto on a prestigious one-year Rockefeller Traveling Fellowship, which was to have allowed him a year to study in Toronto, London (U.K.), and New York. He began studying the effect of pH on blood sugar under the renowned authority on carbohydrate metabolism Macleod, whom he revered and because of whom he had chosen to work in Toronto. Prior to Macleod's departure for Scotland, he had introduced Collip to several people, including Banting.

Over the summer, Collip had expressed his interest in the isletin work. It seemed perfectly logical to Banting that Collip should join the effort, his skills being exactly those required for the next phase, but Macleod declined. It was not yet time to expand the team, he said, and he cautioned Banting to avoid thinking too far ahead. Frustrated, Banting returned to the lab to try to produce results that would convince Macleod of the validity of their work and its worthiness of additional resources.

In October, Banting appeared on the payroll as a special assistant in pharmacology, courtesy of Velyien Henderson. His pay was $250 per month. Macleod arranged for retroactive pay for the summer's work of $170 for Best (the normal pay for a student assistant) and $150 for Banting, who had no official affiliation with the university.

In mid-November 1921 Banting contributed a new idea to the long history of attempts to isolate insulin. He remembered from his days on the farm that fetal calves received nourishment from the mother and therefore required no digestive glands until after birth. He also remembered that cows were often made pregnant before being slaughtered, because it fattened them and made them better eaters. In early December Banting and Best visited a local abbatoir where they cut out the pancreases of nine fetal calves and brought them back to the lab. From these they prepared an extract from the whole pancreatic gland of a fetal calf and injected this into a previously depancreatized (and thus diabetic) recipient dog. The result was an unmistakable decline in the blood sugar. They repeated the experiment and achieved the same result. Now they had a more reliable source of isletin. Banting reported his findings. For the first time Macleod seemed impressed.

Macleod invited Banting and Best to present a summary of their summer experiments in November at a gathering of the Journal Club of the

University of Toronto Department of Physiology. Banting was not fond of public speaking, but he was fired by the desire to claim his discovery and to prove that his gamble hadn't been a complete waste of time.

This would be the first semipublic announcement of Banting's and Best's work over the summer of 1921. Auspiciously, the Journal Club meeting was to take place on November 14—Banting's thirtieth birthday. It was agreed that Banting would present the paper, Best would be responsible for showing charts and illustrations, and Macleod would introduce them. Banting asked Macleod if his name should appear on the paper. Macleod chose not to have his name included among the authors.

The day arrived at last. Macleod began his introduction, and, according to Banting, he continued past the introduction to describe the work. Essentially, Macleod presented the paper, saying all the things that Banting had intended to say. When Macleod finished and turned the meeting over to Banting, the latter was flummoxed and humiliated. (Later, Banting claimed that Macleod used the pronoun "we" throughout the introduction, although he had been in Scotland for nearly the entire duration of the experiments he was describing.) This experience cemented Banting's resentment of Macleod. He ended the day feeling frustrated and anxious. Unable to sleep that night, he wrote in his diary, "Half my life is over." As it turned out, he was much closer to the end of his life than that.

The paper was published in February 1922 in the *Journal of Laboratory and Clinical Medicine* under the title "The Internal Secretion of the Pancreas." The authors were listed as F. G. Banting, M.B., and C. H. Best, B.A. The only mention of Macleod was in the bibliography.

Even before the paper was published, news of an important discovery in Toronto had begun to spread through the medical research community. Macleod had begun to receive letters from doctors desperate to save their doomed patients. That November, Dr. Elliott Joslin wrote:

> *At the meeting of the Southern Medical Association in Hot Springs, Arkansas, from which I have just returned, I heard Dr. Barker refer to experiments which you had conducted with extracts from the Islands of Langerhans. . . . Naturally if there is a grain of hopefulness in these*

*experiments which I can give to patients or even can say to them that you
are working upon the subject, it would afford much comfort, not only to
them but to me as well, because I see so many pathetic cases.*

Three weeks later Dr. Leonard G. Rowntree of Mayo Clinic in Rochester, Minnesota, wrote:

*I have heard indirectly that you have very recently made some important
discoveries in relation to the islands of Langerhans and diabetes. . . .
We have a little chap four years old, who, despite everything that we have
tried, is slipping away from us, and if there is anything in your work which
bears on the treatment of diabetes, we would greatly appreciate hearing
from you.*

Dr. N. B. Taylor of the University of Toronto, who attended the
November meeting at which Banting spoke, suggested that Banting
demonstrate the efficacy of his extract by attempting to prolong the life
of a diabetic dog. Banting, Best, and Macleod agreed. Less than a week
later, on December 6, 1921, a longevity experiment began involving
Dog 33, later to be renamed Marjorie.

All this time the substance was known as isletin, as Banting and Best
had dubbed it during their desperate summer striving. Macleod insisted
that the name be changed to insulin so as not to change "terminologic
horses [in the] mid-investigational stream." He pointed out that the term
insulin had been suggested by de Mayer in 1909 and was subsequently
endorsed by Sir Edward Sharpey-Schäfer in 1913 for the then hypo-
thetical secretion. To Banting, Macleod's insistence on renaming isletin
was just another illustration of his own disempowerment at the hands
of the great scholar.

Banting was impatient and increasingly desperate to prove himself.
Even with these endless experiments confirming the active extract, were
they really any closer to a clinical solution for humans? On November
23, Banting told Best that he was going to inject himself with the extract and asked Best to witness and record any results if Banting were
incapacitated. Banting wrote a brief note of explanation and apology to
his mother and father and pinned it to the front of his lab coat. Then he
self-administered a subcutaneous injection of 1.5 cc of the extract.

There was no effect. Banting recorded the fact in the laboratory notebook and left the lab utterly dejected.

When the call went out for papers to be considered for the American Physiological Society's thirty-fourth annual meeting in New Haven, Connecticut, in December 1921, Macleod, who was then president of the prestigious organization, encouraged Banting to submit the summer's work. Banting asked permission to add Macleod's name to his own and Best's as the paper's authors in order to raise its chances of being accepted. Macleod consented. The paper was accepted.

The conference was to take place from Wednesday, December 28, to Friday, December 30, 1921. Weeks before, the rumor began to spread throughout the medical research community that something really promising had occurred in Toronto. The title of the presentation, "The Beneficial Influences of Certain Pancreatic Extracts on Pancreatic Diabetes" was listed as being authored by one member and two guests: J. J. R. Macleod, F. G. Banting (by invitation) and C. H. Best (by invitation). The poorly done experiments of the early summer were omitted from this paper.

The paper was scheduled to be delivered on Friday afternoon, the least advantageous position in the conference, when many of the attendees would be leaving to catch trains. At least three people resolved to be present to hear the paper on December 30 in New Haven, even if that session began at midnight. They were Dr. Elliott Joslin of Boston, Massachusetts; Dr. Frederick Allen of Morristown, New Jersey; and Dr. George Henry Alexander ("Alec") Clowes, research director of Eli Lilly and Company in Indianapolis, Indiana.

NINETEEN

The Crossroads of America, Indianapolis, Indiana, 1919–1921

ALEC CLOWES WAS A DAZZLING TORNADO OF A MAN. WHETHER careening around Indianapolis in his luxurious Duesenberg automobile or pelting a fellow scientist with questions, he was constantly in motion, late for every meeting, often beginning conversations midsentence. He was impatient with details but did not like to delegate them. He wrote so rapidly that he had trouble deciphering his own handwriting. He ignored organizational hierarchy and abhorred committees. He was equally prone to outbursts of frustration and gestures of generosity. His handsome face was dominated by beetle brows under which his intense blue eyes often twinkled with ideas or mischief or both. Although he was not a medical doctor, those who knew him well called him "Doc." He parked wherever he liked and played golf holes in the order that appealed to him, often beginning with the hole nearest to where he parked. Eli Lilly said of him, "He lived more hours in a day than any man I knew."

Clowes (pronounced "Clues") joined Eli Lilly and Company in 1919, charged with identifying medical research projects having commercial potential for Lilly. In this unusual capacity Clowes was at liberty, and had the professional obligation, to explore the rarefied world of medical research as his interest drew him. At that time, it was widely accepted that the interests of medical research and the pharmaceutical business were utterly and irreconcilably incompatible. Researchers were primarily concerned with contributing to a body of research by writing, presenting, and publishing scientific papers. Pharmaceutical firms were primarily concerned with making money by means of manufacturing and selling products. Any research effort conducted by a pharmaceutical manufacturer was viewed with contempt by physicians and university scientists. In 1915 the Council on Pharmacy of the American Medical Association opined "it is only from laboratories free from any relation with manufacturers that real pharmaceutical advances can be expected." Certainly Banting and Macleod subscribed to the belief that a profit motive could only impair research. Furthermore, many biochemical research scientists, including Banting and Macleod, were also medical doctors who had taken the Hippocratic oath and were therefore proscribed from using their knowledge for purposes, such as profit, which might interfere with the physical benefit of humankind.

In the early twentieth century, pharmaceutical companies were much like the apothecaries and patent medicine makers of the nineteenth century. They generally sought to secure proprietary claims by improving products already on the market, rather than inventing new medicines. Around 1920, Eli Lilly and Company's popular products included: Charcoal Lozenges for indigestion, Cape Aloes for constipation, Passolaria for insomnia and anxiety, Liquid Blaud for anemia, and Elixir #63, containing catnip and fennel, for colds, headaches, colic and fever.

Eli Lilly, grandson of the company's founder, thought that the future hinged on patenting fundamentally *new* ideas, not improvements of old ideas. Had not George Westinghouse and Thomas Edison proved that cooperation between inventors and industry could catalyze the development process and improve the product? An internal research and development division, Eli posited, would enable the company to develop and patent entirely new proprietary drugs. He held that the future of pharmaceutical manufacturing was in fundamental biological research. It was a radical idea. In essence he envisioned the model that would become the industry standard among Big Pharma companies for decades to come, even to the present day.

As Eli Lilly saw it, he faced two hurdles in creating a creditable new internal research group, and they were two sides of the same coin. The first hurdle was to persuade the company's board of directors to invest in a fundamental research department. The second hurdle was to persuade a research scientist to climb down from the ivory tower to work in the world of commercial enterprise. In the first challenge Eli had a powerful ally—his father, J. K. Lilly Sr., president of the company.

J. K. Lilly Sr. was a man of uncommon judgment and beneficence who inspired respect and affection in almost everyone he encountered. He had been only fourteen years old when his father, Colonel Eli Lilly, founded Eli Lilly and Company in 1876. J.K. Sr. joined the company after graduating *cum laude* in 1882 from the first pharmacy school in North America, the Philadelphia College of Pharmacy. After the Colonel died, J. K. Lilly Sr. became president of the company in 1898. The development and introduction of North America's first lifesaving drug could hardly have been entrusted to a better man.

Eli had been promoting novel ideas ever since his introduction into the family business in 1907 as a one-man finance department. Eli's careful analysis of the Fluid Extract Department had resulted in the company saving fifteen thousand dollars annually by replacing wooden barrels with copper-lined barrels, eliminating loss through absorption of the product. He designed a slope-shouldered bottle for powdered extracts that helped pharmacists avoid wasted product trapped in the bottle's interior. And taking a cue from Henry Ford, Eli introduced straight-line mass production to the pharmaceutical business with the help of a specially designed building and a complex system of conveyor belts, chutes, pulleys, and pipes.

There were many long discussions in the boardroom. Leading the charge for innovation was Eli. The conservative argument was often led by Charles Lynn, general manager and trusted right-hand man of Lilly Sr. Lynn held the distinction of being the first nonfamily member to direct the company. He was a ham-fisted, cigar-smoking pragmatist who was innately skeptical of innovative ideas, often with sound reasoning. In the end, Eli won the debate to establish a research department to seek out new products and begin the search for its director. Lynn bit down on his cigar with a savage intensity but he could say nothing. J. K. Lilly Sr. was gradually turning the business over to his eldest son, Eli.

Eli set out to find an experienced, well-respected medical researcher who would be willing to cross over to commercial industry. But who? Clearly it would be a man of such intellectual confidence, ambition, and curiosity as to be unintimidated by the potential disapproval of his peers in research, someone whose accomplishments were impressive enough to prevent those disapproving peers from dismissing him, someone able to bridge two very different cultures and see through those differences to practicable solutions. To accomplish all that, this someone would have to possess inexhaustible energy. Above all, this someone would have to be not just knowledgeable but imaginative. Lilly thought Clowes might be that man.

Clowes completed his medical studies in chemistry at the Royal College of Science in London, and went on to pursue his doctoral degree at the University of Göttingen. (In the late nineteenth and early twentieth century, England and Germany were considered the scientific leaders of the world.) In 1901 Clowes had fled the hidebound academic and professional hierarchies of Europe for America, where his intellectual ingenuity might find more opportunity for expression. For eighteen years he worked at Roswell Park Memorial Institute, a cancer laboratory in Buffalo, New York. In Buffalo he married Edith Whitehill Hinkel and started a family. During the war he joined the Chemical Warfare Service in Washington, D.C. When the war ended in 1918, Clowes was living at the Cosmos Club in Washington, D.C., casting about for a new direction. He was forty-one years old, not an age when the average man would consider making a risky career change, but Clowes was not an average man. Would he return to Buffalo or look for something new? Just then the Lillys invited him to Indianapolis for lunch and an interview. The timing could not have been better.

From the moment that he stepped off the train in December 1918 into the glorious Romanesque style Union Station, Clowes was favorably impressed with Indianapolis. The barrel-vaulted ceilings soared above him, and beams of sunlight streamed through skylights down onto the marble-inlaid floors. It reminded him of the great train stations of London. Built in 1852–53, Indianapolis's Union Station held the distinction of being the nation's first centralized train station. The growth of railroads led to building an even larger version in 1888.

Indianapolis then was home to several major industries, including automobile manufacturing and auto parts, railroad cars, and meat packing. The huge number of workers who kept these industries functioning relied on the world's largest intercity electric railway system, the Interurban. In the year 1918 more than 7.5 million passengers were carried in 128,145 of these clean, convenient, and inexpensive trains. Interurbans traveled hundreds of miles in nearly all directions, from six o'clock in the morning to midnight, express and local, parlor and sleeper, all across the state's twenty-three million acres and beyond.

The city's architecturally appealing downtown area bustled with energy. There was the elegant Opera House, the striking State House and the solemnly beautiful 248-foot-tall Soldiers and Sailors Monument, anchoring the Circle at the center. In 1920 the state's employment growth numbers would show that manufacturing and industry had surpassed agriculture for the first time. By 1925 Indianapolis would be dubbed "the Crossroads of America" by the National Geographic Society. Clowes could see that the city had much to recommend it, which would be important when he had to make a case to Edith Clowes that the family should relocate from her hometown of Buffalo, New York.

J. K. Lilly Sr., then fifty-seven years old and his son Eli, then thirty-three met Clowes at Union Station. They took him by chauffeured car on a forty-five-minute tour of Indianapolis, narrated in large part by an enthusiastic Eli Lilly, except when the elder Lilly could get a word in. Clowes loved cars and Indianapolis was steeped in American car culture. Eli informed his recruit that sixty or so different automobile makes were manufactured in Indianapolis, including Overland, Cole, Marmon, Stutz, Duesenberg, Atlas-Knight, Economycar, Hoosier Scout, and Pathfinder. The city competed with Detroit and Cleveland in automobile manufacturing. But only Indianapolis could claim the Indianapolis Raceway and the Stutz Bearcat, world champion of America and Europe in speedway, road race, and long distance competitions. Cannonball Baker had driven a Bearcat from San Diego to New York in eleven days, seven hours, and fifteen minutes. Ford's large plant in Indianapolis manufactured twenty-five thousand Model Ts annually. Theodore Dreiser penned *A Hoosier Holiday* (1916), in which he described a car trip from New York to Indiana, and thus helped to spread the religion of the automobile to Americans everywhere.

Indianapolis also happened to be the home of Charles W. Fairbanks, who had served as a U.S. senator for eight years before becoming vice president under Theodore Roosevelt and later the running mate of Charles Evans Hughes in the 1916 presidential election.

The three men dined at the Indianapolis Athletic Club, where the menu had been arranged in advance by the Lillys, specifically to indoctrinate their visitor's palate to Hoosier cuisine. Over lunch the three men discussed the development of drugs, using aspirin as a case study. All three were familiar with the basic facts of the story; Clowes would have studied it thoroughly at Göttingen. In 400 B.C., Hippocrates used the powdered bark and leaves of the willow tree to help relieve pain and fever. By 1829, scientists had identified willow's beneficial compound as salicin. Then French chemist Henri Leroux improved the extraction process and Italian chemist Raffaele Piria refined salicin, isolating salicylic acid. Salicylic acid is highly effective but it irritates the stomach. In 1853 another French chemist, Charles Gerhardt, succeeded in buffering salicylic acid without diminishing its efficacy. Like a true academic, Gerhardt published a paper to document his results and thought no more about it. It wasn't until 1897—forty-four years after Gerhardt's discovery—that a chemist named Felix Hoffman at Germany's Friedrich Bayer & Co. began working with the compound in order to alleviate his father's arthritis pain. By 1899 Bayer aspirin was selling around the world.

The younger Lilly practically crowed. "How many thousands of people suffered needlessly during the forty-six years between Gerhardt's discovery and Bayer's distribution of aspirin?"

Clowes nodded. The younger man's enthusiasm appealed to him. It was true that if Bayer had been involved in the process in 1853, a clinical application would almost certainly have been available to patients sooner. "Ideas don't cure people. *Drugs* cure people." Lilly continued, "That's why we *must* bring the research scientists and the drug manufacturers together."

To do so would require considerable risk for both parties. As Clowes's longtime secretary once put it, at that time a man dedicated to theoretical research who shifted to commercial objectives was somewhat in the position among his fellow scientists of having sold his birthright for a mess of porridge. For the Lillys it would require an enormous financial investment with no guaranteed return. Such entrepreneurial ventures were not entirely new to the Lillys. When Colonel Lilly saw that what deterred the ailing individual from taking medicine was that most of it was so unpalatable, he sought a new delivery mechanism that would solve the problem. While his peers were sweetening and flavoring their medicines, Colonel Lilly built its first gelatin capsule plant in 1895. In 1898 empty, easy-to-swallow gelatin capsules, in seven sizes, appeared on the Lilly price list. They were hugely successful. In 1905, company sales passed the $1 million mark.

And so the three men reached an agreement and the gamble that Clowes began in 1901 with his immigration to America would continue with his leaving the familiar world of research to join a commercial pharmaceutical company in 1919. Alec and Edith Clowes and their two sons moved from Buffalo to Indianapolis in the spring of 1919. At Clowes's behest, the Lillys funded a research facility in Woods Hole, Massachusetts, so that Clowes could continue to pursue his interest in marine biology. Every summer he invited guest scientists to join him there and so facilitated partnerships between Lilly and the research world. He enjoyed sailing, and the sea breezes relieved his hayfever. He often lingered at Woods Hole until early October. For two and a half years the Lillys had treated Clowes with the greatest generosity, creating a pure research position and allowing him full freedom to work wherever and whenever he pleased. All this openhanded munificence only drove Clowes harder toward the objective of finding a golden opportunity. And yet, there had been no dramatic discoveries or developments in his two years in Indianapolis. The stakes were no longer his alone. The Lillys had taken the leap of faith, and, of course, Edith had also, having moved across the country. Now it all came down to Christmas day, 1921.

Admittedly his decision to attend the American Physiological Society meeting was based on a hunch, but it was a hunch with J. J. R. Macleod's name attached to it. The history of diabetes research had been particularly riddled with false claims and near misses and Clowes felt sure that J. J. R. Macleod was both too proud and too savvy to attach his name to an idea he wasn't completely sure of. Still, Canada did seem an unlikely location for a medical breakthrough of such sweeping importance. What had driven a man of Macleod's standing to move to Toronto was certainly a mystery to Clowes, but he supposed Macleod would say the same about Clowes's choice to defect to the even more exotic territory of commercial industry.

Nearly everything about Clowes's attendance at the meeting in New Haven, Connecticut, in December 1921 was unlikely. He was an Englishman working in America. He was a researcher working in industry. His focus was cancer, not diabetes. Charles Hughes and Alec Clowes did not know each other, but they would soon have a powerful impact on each other's lives. They had one thing in common—they each had lost a child to disease. Hughes had lost Helen and Clowes had lost a three-year-old son to leukemia in Buffalo. So it was no small sacrifice that attendance at the meeting meant that he could not spend Christmas Day with his family. But if the rumors from Toronto were true then millions of mothers and fathers would be spared the suffering of losing a child.

While Banting and Macleod prepared to make their announcement in New Haven, the world's diplomatic powers continued to negotiate disarmament in Washington. In December 1921 the front page of *The Indianapolis News* regularly featured articles on the progress of the Washington Conference. One headline read "Conference Takes A Day Off At Last: Insatiable Mr. Hughes Permits a Lapse for Christmas but All Would Work Monday." The inner pages were crammed with advertisements. The Circle Talking Machine Shop offered "Victrolas for everybody. $25 to $1,500." Children both naughty and nice would be delighted with sleds from one dollar to five dollars fifty cents. The "Photoplay Attractions" for the week listed the movies featuring Mary Pickford, Norma Talmadge, Jackie Coogan, and Buster Keaton. The Spinks-Arms Hotel was celebrating its first anniversary with an old-fashioned, mid-day Christmas dinner for one dollar and fifty cents per plate. No fewer than fifty-seven churches announced the times of their Christmas Day services and the topics of their sermons. Alec and Edith rarely missed a Sunday at the Christ Episcopal Church on The Circle, where they usually saw fellow parishioners Eli Lilly with his wife Evelyn and daughter Evie.

Every December Edith Clowes took her sons, George Jr. and Allen, to see the Christmas displays in downtown Indianapolis. With a child in each graceful, gloved hand, the threesome strolled along the Italianate storefronts on Meridian Street to the southwest corner of Meridian and Washington streets. There stood L. S. Ayres, the finest of the Indianapolis department stores, which rose eight stories high with six elevators and two hundred and fifty feet of windows. At Christmastime, each window was transformed with an elaborate diorama. Inside, on a balcony above the main floor, a white-robed chorus serenaded the shoppers with cheery carols and the entire sixth floor was transformed into "Toyland," where towering displays of toys fitting every description waited to dazzle small, wide-eyed visitors. For the Clowes family, Christmas of 1921 would be different from all the rest. Before the sun rose on December 25th, Alec Clowes would leave the Duchess—his fond nickname for his clever and refined wife—and their two boys to board a train bound for Pennsylvania Station in New York City, where he would walk across town to Grand Central Terminal to board another train to New Haven.

Clowes was not a particularly good sleeper anyway. Sometimes he went out walking before the sun was up, accompanied by his walking stick and the family dog, a collie named Roddy. These last few months he had seemed particularly restless, often rising at four o'clock in the morning to read and to think. But on Christmas morning, attired in his habitual un-pressed British tweed, Alec Clowes would find himself at Indianapolis's Union train station, where his adventure with Eli Lilly had begun two years before. He could not possibly imagine how frequently he would walk across that marble floor over the following eighteen months. During that time Clowes would travel so often that it would not be uncommon for him to arrive at a station, step dazedly onto the platform, go to a telephone, and place a call to Frances to ask her where exactly he was going.

On Christmas Eve the temperature in Indianapolis dropped thirty degrees. The following morning Union Station was so empty that Clowes could hear his footsteps echoing as he strode to his train. Settling into his seat in a first class train compartment, he put his briefcase on the empty seat across from him and closed his eyes. His mind wandered to the brick Tudor house he'd just left. He imagined the first sun glittering in the icy branches of the poplar trees in the front yard. He imagined his sons racing each other down the front stairs to the Christmas tree.

The train lumbered through the city and picked up speed across the great white plains, deep with snowdrifts. Clowes thought of the upcoming conference and the odds that the news from Toronto was true. Just because no one had been able to isolate the pancreatic extract yet didn't mean that they couldn't do it now. Was it so unreasonable to imagine that on Christmas 1922, one year hence, J. K. Lilly Sr. would receive dozens of cards and letters from strong, active diabetic children thanking him for their very lives and describing in delirious detail the foods that they could now consume? Was it absurd to dream that within twenty years, the life expectancy of a ten-year-old diabetic child would be more than twenty-five times greater than it was on that lonely Christmas Day 1921?

Perhaps, but that is exactly what happened.

TWENTY

The American Physiological Society Meeting,
New Haven, Connecticut, December 28–30, 1921

THE FRANTIC EFFORT IN TORONTO CONTINUED RIGHT UP TO THE hour of departure for the American Physiological Society meeting. Less than a week before an exhausted Banting boarded the train for New England, Macleod gave in to Banting's insistent pleas and Collip officially joined the insulin team. Apparently Macleod was finally convinced that Banting and Best's discovery was worthy of additional resources, because he enlisted not only Collip but also Almon A. Fletcher, John Hepburn, J. K. Latchford, and Clark Noble. They, too, participated in the race to achieve two objectives: first, to produce an extract pure enough for human trial, and second, to develop a procedure that would consistently produce effective extract in large quantities.

Reining in the new team's exuberance, Macleod attempted to organize the effort. He assigned specific duties to each team member. Clark Noble would focus on the extract's stability and potency by assisting Collip with assays using rabbits. Collip was to focus on making an extract pure enough for human trial. Dr. John Hepburn, who had initially come to Toronto to study with Macleod under the auspices of the American Physiological Society's first fellowship, was assigned to work with Charley Best on respiratory quotient tests. (At that time it was thought that you could learn whether carbohydrates were being burned in the body by measuring the ratio of carbon dioxide exhaled to oxygen inhaled.) Last but not least, Banting was charged with performing any surgery that might be required by the group.

Most of the pressure fell directly on the shoulders of Bert Collip. He was a particularly talented and intuitive biochemical savant, well suited to the task. That he happened to be available to join the insulin team was a great stroke of luck. By December 1921 he should have moved on from Toronto to begin the next part of his Rockefeller Traveling Fellowship in London or New York. Instead, he quarantined himself in his lab in the pathology building on the grounds of the Toronto General Hospital and worked around the clock, pushing himself to his limits. Acutely aware of the enormous significance of his assignment, he had decided to forego the rest of the fellowship and remain in Toronto for the duration.

At this time, Collip was working very closely with Macleod, which was another reason for his decision to remain in Toronto. The two professors met for lunch nearly every day. The work made fast and significant progress. A diabetic Airedale injected with Collip's extract passed sugar-free urine.

Collip used rabbits to assay the potency of the extract. He determined that one unit would be the amount sufficient to send a rabbit into convulsions, hypoglycemic coma, and death. This proved to be an expensive method. With rabbits billed to the Department of Physiology at $1.25 each, Collip was going through rabbits at an alarming rate. It was Macleod, observing Clark Noble drawing blood from the rabbits for blood sugar analysis, who first suggested that they might restore comatose rabbits with glucose, thereby preserving the subject for further testing.

In addition to their officially assigned roles, Banting and Best continued to experiment with whole-pancreas extract and fetal calf pancreas extract as well as various methods of preparation. They adopted methods that Collip had worked out, such as the use of a vacuum still. They tried different ways of administering the extract, including through a stomach tube. They even injected dogs with extracts of liver, spleen, thyroid, and thymus; none but the pancreatic extract lowered blood sugar. For the first time, they began to experiment on normal dogs, perhaps because they were running out of diabetic subjects and time to prepare them. Banting and Best turned what was supposed to be a collaboration into a competition. They were determined to purify the extract before Collip did, which only served to infuriate Collip.

On December 20, 1921, Banting's old friend and colleague Dr. Joe Gilchrist became the first human diabetic to receive insulin. Banting had hoped that this historic moment would allow him to make a dramatic announcement at the conference, an announcement that he would not tell Macleod about beforehand. Because the extract was not pure enough for injection into a human being, Joe was given an oral dose. There was no benefit.

Now that most of the work was in the hands of the chemists, Banting began to feel tangential and insecure. All around him people were merrily preparing for the holidays with wives and sweethearts. Charley would go home to Maine and Margaret. Collip would celebrate with his wife, Ray, and their young family. Jake and Mary Macleod would celebrate in their cozy, comfortable English country-style home in the Rosedale section of Toronto.

Banting isolated himself in his bivouac in the boardinghouse and glared through the soot streaks on the window at the happy shoppers on the street below. He dreaded returning to his family in Alliston, from whom he felt increasingly estranged. There, he knew, he would face the inevitable questions, questions for which he had no answers. They would be the questions of farmers, steeped in the practicalities of financial and physical survival from harvest to harvest.

Banting's life made no sense to them. How could it? He was thirty years old, unattached, and only marginally employed. He had given up everything to pursue an idea the merit of which few seemed to recognize—until now. Now that others finally saw the potential, he felt like they were elbowing him out of the way in order to take credit for the idea. He made his apologies to his family and remained in Toronto, ostensibly to prepare for what would be his first public presentation of a scientific paper. In reality, he did little more than take long cold walks on the abandoned campus. In the afternoon he often found himself at the Christie Street Hospital, visiting with the veterans, or at the lab with his devoted companion, Marjorie, who on Christmas Day had lived for thirty-seven days without a pancreas.

Just when he thought his circumstances could not possibly get worse, they did.

★ ★ ★

Once he reached New Haven, Banting's sense of isolation grew more acute. The American Physiological Society in 1921 was an exclusive group of three hundred eminent men, nearly all of whom knew one another. From a distance Banting observed with disgust the groups of distinguished scientific luminaries tripping over themselves to shake Macleod's hand. A few times he overheard them telling him how much they were looking forward to "his" presentation—and he noted that Macleod did not hasten to correct them. Among those whom Macleod sought out at the conference was Alec Clowes. He was particularly interested in his fellow Briton's work at the Lilly marine biological laboratory Woods Hole. Banting had yet to recognize a single familiar face among the attendees; Charley was to arrive later, coming directly from Maine.

The conference began on Wednesday, December 28. Banting attended the lectures and presentations, hoping to gain some insights into how to make the best show of his own presentation. He loathed public speaking, and as the dreaded hour drew closer, Banting's anxiety grew until he began to have second thoughts about the whole idea. He sat in on a talk by N. B. Taylor from Toronto, who had been present at Banting's talk to the Canadian Journal Club. He also listened to two papers by Ernest L. Scott. Not only had Scott ligated the pancreatic ducts of dogs as part of his master's degree at Columbia University, he had also used alcohol to extract insulin from the whole pancreas, a procedure that had recently been adopted at the University of Toronto. Although Scott himself believed he had discovered insulin, his results were not easily replicated. His 1912 article described his work in such cautious terms that the significance of his findings was not recognized. Scott ultimately abandoned the work, and his presentation that December addressed an entirely different subject.

What everyone really came to New Haven to hear that December was the paper on pancreatic extract by Jake Macleod and his associates, which the conference planners made sure to schedule for the afternoon of the final day of the conference so that no one would leave early. When the fateful Friday came, the room was packed with a discerning audience of scientific experts, including Frederick Allen, Elliott Joslin, Alec

Clowes, Israel Kleiner, Anton Carlson, and Ernest L. Scott. The slightest flaw in the experimental work would be noted by these men.

As neither Banting nor Best was a member of the American Physiological Society, Macleod began by introducing them and describing the work they had done over the summer. Macleod, having observed Banting's mounting trepidation, provided a rather thorough description of the experiments in case Banting proved unable to do so. Banting noticed that Macleod repeatedly used the word "we" in describing the work. Banting's neck turned red with rage as he reflected on the long weeks in July and August when he had labored alone, hungry, and desperate, in the stench of the lab. Lost in these bitter ruminations he did not hear Macleod invite him to the podium.

"Dr. Banting?" Macleod repeated his invitation, gestured to the podium and stepped aside.

Banting rose and crossed to where Macleod had stood. As he turned to the distinguished crowd, he gripped the podium with such intensity that his knuckles turned white.

He commenced haltingly, managing to say that on that very day, December 30, 1920, there was a dog in Toronto who had lived without a pancreas for an unprecedented forty-two days by being given daily injections of pancreatic extract. The goal now was to prepare a refined extract suitable for human use. As Banting continued, his face grew redder and his voice grew quieter, until he was muttering. Those in the back of the room could not hear him at all. He concluded by saying that his colleague, Charles Best, had prepared some charts and graphs that illustrated their work. Then he crossed to the empty chair beside Charley and sat down.

It was not clear to the audience whether Banting intended to retrieve the charts and graphs and continue or was finished speaking, so no one clapped. Banting looked at his feet. Charley looked at Macleod. Macleod cleared his throat and went to the podium. The presentation had ended early. There was still quite a bit of time before the next presentation began.

"Thank you, Dr. Banting," Macleod said authoritatively, rescuing the room from awkward silence. There was brief applause before everyone stood up and moved en masse toward Macleod, some to question his data and others to offer cautious congratulations. Scott was among the first to reach him. He wanted to be sure that Macleod knew he had performed essentially the identical experiment as they had in Toronto with mixed results. Allen, who had come to the meeting in part to recruit contributors to his scientific periodical *Journal of Metabolic Research,* buttonholed Macleod and invited him to be a contributing editor in the upcoming issue. Each issue compiled the research writing of a large and impressive list of scientific investigators. The names of Banting, Carlson, Clowes, Macleod, Murlin, Paullin, and Woodyatt would appear at various times on the masthead. As he waited for his turn to talk with Macleod, Allen thought of Elizabeth Hughes. How right he was to dissuade Antoinette from sending her to Bermuda. Now, vindicated at last, he could go to her with concrete evidence that a breakthrough *had* come and that he had personally shaken the discoverer's hand.

While the crowd continued to shuffle around Macleod, Clowes approached Banting and Best, who remained seated to the side of the podium, alone and bewildered. He extended his hand, smiling down at Fred Banting.

"Well done, Dr. Banting. Well done." he said in a clipped, upper class British accent. "Thank you for sparing us a long academic review of previously published experiments when we all know that the only thing that matters is what progress we can make from here forward."

Banting blinked and looked questioningly into the piercing blue eyes of Alec Clowes.

"Alec Clowes. Eli Lilly and Company." He spoke in a booming voice.

Clowes held out a business card to Banting. Banting took it and said, "I'm very impressed with your card, Dr. Clowes. I regret that I don't have one to offer you in return. Anyway, it's not just my work. It's Charley's work, too."

Best jumped to his feet and shook Clowes's hand. Clowes handed him a business card.

"As I see it, the challenge ahead is to scale up production. Agreed?"

Banting nodded.

"Then I intend to recommend that Mr. Lilly provide full support for that effort: funding, purification, dosage, manufacturing, marketing, the works. You're going to need it. This will take corporate horsepower.

If you leave a discovery this important in an academic setting, you'll spend too much time in committees and conferences and not enough time saving diabetics. You'll hear from me again soon." And then he was gone.

Later, Clowes left a note for Macleod at his hotel to the effect that Eli Lilly and Company would like to assist in the effort to produce a pharmaceutical-grade product. As much as Macleod respected Clowes, he was suspicious of commercial interests, particularly that of an American corporation. Besides, the university had the resources to manufacture insulin without help from south of the border. Macleod promptly scribbled a reply on the back of the note: "Many thanks for your interest and generosity but the University of Toronto is equipped with a commercial manufacturing facility—Connaught Laboratories."

Macleod was referring to the unique medical research and public service enterprise affiliated with the University of Toronto. It had begun years before in the basement and subbasement of the same building in which Banting and Best made their discovery. It had been established to prepare a Canadian supply of diphtheria antitoxin for free distribution through provincial health departments. It was the brainchild of Department of Hygiene professor John G. FitzGerald. A global tetanus antitoxin shortage in 1915 during the height of the war prompted the expansion and relocation of Connaught to a fifty-eight-acre farm site twelve miles northwest of the campus. Macleod had thought all along that, when the time was right, Connaught could be tapped to launch the large-volume production of insulin. He had already discussed this with President Falconer, who heartily endorsed the idea of claiming credit and control of the development and manufacture for the University of Toronto.

Macleod remained in New Haven for a few days on American Physiological Society business. He spent the evening after the presentation dining at a fine steak house with his fellow APS officers, oblivious to any ill feelings toward him from Banting. As far as he knew, all was proceeding splendidly, and the meeting had been a tremendous success.

Banting and Best left that night. They couldn't afford to stay another night in New Haven, financially or emotionally. They had reserved a sleeping car on the overnight train back to Toronto, but Banting never even folded down his berth. He stayed up all night in the smoking car, reflecting on what seemed to him yet another humiliation at the hands of his nemesis.

"They're all vultures and vipers," Banting muttered as he and Best settled into their seats. "I tell you one thing Charley. If I'm going down, you can be sure I'm taking Macleod with me."

"Going down? You just discovered insulin!" Charley erupted in a rare display of emotion. "Aren't you always telling me this is the biggest medical breakthrough since Pasteur discovered the rabies virus?"

"Bigger than that, Charley. A lot more people get diabetes than get rabies."

"Well?"

"Sure, sure, but now that I've served my purpose and the semester is over, Macleod is hoping I'll just shuffle quietly back to Alliston to milk cows."

"But you have Henderson's position in pharmacology. Your name is on every publication. By the time we get back, Collip may have a pure enough extract for human trial. And let's see what this fellow from Eli Lilly can do."

"Forget him. He's a friend of Macleod's. I saw them talking in the lobby of the hotel."

"It's too bad you feel that way, Fred, because he seems to believe in you."

"No one believes in me but me. Not my family, not Edith, not Macleod. From now on, it's war, Charley. And that's one subject I daresay I know more about than Macleod."

Charley retreated to the sleeper, worrying about how he could possibly avoid being sliced to ribbons in the crossfire between the two main influences in his academic career.

Back when Clowes had worked in Buffalo, he studied the natural repellency between oil and water. It would be the best preparation Clowes could have undertaken for his future dealings with Jake Macleod and Fred Banting.

Not the slightest bit discouraged by Macleod's initial rejection of Eli Lilly's assistance, Clowes walked briskly to the nearest Western Union office and wired Lilly a three-word report on the APS meeting: "This is it."

TWENTY-ONE

Success and Failure, The University of Toronto, January 1922

AFTER BANTING AND BEST RETURNED FROM THE AMERICAN PHYS-iological Society meeting, their race with Collip intensified. As the reality of a human trial became more plausible, Duncan Graham discussed the practicalities with Macleod. Graham was the recently appointed Eaton Professor of Medicine at the University of Toronto with jurisdiction over the teaching wards of Toronto General Hospital. It was decided that Collip, as the best biochemist, would supply the purified extract. Since neither Macleod nor Collip was a practicing clinician, Dr. Walter Campbell was chosen to oversee the clinical administration of the trial, under the direction of Graham. The test would take place in Ward H, the diabetic clinic of Toronto General Hospital. Graham occasionally dropped by Collip's lab on the top floor of the pathology building to check on his progress and then joined Macleod and Collip for lunch.

When Banting caught wind of this plan he was predictably furious. He had assumed he would be the one to administer the first clinical test. After all, it was his idea, and the clinical application had been his focus from the start. But Duncan Graham would not allow it. Banting had never treated a human diabetic. Further, he had no affiliation with Toronto General Hospital and only a temporary affiliation with the university.

Banting stormed into Macleod's office and demanded that Graham use his and Best's extract rather than Collip's for the first human trial and that Banting himself administer it. Macleod argued that where human life was at stake, precedence was irrelevant. He tried to persuade Banting that everyone on the team would benefit from a successful trial. But Banting bellowed that for these very reasons his extract should be used—the extract that had kept the dog Marjorie alive for two months, the only extract that had been proven safe and effective over time. Macleod was grateful for the enormous desk between him and Banting. He wondered what his secretary, sitting just outside the door, must be thinking. He told Banting he would consider it.

Although it galled him to do so, Macleod tried to persuade his good friend Duncan Graham to acquiesce to Banting's wishes, just to keep the peace. Graham insisted that Dr. Campbell administer the human trial. Furthermore, neither Banting nor Best would be granted hospital privileges as long as he was in charge. However, as a personal favor to Macleod, Graham reluctantly agreed to use Banting and Best's extract, despite its being less pure than what Collip could prepare. Macleod was so mortified by this turn of events and his role in them that he couldn't bring himself to talk to Collip before the trial began.

Amid this high drama and posturing, a listless, slack-jawed fourteen-year-old, sixty-five-pound diabetic boy was admitted as a charity case to Toronto General Hospital on December 2, 1921. Leonard Thompson had been the patient of Dr. Campbell, who, recognizing that the boy was now entering the final, fatal stage of juvenile diabetes, asked Graham for help. Leonard was so weak and wasted that his father carried him into Graham's office. He had lost most of his hair, and his stomach was grotesquely distended. His breath smelled of acetone. His blood sugar ranged from 3.5 to 5.6 milligrams per cubic centimeter versus the normal range of 1 mg per cc. He was immediately placed on a severely restricted diet of 450 calories, but he continued to fail, spiraling into the pitiless and irrevocable pattern that Dr. Campbell had witnessed many times before. Dr. Campbell was compelled to tell Mr. Thompson that, barring a miracle, there was no hope.

On January 11, Dr. Ed Jeffrey, an intern under Dr. Campbell's supervision carefully sharpened a 26-gauge steel needle on a whetstone. Then he assembled the syringe by screwing the needle into the glass barrel. Finally, he drew the opaque, brown extract into the barrel and entered the room where Leonard Thompson lay. Dr. Jeffrey injected the boy with 15 cc of extract—7.5 cc into each buttock. This was roughly half the dose that a dog of equal weight would get. On Thompson's hospital chart, the medication administered was recorded as "Macleod's serum." The result was inconclusive: There was a modest lowering of blood sugar and the formation of large abscesses at the injection sites.

When Collip learned of the reversal of the established plan, he considered it a personal betrayal by Macleod. Meanwhile, Banting told everyone that the trial had failed because the quantity was insufficient. Banting voiced his tale of injustice and tribulation loudly and without discrimination to whomever he could trap long enough to listen. With each telling he became more convinced of his own maltreatment at the hands of Macleod. Unwisely, he confided his views to Duncan Graham, who was alarmed to discover just how unhinged Banting really was. He immediately reported the conversation to Macleod, encouraging him to terminate Banting's appointment right away and put as much distance as possible between Banting and the university. But how?

Unfortunately for Macleod, it was impossible to dismiss Banting. His constant caterwauling about his relegation to the status of a bystander had begun to win some sympathizers. Velyien Henderson was Banting's primary confidant, and Henderson's own personal dislike of Macleod influenced his perspective on Banting's situation. There was Banting's cousin Fred Hipwell who was predisposed to favor Banting's point of view. There was his old University of Toronto classmate Joe Gilchrist and his former instructor Dr. George W. Ross, better known as Billy Ross.

Dr. Billy Ross was the son of the Honorable Sir George William Ross, who had been until recently the Liberal premier of Ontario. As such, Dr. Ross was extremely well connected and not in the least bit shy about plying that influence to achieve a personal or political agenda. He was also a passionate nationalist. Ever since the decisive battle at Vimy Ridge, in 1917, which the Canadians had won for the Allied forces, there had been a renewed push for a unified and independent Canadian identity, separate and distinct from the British Crown. Vimy intensified the Canadian desire for political self-government that began with the Constitution Act in 1867 and culminated first in the Statute of Westminster in 1931, which granted Canada (and other commonwealth realms) legislative autonomy, and later affirmed in the Canada Act of 1982 which definitively dissolved legislative dependence on the United Kingdom. In Frederick Banting, Billy Ross saw an opportunity for Canadian glory and distinction. To Ross's mind, Banting's subjection at the hands of Macleod was emblematic of Canada's subjection to the British Crown, and he was eager to take up the cause of his defense.

One of Ross's patients was a young reporter for the *Toronto Daily Star* named Roy Greenaway. Seeing an opportunity, Ross mentioned to Greenaway Banting's tale of woe and its latest manifestation of the disappointing clinical trial, making sure to emphasize Banting's perspective. Now Greenaway had a scoop and an underdog hero.

In short order Greenaway made his way to the Physiology Building where he found Charley Best working alone. Best was amused to see Greenaway recoil at the odor of decaying offal and dog feces that permeated the laboratory.

"Not your brand of cologne?" he joked.

Charley, ever politically cautious, walked Greenaway over to Macleod's office. Greenaway, seeing the story as his big break, was eager to talk with anyone and everyone connected with the story. Macleod was appalled at the idea of the popular press prematurely releasing information about their experiments. As if his professional life wasn't complicated enough, he could hardly imagine the deluge of trouble that such a news release might bring down upon the university. He warned Greenaway that the only successful experiments had been performed on animals and that it would be irresponsible, even unconscionable, for Greenaway to suggest otherwise. He was reluctant even to say this much for fear of bringing a picket of antivivisectionists to the campus.

"Medical progress is a slow process," he advised sternly. "All I can say is that since the summer we have been working with a pancreatic extract that appears to show some promise in alleviating the symptoms of diabetes in animals. To raise people's hopes that a cure is at hand would be a cruel and self-serving exercise."

The article appeared in the *Toronto Daily Star* on January 14 under the headline:

WORK ON DIABETES SHOWS PROGRESS
AGAINST DISEASE
Toronto Medical Men Hoping That
Cure Is Close at Hand

A Boy Is Treated

Effect of First Treatment Is So Good That
Injections Are Continued

For the most part Greenaway had honored Macleod's advice, and the language was considerably more subdued than what he had originally planned. Macleod and Banting were the only two directly quoted.

Banting read the article and focused on just two words—"we" and "our"—both of which were used by Macleod to describe the eight months of experiments. Banting's ire rose as he remembered the summer months when Macleod was vacationing in Scotland. It did not occur to him that Macleod might be protecting him, protecting the interests of the university, and even protecting the work itself.

In Indianapolis, Eli Lilly and Alec Clowes read the article and together marched into J.K. Sr.'s office to read it to him. J.K. instructed Clowes to do whatever he had to do to secure a role for the company in the development of insulin.

Between January and April Clowes made four trips to Toronto. He usually met with Macleod and rarely spoke with Banting. President Falconer urged Macleod to "keep it Canadian" and so Macleod painted a bright picture of the team and the process for Clowes, constantly reassuring him that they were getting along just fine without help from Indianapolis.

The reality was quite different. It was increasingly difficult for Macleod to take himself to the office in the morning. Mary watched helplessly as her husband became brittle and withdrawn, and the dark days in Cleveland seemed to be beginning all over again in Toronto. His health began to deteriorate. His joints were stiffening with arthritic pain, and he rarely felt well enough to golf. One morning as Macleod lingered at the breakfast table with Mary for an especially long time, he muttered that he felt he should take a chair and a whip to work like a lion tamer.

That morning he and Mary quietly decided to look toward moving back to their beloved Scotland.

On the night of January 16 Collip was working in his lonely aerie, conjuring batch after batch of extract at a pulse-accelerating pace. He no longer paused to make notes about his process. It was as if he had entered into the process, become a part of it. His mind and body were directed by an unseen force, perhaps the will of the extract itself to be discovered.

He was performing a series of methodical tasks called fractionation. He mixed whole, macerated pancreas with increasing amounts of alcohol and centrifuged each incrementally concentrated mixture to precipitate out all the impurities that were not soluble in that percentage of alcohol. For example, Collip would mix pancreas with alcohol to a 30 percent concentration, place it in a test tube and spin the tube in a centrifuge. Thirty or so minutes later, the centrifuge would stop spinning. Inside the tube he would find a pellet of insoluble proteins or impurities and the supernatant liquid. He would discard the pellet and dilute the liquid with alcohol until it reached a 40 percent concentration. Then he would place a test tube containing this mixture into the centrifuge and repeat the process. When the spinning stopped he would have a pellet of proteins insoluble in alcohol of 40 percent concentration. Again he would dilute the supernatant liquid with alcohol incrementally increasing the concentration to 50, 60, 70, and 80 percent.

When he reached 90 percent, Collip discovered that the active principle of the extract was insoluble in a 90 percent alcohol solution. In other words, when the centrifuge stopped spinning on the test tube of 90 percent alcohol solution, Collip had trapped the active principle—the insulin—in the pellet. Moreover, the insulin was in a relatively pure state, as most of the impurities had been precipitated out through the fractionation process. This he would later confirm through rabbit assay tests. Years later Collip would say, "I experienced then and there all alone on the top floor of the old pathology building perhaps the greatest thrill it has ever been given me to realize."

Sometime within the following days, Collip went to the second floor of the Physiology Building to tell Charley Best the news. There he found both Banting and Best in the lab. He told them that he had purified the extract but wouldn't tell them how he'd done it. His refusal to reveal his secret—whatever his reasons—sent Banting into a rage. According to *Time* magazine in 1941, "Banting leaped on Collip in the university halls, threw him down, banged his head on the floor and bellowed: *So, you will call this Collip's serum will you?*" Charley grabbed Fred by the neck and struggled to pull him off. As soon as Collip could scramble free of Banting's grip, he stood up and stormed out of the building without a word.

The next day Collip went directly to Macleod to report the incident. Macleod went to speak to Falconer, for now he would certainly have Falconer's support for ejecting Banting. But instead of finding an ally, he ran headlong into a barrage of blame. Falconer held Macleod responsible for the dysfunction of the department and the disgrace to the university.

"Collip will return to Alberta in a few months," he said. "What do you think he will say of his time here?"

Macleod was too stunned to respond.

Falconer suggested that Macleod call a meeting and try to work things out, and he recommended that Macleod ask someone *else* to run the meeting, someone who had the authority to control the situation. Falconer proposed Dr. FitzGerald of the Connaught Antitoxin Laboratories. Macleod swallowed his pride and asked FitzGerald to help mediate the personal tensions that had arisen among the discovery team. FitzGerald agreed and also offered to help with the larger-scale production methods and costs of preparing the new extract for clinical trial. The meeting was set for January 25, a Wednesday.

During all this tumult, the science somehow managed to continue, on two tracks—research and clinical. On January 21, Banting and Best discontinued the dog Marjorie's injections in order to reserve their extract for another chance at a human trial. Predictably, their affectionate laboratory mascot began to weaken and fail.

On Monday, January 23, at eleven o'clock in the morning, Dr. Walter Campbell gave Leonard Thompson his second insulin injection—5 cc of Collip's extract. Six hours later, the boy received another injection of 20 cc of Collip's extract. The following day there were two injections of 10 cc each. Thompson's glycosuria nearly disappeared. His blood sugar plummeted from 5.2 milligrams to 1.2 milligrams per cc. It was nothing short of miraculous.

By this time, Marjorie could hardly stand. Unable to watch her deteriorate further, Banting injected Marjorie with some of the precious remaining extract. She immediately rebounded and was her old affectionate self again, following him around the lab and willingly subjecting herself to blood draws.

On January 25, Banting, Best, Collip, Macleod, FitzGerald, and Falconer assembled for the meeting. Collip's face bore the plum-colored vestige of a black eye. Banting arrived unshaven and dressed in a crumpled wool jacket, his ungloved hands raw from the cold. His trousers were riddled with burn holes from cigarette ashes. Until this meeting, the true extent of Banting's mental disintegration had not been apparent to anyone but Charley Best.

Banting accused Macleod of trying to steal credit for his discovery, using the example that the extract was listed on Thompson's chart, the document of historical record, as "Macleod's serum." With a cold, sickening dread, Macleod wondered how Banting could have known that detail except through Graham.

"Perhaps it has nothing to do with credit. Perhaps it has to do with blame," FitzGerald offered quietly. "If Thompson had died, someone would have to take responsibility; someone with official standing at the University. I doubt Graham would have allowed your name to go on the chart. It's not that you aren't deserving; it's that you can't answer for the university in case of failure. If anything, Macleod put his name on the record to protect you. Am I right, Professor Macleod?"

Macleod nodded stiffly.

Neither Macleod nor Falconer would say more than a few words during the meeting; Falconer because he wouldn't, and Macleod because he couldn't. Anything Macleod might have said would be misconstrued as a slight against the myopic Banting. He had been effectively silenced.

There were several results of the meeting. The most concrete was a document, signed by Banting, Best, Collip, and Macleod. It bore the rather unwieldy title of "Memorandum in Reference to the Co-operation of the Connaught Antitoxin Laboratories in the Researches of Dr. Banting, Mr. Best, and Dr. Collip—Under the General Direction of Professor J. J. R. Macleod to Obtain an Extract of Pancreas Having a Specific

Effect on the Blood Sugar Concentration." There were two key points. The first was that during the period in which the discovery team would be cooperating with Connaught, neither Banting, Best, nor Collip would endeavor to obtain a patent or seek a partnership with a commercial firm to produce or exploit the extract product or the process by which it was made. The second point was that any modification in this policy could not be made without prior consultation among Banting, Best, Collip, Macleod, and FitzGerald. Around this time it was also agreed that going forward, the names on all research papers would appear in alphabetic order: Banting, Best, Collip, Macleod.

While Collip returned to the lab to make more extract on January 25 and 26, Leonard Thompson did not receive any extract, but injections resumed on the 27, as did his steady recovery. He was more alert and animated. His blood sugar continued to show suppressed values. Best of all, as Collip's batches became more pure and potent, Leonard Thompson's daily dose was reduced to two injections of 4 cc per day.

All appeared to be back on track with Collip's serum producing good results at Toronto General Hospital and Best working closely with FitzGerald at Connaught to make the extract in high volume. But Banting continued to feel sidelined. He was more desperate than ever to secure some way to indelibly document his rights and primacy as the idea's originator.

He came to see Marjorie as his answer. She had survived for seventy days without a pancreas—longer than any living creature. The fact that daily doses of the extract had sustained her was clear evidence that Banting and Best had produced effective, nontoxic pancreatic extract.

On January 27, Banting went to the lab early in the morning, alone. He opened Marjorie's cage and cut her a slice of the raw pancreas that he had stored on ice. Then he pretended to busy himself in the lab. She stayed close at his heels, nearby but never underfoot. Whenever he glanced down in her direction she wagged her tail. He tried not to let her see the tears in his eyes. He picked her up and placed her gently on the table. He was careful to avoid her abscesses; she never complained. He stroked her speckled fur and she looked back at him with an uncanny understanding of what was about to happen. He wiped his nose on the sleeve of his lab coat.

He asked her to sit and then lie down. She obeyed as she always had, and for the last time. As Banting administered a fatal dose of chloroform he spoke softly to her, thanking her for her loyalty and kindness, her bravery and generosity. He apologized for all the pain that she had endured and for the unhappy fact of her final sacrifice. He promised her that her death would not be in vain, that he would redeem it with the lives of children, and that each child he saved would know her name. When he was sure that she was gone he wrapped her in a blanket and carried her across the campus to Toronto General Hospital. He hugged her body to his chest, even as he felt the warmth leaving her. He bowed his head into her soft fur to blot his tears. It seemed to him that the dogs were the only civilized creatures on the insulin discovery team and the humans treated them more humanely than they treated each other. Now he had killed the best of the best. How much more sacrifice could possibly be required to bring this inkling of an idea into practical use?

He would soon have an answer. Macleod had always questioned whether Marjorie's pancreas had been completely removed. In order to dispel these doubts Banting had arranged for a disinterested pathologist at Toronto General Hospital to perform an autopsy. Banting delivered Marjorie's body to Dr. W. L. Robinson.

Later that day Banting was to learn, much to his disbelief and distress, that Robinson had found that Marjorie did indeed still have a small nodule of pancreatic tissue, about three millimeters in diameter, under the lining of her duodenum. Although he found no islet cells in it, the presence of the nodule was enough to cause skepticism about the conclusiveness of Banting and Best's most successful longevity experiment.

Banting was now utterly crushed.

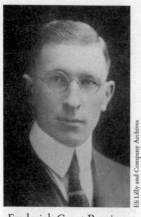

Frederick Grant Banting

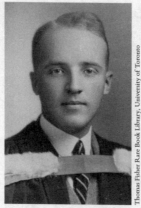

Charles Herbert Best

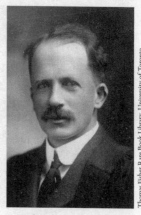

John James Rickard Macleod

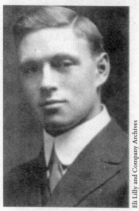

James Bertram Collip

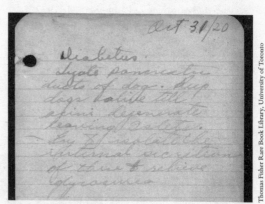

Banting's note after reading Moses Barron's article, October 31, 1920.

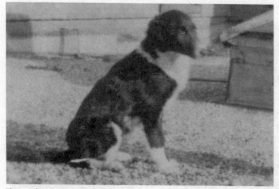

Dog 33, "Marjorie," on roof of Medical Building, circa November 1921.

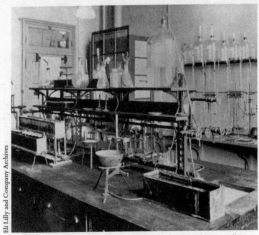

University of Toronto lab where Banting and Best carried out their research in 1921–1922.

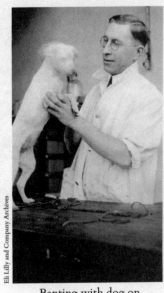

Banting with dog on operating table, 1923.

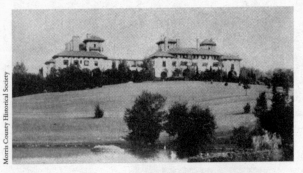

The Physiatric Institute. View of main building from second hole of golf course.

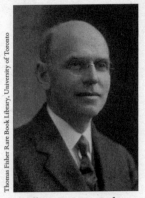

Elliott Proctor Joslin

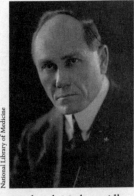

Frederick Madison Allen

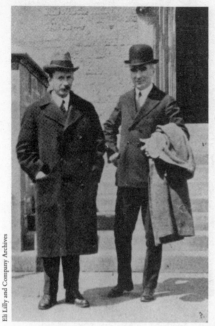

Macleod and Clowes, 1922

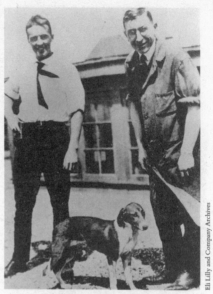

Best and Banting on roof of Medical
Building at the University of Toronto,
August 1921.

The Hughes family, 1916.
From left: C. E. Hughes, Elizabeth,
Catherine, Helen, Antoinette.

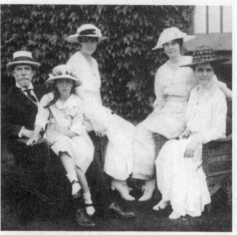

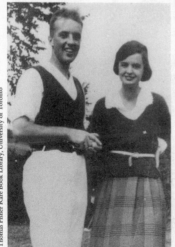

Charles Best and his fiancée,
Margaret Mahon, 1921.

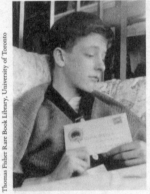

G. H. A. Clowes, 1926

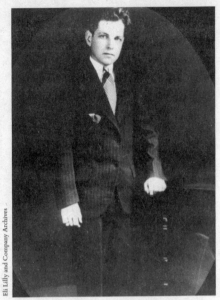

Leonard Thompson, the first patient
successfully treated with insulin,
in Canada.

James Havens, the first
patient successfully
treated with insulin,
in the United States.

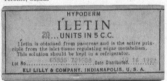

Bottle of I'letin® in cardboard
box, Eli Lilly and Company,
October 16, 1922.

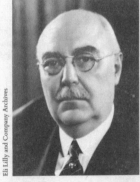

J. K. Lilly Sr., circa 1932

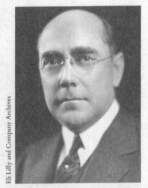

Eli Lilly, circa 1934

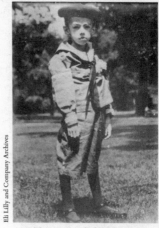

Teddy Ryder before insulin.

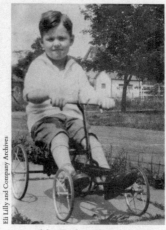

Teddy Ryder after insulin.

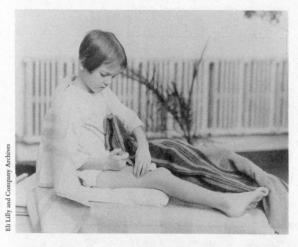

Girl injecting herself
with insulin, 1930.

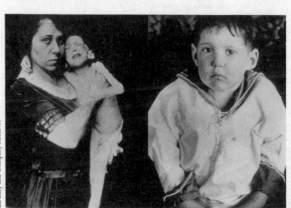

Diabetic child
identified only
as "J.L." before
and after insulin.

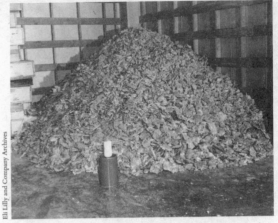

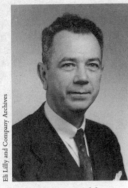

Ten thousand pounds of pancreases needed to make one pound of insulin crystals (foreground), 1951.

George Walden

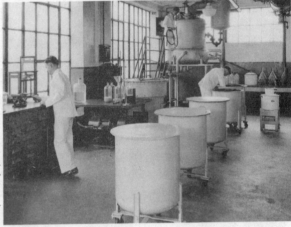

Purification by isoelectric precipitation, 1923.

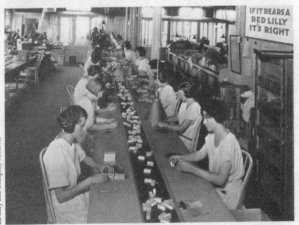

IF IT BEARS A RED LILLY IT'S RIGHT

Insulin finishing line, 1923.

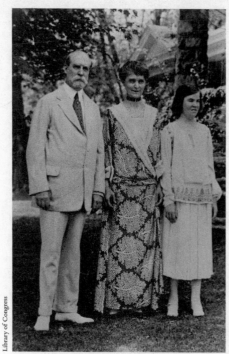

Elizabeth with her parents,
dated between 1917 and 1925.

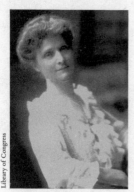

Antoinette Hughes,
1916

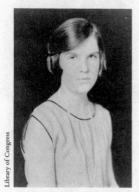

Elizabeth Hughes,
circa 1924

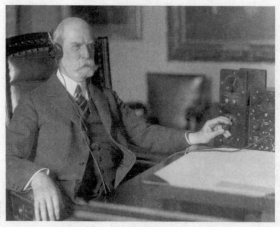

Charles Evans Hughes
with wireless radio
phone, 1922.

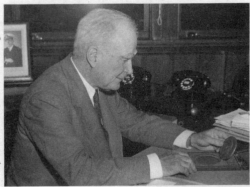

Grinding glands for insulin, 1923.

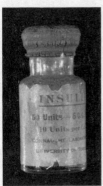

Bottle of insulin, Connaught Medical Research Laboratories, November 5, 1923.

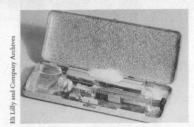

Early insulin kit, 1920s.

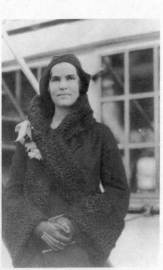

G. H. A. Clowes with Banting Medal, 1947.

Elizabeth Hughes on December 22, 1930, shortly after her marriage to William T. Gossett.

TWENTY-TWO

Failure and Success, The University of Toronto,
February to April 1922

At Toronto General Hospital, Doctors Walter Campbell and Almon Fletcher admitted six more patients to Ward H and treated them with Collip's extract. Every one of them improved. One of these patients was an emaciated girl, a friend of Charley Best from a Toronto suburb. Within hours of receiving insulin she became herself again—a happy, playful child. Instead of being pleased, Banting could not help but resent that it was Collip's extract that had helped Best's friend.

The fact that he had lost the humanity to feel happy for a little girl's life sent him into a sickening spiral of self-recrimination. In February, Banting began to drink heavily, stealing the 95 percent pure ethyl alcohol from the lab. He plunged into an emotional vertigo that he felt he could not survive. He was like the poor chap he'd encountered in England when he was waiting for his arm to heal. Shell shock, they'd called it. Like that soldier, Banting had caught a glimpse of the indifference and injustice of the universe, and now that he had seen it, he could not *unsee* it. Best could do nothing to pry Banting from his crippling malaise.

Later in February, a paper authored by Banting and Best was published in the *Journal of Laboratory and Clinical Medicine*, and another authored by Banting, Best, Collip, Campbell, and Fletcher was submitted to the *Canadian Medical Association Journal*. But Banting's participation in these efforts was minimal. His heart was no longer in it.

Just as the light of hope was dawning on the world, the original spark began to gutter and fade. Banting spent the entire month of March in an inebriated stupor, ignoring telegrams and phone calls and hardly venturing to campus. The pages of his diary suggest that he had begun to read and think about other research projects; there are several vague notes about potential cures for cancer. Reflecting on this time some years later, Banting admitted that there was not a single night during the month of March that he went to bed sober.

Banting had retreated, but others continued to work on his behalf. Billy Ross continued to talk to Roy Greenaway, and on March 22, the first major press coverage of a "diabetes cure" appeared in the *Toronto Daily Star*. The article spanned seven columns under a dramatic headline:

TORONTO DOCTORS ON TRACK OF
DIABETES CURE
Diabetes Sufferers Given Message of Hope
Banting Stakes His All on the Result

On the same day the *Canadian Medical Association Journal* published "Pancreatic Extracts in the Treatment of Diabetes Mellitus" by Banting, Best, Collip, Campbell, and Fletcher. Banting probably hardly registered either publication. Not only was he not writing the papers, he wasn't reading them either.

Collip inexplicably lost his ability to produce the extract in March. Suddenly, there was no more insulin to give to the six patients at Toronto General Hospital. Working independently, Best and Collip strove to produce even an ounce of extract, but despite their frantic efforts Charley Best's young friend, who had made such a heartening recovery on Ward H, slipped into a coma and died. Unless they could recover their ability to make the extract, the same fate awaited all the patients on the Ward.

On the evening of March 31, Best broke. He visited Banting's boarding-house room and let loose his fury and frustration as he had never dared to before. He attacked Banting for allowing himself to languish in morbid self-pity when so many around him were working hard toward a solution. Banting drank stolen alcohol from a beaker and listened impassively.

"You said we'd do whatever it takes!" Charley howled.

Banting shrugged. "Changed my mind."

"It's too late to change your mind. You sold your house. You sold your car. We stole dogs!"

"It takes a brave man to know when to surrender." Banting raised his glass and drank to bravery while Charley watched in disbelief. "Collip's process worked. Ours didn't. Here's to the continued success and glory of James Bertram Collip! I salute you—you prig bastard."

"So he won the purification round. So what. We still have to find a way to make large quantities. Aren't you the one who's always reminding everyone that this is about the diabetics?"

"To the diabetics!" Banting raised the beaker, drained it, and threw it across the room. It shattered against the wall.

Charley reached into his book bag and pulled out a notebook.

"I went through all of our lab books and diaries and I've written out a precise description of our process. If we go over it together maybe we can see how to increase quantity without losing potency."

"I don't care."

"I'm going to read it anyway." Charley opened the notebook. Banting lay back on the bed and closed his eyes.

"Finely mince beef or pork pancreas. Add 5 cc's sulphuric acid per pound of gland. Stir this mixture for three to four hours. Add a solution of 95 percent alcohol until the overall concentration of alcohol is 60 to 70 percent. Centrifuge the mixture and filter through paper. Neutralize the filtrate with sodium hydroxide. Concentrate to one-fifteenth of original volume *in vacuo* and heat the concentrate to fifty degrees centigrade to separate the lipoids. Remove lipoids and other residue by further filtration. Add 37 grams of ammonium sulphate per 100 cc's of concentrate. Skim off protein material as it floats to the top of the liquid."

Banting interrupted. "This is pointless, you know."

"Then what do you suggest?"

"Well, my plan has been to get drunk and stay drunk long enough for an epiphany to bubble up from the subconscious."

"I almost think you're serious."

"I am. Join me?" Banting took a swig from the bottle of laboratory alcohol.

Charley looked on in disgust and continued reading.

"Mix it with hot acid alcohol until completely dissolved. Add 10 volumes of warm alcohol. Neutralize this solution with sodium hydroxide. Cool to room temperature. Store for two days at five degrees centigrade. After two days, pour off the dark-colored supernatant alcohol. Dry the precipitate to remove all traces of alcohol."

"Charley?"

"Yes?"

Now Banting spoke with a chilling calm.

"There is nothing you can say to make me stay in this. I'm through."

Charley took a cold, hard look at his friend and colleague. There was one thing that he could have said to make Banting change his mind, and somehow he said it.

"If you get out, I get out," Charley said.

"Don't be stupid!" Banting spat. "*Your* future is secure. Macleod will take care of you."

"He won't have to. I quit."

They glared at each other, but Banting was too drunk to sustain it and his eyes slid shut. After a few moments, Banting's breathing became deep and slow. Partly to see if he was asleep, Charley asked quietly, "What will you do now?" Without opening his eyes, Banting smiled.

"Paint, I think."

"Paint? Paint what?"

"Landscapes. Nature. Canada. I know a guy by the name of Jackson, a real artist, who wants to take a painting trip to the Canadian Rockies."

"So you'll give up research altogether?" Banting didn't answer. "I've never heard you mention painting. Are you any good?"

"Nope. But I'm no good at medical research either."

Charley looked down at the notebook still open on his lap. He scanned the remaining pages of notes that he had meticulously copied into the pages. Banting began to snore. Charley closed the notebook and placed it on the small table beside the bed. He stood up.

"Goodbye, Fred. I hope painting makes you happy." Charley left.

★ ★ ★

The next day Banting awoke to find Charley's notebook on his bedside table and slowly the events of the previous night came back to him. He cared little for his own future, but he could not allow Charley to scuttle his. He rebounded with a vengeance from his dark night of the soul. It was April 1: the beginning of a new month, the beginning of a new start.

Banting saw now that his retreat into depression and drink only helped prove that Macleod and Graham were right about him all along. In his wallow of misery he had not seen how his behavior had played directly into the hands of his detractors. But Charley had seen it. Many times over the past months Charley had tried to tell him, beginning with the train ride back from New Haven in December. Banting thought of the desperate times they had endured together the previous summer. And he thought of Marjorie and of her sacrifice, and of the promise he had made to her. He must repay loyalty with loyalty.

For months his friends and advisors had suggested that he establish a clinical practice. The fact that he was not a practicing physician and had never treated diabetics was Graham's primary justification for denying him a role in the human trials at Toronto General Hospital. But having been rejected by both Toronto General Hospital and the Hospital for Sick Children, how was he to acquire such clinical experience? Banting suddenly saw a simple solution to what had so recently seemed an intractable problem. He opened a private practice at 160 Bloor Street West to treat diabetics. His cousin and fellow doctor, Fred Hipwell, joined him in the practice.

In April, a representative of the Canadian government's Department of Soldiers Civil Re-Establishment came to Toronto to discuss how the department might be helpful in further developing insulin. It was decided that a diabetic clinic would be established at Toronto's Christie Street Military Hospital. The soldiers who had fought the Germans would now enlist to fight diabetes. Banting was to be in charge of the program. Banting's old friend and classmate Joe Gilchrist would have a role too.

By this time Charley Best had taken over as lead chemist on the team because Collip's appointment at the University of Toronto was to expire on May 31. While there had been some discussion about Collip's being invited to stay on, the enmity among the discoverers—and particularly the threat of physical violence from Banting—dampened his interest.

Banting's luck had changed abruptly. He now found that he had better facilities and potentially more access to insulin than anyone—except that there *was* no insulin. For several weeks, no one had been able to produce a single drop of effective extract. After weeks of frustration and failure, Toronto's resolve to keep the Americans out was weakening.

On April 3, Macleod wrote to Clowes:

> *We have not as yet succeeded in working out to our satisfaction all the steps necessary to prepare a non-toxic potent extract. . . . We are working intensively on this problem in the hope that in a month or two we may be able to publish our method in sufficient detail so that the extract can be prepared satisfactorily elsewhere.*

Banting's friends urged him to patent the insulin formulation and method of purification. Banting refused to have anything to do with the idea, feeling that it was in conflict with the Hippocratic oath, but he recognized the need to protect the discovery from unscrupulous opportunists. In April, Banting, Best, Collip, Macleod, and FitzGerald composed a joint letter to Falconer. The letter proposed that a patent be sought by Best and Collip, neither of whom had taken the Hippocratic oath, and that the rights then be assigned immediately to the board of governors of the University of Toronto in return for the sum of one dollar.

Even as insulin production faltered in Toronto and the enmity among the discovery team intensified, reports of extraordinary success in Toronto appeared in American newspapers. Many read like fairy tales. One story began: "So impressed with the feasibility of Dr. Banting's hypothesis was Professor J. J. R. Macleod, an investigator himself in this field of research for over 15 years, that every opportunity was given to the young doctor from London to push on [with] his experiments." Another described diabetic children frolicking in hospital wards, eating dates, and sipping tea with milk and sugar.

Dr. Frederick Allen read these articles with great interest. Here at last was the fulfillment of a promise that he had been making to his patients for years, entreating them to believe that a cure *would* come. Although he was originally cautious about trying insulin on his starvation-depleted patients, he would ultimately provide insulin to more patients than anyone during the first year of human trial. In 1922 a total of 161 patients would receive insulin through Dr. Frederick Allen.

Elizabeth Hughes would not be among them.

TWENTY-THREE

Honeymoon Cottage, Hamilton, Bermuda, January to July 1922

B Y THE TIME FREDERICK ALLEN RETURNED TO MORRISTOWN AND contacted Antoinette Hughes with the news of a cure, it was too late. Elizabeth and Blanche had sailed from New York City to Hamilton, Bermuda, on the *Fort Hamilton,* an oil-burning, steel twin-screw steamer. At 420 feet long and 50 feet wide, it was a small transatlantic liner with accommodations for 240 first-class passengers. They stayed in cabin number 18, which was comfortably situated in the middle of the ship, where the nausea-inducing motion would be minimal. Just in case, Blanche warded off possible seasickness with a preventive prescription of her own design: Epsom salts on the morning of the day before travel followed by two doses of calomel at bedtime.

It was an easy journey. Although Elizabeth was not in good health, she was in good spirits, cheered by the thought that with every mile she was leaving behind the potentially fatal threat of colds, influenza, and tonsillitis. Unknowingly, of course, she was also sailing away from the only hope for her survival.

In January, the temperature in Bermuda generally hovered in the sixties, with a brief tropical rainstorm in the afternoon, just to keep things interesting. Elizabeth and Blanche tried to venture out once a day, timing their outing to the predictable weather pattern. They often took a steamer rug and a picnic basket to a remote overlook and settled in for an afternoon of reading, napping, and watching white and brown pelicans wheel and dive over the broad blue water. On the island of Bermuda there was much to engage Elizabeth's active mind: unfamiliar flora, coral rock atolls, tropical sea gardens, and caves studded with stalactites and stalagmites. And even when they were at home in their cottage, which was built in 1653 by a "buccaneering captain," Elizabeth loved to daydream about the pirates and sailors of local legend.

Elizabeth set about trying to identify and catalogue the flora she encountered on her daily expeditions. Her letters to Mumsey were full of elaborate descriptions of oleander, loquat, royal poinciana, screw pine, paw-paw, cassava, and banana trees. She sometimes would tuck an oleander blossom into the envelope, hoping that the fragrance might last until her mother opened it. The avian life was especially fascinating to Elizabeth. After breakfast she loved to lie in the hammock and watch the cardinals chase the sparrows away from the seed cups she had arranged on the patio. How Eddie would have enjoyed these avian antics! She forced herself to forget about him, driving all thoughts of him, the canary, and the entire institute from her mind.

Her ambitions as an amateur naturalist were in conflict with the abundant social invitations proffered to the daughter of the U.S. secretary of state. Many of those extending the invitations were connected in some way to government or diplomatic service and were impossible to refuse. During the high season the entire social registry seemed to pass through the island in a steady stream. The arrival of these notable figures was such a regular event that crowds gathered at the dock in their white flannel suits and their gowns and hats to greet the arrival of the ocean liners the *Fort Hamilton* and the *Fort Victoria*. The more permanent residents included Governor General Sir James Willcocks and Lady Willcocks, Colonial Secretary H. M. M. Moore, Chief Justice Sir Colin Rees Davis, Vice Admiral Sir William Pakenham and Albert W. Swalm of the American Consulate.

Elizabeth reacted:

> *I didn't come to Bermuda to go to teas and go calling on your friends every minute and yet every day almost I get asked to tea . . . and although they're all sweet and all and I like to visit with them, still can't you imagine my position somewhat, and can't you see what a bore and nuisance it is, for I really ought to return their calls, I suppose? I thought*

after I'd seen them all once or twice it would be enough, but heavens they
keep on pestering the life out of me and I don't know what to do, for I
simply detest spending all these lovely aft[ernoons] dressing up and call-
ing on old ladies, pardon me, but they do seem old for a girl of 14 to keep
up with all the time.

When the social invitations revolved around a concert or a tour or a sail,
Elizabeth quite welcomed them, but she found the luncheons, dances,
and teas tedious and stressful. These affairs inevitably involved huge,
elaborate displays of food—dainty crustless sandwiches, berries with clot-
ted cream, tea with sugar—all of which was strictly off-limits. Her diet
was 45 grams of protein, 56 grams of fat, 12 grams of carbohydrates, for
a total of 750 calories for four days of the week, and then two days before her fast day the carbohydrates were reduced to ten grams.

At the luncheons what really tried her patience was the furtive and
pitying glances of those partaking in the sumptuous repast. And then
there was the banal ritual of polite questions, always the same ones:
How is your mother? How is your father? How is your sister? What do you think
of Chauncey? Will you be in the wedding? What is your brother doing now? Such
a terrible tragedy about Helen.

However, it was at one particularly tiresome luncheon in January
that she had the great good fortune of meeting Colonel Albert W. Swalm.
She was sitting at a table with an untouched plate of artfully prepared
food in front of her. Behind her she heard a booming voice.

"May I?"

Elizabeth turned to see a courtly, seventy-seven-year-old Civil War
veteran with a twinkle of mischief in his eye.

Elizabeth looked to Blanche, who was seated off to the side, ever
watchful of her charge. Blanche winked at Elizabeth, indicating the el-
derly gentleman posed no threat. So, assured, Elizabeth invited him to
join her at the table.

"Greetings and salutations, Mademoiselle!" He said, sitting down.
"I am Colonel Albert Swalm at your service. And who might I tell my
wife I had the pleasure of sitting beside this afternoon?" The Colonel's
jocularity reminded her of dear old William Taft.

"I am Miss Elizabeth Hughes."

Colonel Swalm certainly knew exactly who Elizabeth was, and as

U.S. consul to Bermuda, he even had an official relationship to her father, but he never mentioned it.

They chatted pleasantly for a few minutes and then Colonel Swalm asked Elizabeth the exact question that no one ever asked her. It was a common question, a question that most adults ask most children upon meeting them for the first time, but no one ever posed the question to Elizabeth. They were entirely too discreet, too witheringly kind. The unspoken reality was that the question would be irrelevant in her case.

"What would you like to be when you grow up?"

She was so surprised that it took a moment for her to answer.

"I want to be a writer," she said.

"A writer! Excellent! In that case you may be interested to learn that you are sitting beside the former editor of the *Grand Junction Headlight,* the former editor of the *Jefferson Bee* and the owner-publisher of the *Fort Dodge Messenger* and the Oskaloosa *Herald.* What kinds of things do you write?"

"Well, these days I mostly write letters, but I have had a few stories published in *St. Nicholas,*" she said brightly.

From that first meeting they sought each other out at all social affairs, and each was relieved to find the other in attendance. Although they often represented the oldest and youngest guest at any gathering, they gravitated to each other, even taking the liberty of rearranging place cards so that they could sit beside each other.

Colonel Swalm could be relied on to tell entertaining stories about his twenty-five-year career in the United States Consular Service. As far as Elizabeth was concerned, however, his greatest talent was to take the sting out of the dreaded comestible aspect of obligatory social engagements. Seated beside her, he would sometimes eat his own sandwiches, wink at her, and switch plates so that the empty plate would be in front of her. Then he would nibble at the food on what had been her plate and tell the hostess he was trying to reduce. There was never any fuss about the food when Colonel Swalm was present. By one strategy or another, what had been onerous became fun.

Soon Mrs. Swalm had adopted Elizabeth, too. Pauline Swalm was an accomplished journalist and speaker with an avid interest in politics and was very much an equal partner in her husband's publishing enterprises. The Swalms appointed themselves the official editors of Elizabeth's eventual autobiography. They promised her that if she wrote it, they would shepherd it to their publishing contacts. In a letter dated March 24, 1922, Elizabeth wrote that the Swalms had given her the courage to commit herself to her highest ambition—to write.

One afternoon Mrs. Swalm invited Elizabeth to accompany her to the semiannual sale at Trimingham's, *the* department store in Bermuda, to buy some yarn. Elizabeth had stopped buying yarn in the unspoken understanding that any project she began now would likely remain unfinished. But when Mrs. Swalm called to arrange a time to take Elizabeth to Trimingham's, neither Elizabeth nor Blanche had the heart to object. And so Elizabeth and Mrs. Swalm spent the afternoon scrutinizing skeins of fine Scottish yarn. Mrs. Swalm held shades of aqua and teal and periwinkle to Elizabeth's cheek. Elizabeth decided on three skeins of a lovely marled cornflower blue, and with them she began to knit a cardigan sweater. Neither Elizabeth nor Mrs. Swalm could have known what a frigid climate Elizabeth would find herself in that coming autumn, and how much she would need and use that sweater.

After the conclusion of the Washington Conference on February 6, Charles and Antoinette Hughes had hoped to take a three-week long rest in Bermuda with Elizabeth. Charles was exhausted from the stress of the international negotiations, and Antoinette had hoped to catch her breath before planning Catherine's June wedding, which was to be a grand event and the first cabinet wedding of the Harding administration. Three times they reserved a cabin on a Furness-Bermuda Line steamship from New York to Hamilton and three times they were compelled to cancel the reservation. Finally, on Tuesday, February 13, Charles turned the State Department business over to the care of Under Secretary Henry P. Fletcher and left for New York, where he and Antoinette visited with Charlie and Marjory and their two children, before embarking on the journey to Bermuda. Despite a stinging sleet storm, Charlie and his family escorted his parents onto the deck of the steamer *Fort Hamilton*. There, despite the weather and his own exhaustion, the elder Hughes stood obligingly on deck for thirty minutes so that still and motion picture photographers could document the departure for a public that seemed never to tire of him.

When the Hugheses arrived in Hamilton they were greeted by an unusually large gathering of the regular well-heeled crowd. Other than a few obligatory dinners and receptions, they hoped to spend as much time with Elizabeth as possible.

They were amazed and delighted to find Elizabeth in such good health and fine spirits and even allowed themselves to entertain the hope that some miraculous reversal was occurring. Always adhering to the strictures in the little red volume *Starvation (Allen) Treatment of Diabetes,* Elizabeth was experimenting with many kinds of food now—grapefruit, strawberries, tomatoes, fish (needless to say, not all at the same meal). Her strength and stamina were considerably better than they had been just months before. For two heady, happy weeks Charles, Antoinette, and Elizabeth explored the island by foot, car, and rowboat.

Elizabeth was enthralled with the idea that Charles and Antoinette might be asked to attend the Brazilian Centennial Exposition in August. If they went he would be only the third American secretary of state to officially visit the continent of South America. So enthusiastic was Elizabeth about the Exposition that they entertained the possibility that if her health continued to improve she might accompany them to Rio de Janeiro. By early March they were suntanned and relaxed and so thoroughly restored by both company and climate that the fact that Elizabeth was now nearly two years beyond even the most optimistic prognosis was almost forgotten.

On March 6 Charles and Antoinette returned to New York aboard the *Fort Hamilton.* They arrived in time to catch the 1:10 P.M. train to Washington. Although they had left New York in a sleet storm, they returned to sunshine, which they took as further evidence that things were indeed looking up. On the subject of his daughter's health, Hughes remained characteristically taciturn—so much so that one newspaper headline read: "Hughes Back From Trip: Secretary Arrives From Bermuda, Sunburned and Silent."

Shortly after Charles and Antoinette returned from Bermuda a letter arrived from Dr. Allen. It held a clipping of Roy Greenaway's story in the *Toronto Daily Star* on March 22. Allen hoped that it would prompt Elizabeth's immediate return. At last, it seemed, her trial was over. She could now claim the prize for which she had paid so dearly.

Unfortunately, Elizabeth was too weak to travel. In April she contracted a debilitating case of diarrhea. Blanche tried everything she knew to control the wasting effects, but Elizabeth slid into a dismal feebleness punctuated by frightening fevers and delirium. By May Elizabeth's diet had been slashed to less than three hundred calories per day and her urine was still showing sugar. For the first time her weight, fully clothed, fell below fifty pounds. The idea of Elizabeth's skeletal presence exposed to all the world at Catherine's wedding was unthinkable. Elizabeth was forced to accept that she could not participate in her sister's wedding. Antoinette allowed Elizabeth to think that bowing out was her own idea.

The stalwart Elizabeth insisted on getting outside into the sun and air every day, but by this time she was too weak to venture beyond the hammock on the patio. Each morning Blanche walked or carried her to the hammock between 9 and 11 in the morning. There Elizabeth remained until 6:30 or 7 in the evening, watching the cardinals and drinking in the oleander scented breezes as she drifted in and out of sleep. Ever loyal and devoted, the Swalms continued to call.

The Bermuda Trade Development Board made a gift to Elizabeth of hand-colored photographs of the island by local artist Stuart Hayward. On Thursday, April 14, Colonel Swalm accompanied her to Hayward's studio where she selected eighteen photographs. It was the first time she had left the cottage in weeks. This lifted her spirits considerably and she wrote to her mother that afternoon: "I'm beginning to feel real hopeful now, and we're going to find out my tolerance [then] keep me on that until I get home and have a blood test by Dr. Allen himself."

On Saturday June 10, 1922, at four o'clock in the afternoon Catherine Hughes and Chauncey Waddell were married in the Bethlehem Chapel of the Washington Cathedral. After the wedding ceremony, the reception was held at the Pan-American Union, considered Washington's most beautiful public building. Guests included President and Mrs. Harding, Vice President and Mrs. Coolidge, the entire cabinet and their wives and the members of the diplomatic corps, close friends of the bride's family, and Mr. and Mrs. Edward J. Waddell, who traveled from their home in Greenfield, Ohio, to Washington for the wedding.

After seeing Catherine and Chauncey off to Europe for an extended honeymoon, Charles and Antoinette went to Silver Bay to see the completed Helen Hughes Memorial Chapel for the first time. It was a magnificent reflection of two prominent aspects of Helen's personality:

simplicity and strength. Built of gneiss granite with graceful, Norman-style timber arches, and a slate roof, the chapel was nestled in the verdant heart of the Silver Bay campus in the well-traveled lawn between the cottages and the Inn, where Helen's spirit would never be lonely.

The chapel's interior was furnished with wrought iron sconces and enough plain wooden pews to accommodate two hundred worshippers. The chancel was graced with a slate altar, behind which three tall stained-glass windows shone with vivid hues. These were gifts of the Welsh people of the United States. A framed hand-painted description states that the window's central figure represents Elizabeth of Thuringia (or Elizabeth of Hungary), the patron saint of, among other things, charitable workers and childhood death. At the rear of the chapel was a rose window bearing the simple legend "This Chapel Is Erected in Loving Memory of Helen Hughes 1892–1920." To this day the rose window is lit every night. The altar hangings were given by the Calvary Baptist Church of Washington. On June 25 a choir of forty-five girls from Vassar College, Helen's alma mater, gave a musical program in celebration of Helen's life.

After the dedication ceremony Charles and Antoinette returned to Washington and to an official invitation to represent the United States at the Brazilian Centennial Exposition. It was to begin on September 7, 1922, and conclude on March 31, 1923. The plan was to travel in late August by ship to Rio de Janeiro, an ocean journey lasting nearly two weeks. They would remain in Rio for five or six days of official meetings and receptions before setting sail for the two-week return trip. In all, they would be away for roughly one month. It was obvious that Elizabeth would not be able to accompany them, and they questioned whether they should go themselves. They would be helpless if her final struggle came while they were at sea. In fact, how would they even know if she had taken a turn for the worse?

That spring they had seen one daughter married and one daughter buried. In early July, Elizabeth was finally strong enough to leave Bermuda. She had survived four times as long as the most optimistic prognosis on the Allen diet. Antoinette traveled from Washington to New York to meet the *Fort Hamilton* and take Elizabeth and Blanche to the Physiatric Institute, where Dr. Allen was waiting to see them. Antoinette arrived at the dock early and waited with growing concern as all of the passengers disembarked. Finally, Blanche appeared at the railing on the lower deck, alone and walking slowly toward the gangplank that the last passenger had just descended. Now Antoinette could see that Blanche was wheeling Elizabeth in a wheelchair before her. At the top of the gangplank, however, Elizabeth insisted on rising to her feet and tottering down the ramp to greet her mother on her own twig-thin legs. Antoinette was aghast at the change in her daughter's condition. At fourteen years of age, Elizabeth was five feet tall and weighed forty-eight and a quarter pounds fully clothed. When Elizabeth spotted her mother at the bottom of the gangplank her face broke into a look-Ma-no-chair grin. In that moment Antoinette saw the toothy grimace of her daughter's skull. By the time Elizabeth had teetered to the dock, her lower lip had split and her teeth were slick with blood.

Convinced that this was the end, Antoinette decided to take Elizabeth directly home to Washington instead of to the Physiatric Institute. They took the first train. There was only one thing for Antoinette to do. She sat down at the desk with single-minded determination.

Just as Dr. Allen had struggled to compose his letter to Antoinette six months before asking her to reconsider her decision to send Elizabeth to Bermuda, so Antoinette would struggle to compose her letter to a man who was, at that time, deluged with letters of exactly the type she was writing. She was keenly aware that she might only have this one chance to capture his interest and that Elizabeth's life depended on that chance. She must provide just the right amount of informative detail, just the right amount of pathos, and the letter itself must be neither too long nor too brief.

She took a sheet of gray monarch stationery from the drawer and crossed out 1529 Eighteenth Street, the address at the top of the page. The state of her life was such that she didn't even know where to tell him to send his reply. Would she still be at home or would she take Elizabeth to upstate New York as she had Helen? Would she be on a ship to Brazil? She wrote the return address: c/o The Department of State, Washington, D.C., U.S.A. They would forward his reply to her. Then she worried that he might think she was trying to impress him.

By the time Charles arrived at the hotel that evening, the wastebasket was full of crumpled balls of gray stationery but Antoinette had completed her letter.

July 3, 1922

My dear Dr. Banting:

Because my daughter has Diabetes I have been interested in a very deep and unusual [way] in your reported discoveries in that field. I heard of your work at first only through the press but later from the eminent physicians who expressed their belief that you had made a distinct step forward. I understand that you have passed the steps where you experiment only on animals and are treating patients in your hospital.

I am very anxious to know more of your discovery and your treatment and would greatly appreciate it if you would write me as fully as you deem best.

My daughter, who will be fifteen years of age in August, has had Diabetes for a little more than three years. Her case was, and still is, severe and, though it has been handled skillfully and with the utmost care, her tolerance is still very low and she is pitifully depleted and reduced.

She has been from the beginning under the care of Dr. Frederick M. Allen of New York and for a good share of this period I have named, we have had for her a nurse trained under both Dr. Allen and Dr. Joslin of Boston.

Because of circumstances too numerous to mention and several illnesses—tonsillitis, an ulcerated tooth and a bad attack of diarrhea which she, unfortunately, had in Bermuda last Winter, she has—despite our care, gotten into this exceedingly weak and wasted condition and I am desirous to avail myself of any treatment which would—if no more—increase her tolerance so that she might be able to gain a little.

This attack of diarrhea which I have mentioned was—we believe, a mild epidemic in Bermuda—which, because of her condition, was severe in her case. She ran a temperature and was so completely exhausted by it that it took her some time to get back her strength. I am glad to be able to tell you that she has, practically re-gained her strength and that during this bad upset she did not lose her tolerance; in fact, so far as that is concerned—her winter in Bermuda has been, we feel, a benefit, for, when she went down there, she was taking only 12 grams of carbohydrate and was raised to 20 grams. I am inclosing a diet sheet which will give you a more exact idea of her tolerance.

She is a model patient having never once, in these three years, gone over her diet. The steps backward—when they have come—have invariably been due to no fault of hers and we feel that this strength of character—which her nurse considers quite unusual—is—of course—much in her favor.

Though I realize that the long trip from Washington to Toronto would be—in her condition—hard upon her—yet I would consider bringing her there if you could hold out any hope of a practical gain, and I have written fully so that you might be able to judge a little of the case in advance.

I shall be glad to hear from you at your earliest convenience and thanking you for your attention I am

Very truly yours,

Antoinette C. Hughes
(Mrs. Charles E. Hughes)

It mattered little how carefully Antoinette chose her words or where she directed the letter's recipient to send his reply. Although Toronto had recovered the ability to produce insulin in May, the researchers didn't know why or how they had failed to begin with, and that meant they couldn't be sure they wouldn't lose it again. With the availability of insulin in such a tenuous state it was impossible to take on new patients lest they suffer the same fate as Best's young friend, dying on Ward H for lack of insulin. Banting replied to Antoinette as he did to all such entreaties. He was sorry, but in all of Toronto there was not a single extra drop of insulin to be had.

TWENTY-FOUR

*Patents, Partnership, and Pancreases, Indianapolis and Toronto,
April to August 1922*

IN APRIL 1922, IN THE MIDDLE OF HIS WORKDAY IN THE PURCHAS-
ing Department at Eli Lilly and Company in Indianapolis, Austin
Brown was startled to be summoned to the office of President J. K. Lilly
Sr. He had never been to the president's office, and as he made his way
across the company campus and through the hushed corridors of the
executive building, his mind raced with reasons why Mr. J. K. Lilly could
possibly want to see him. By the time he arrived at the outer office, his
stomach was in knots and his palms were damp and cold. Lilly's secretary immediately ushered him into the inner sanctum, which smelled of
good leather and polished mahogany. There he found not only Mr. Lilly,
but also Clowes and the company treasurer, Nicholas Noyes. Mr. Lilly invited him to sit down in an empty chair, which was handy because his
knees had begun to feel like pudding.

"Thank you for coming," Mr. Lilly said. "I assume you know Dr.
Clowes and Mr. Noyes. Gentlemen, this is Mr. Brown, from purchasing."

Brown opened his mouth but no sound came out. He smiled and
nodded.

"Tell me, Brown," Dr. Clowes asked, "Do you think you could arrange for two thousand pounds of pancreas glands to be delivered to the
Science Building on a weekly basis?"

Brown had never seen a pancreas gland in his life. He tried to imagine where in the body it was located. Was it the gland in the brain that regulated growth? No, that was the pituitary gland. Was it the same as sweetbreads? Was it the same as tripe? As far as purchasing went, he had plenty to say—about paper clips and steno pads, and sure, he knew his way around a laboratory supply catalogue, too, beakers and tongs and microscope slides. But pancreas glands?

"Either beef or pork is fine," Clowes added, as if that would help to clarify things.

Brown nodded. He had no idea where or how to find beef or pork pancreas glands or how difficult or expensive they might be to get. But judging from the expressions on the three faces before him, and the fact that those faces represented the highest echelon of company management, he knew that procuring these glands was a matter of grave importance. He also knew that there was only one answer to the question. It was yes, and that was the answer he gave.

Armed with Brown's affirmative reply, Clowes made his fourth trip to Toronto in as many months. He evangelized to the Toronto team about Lilly's experience in working with glandular products and his confidence in its ability to produce insulin in whatever quantities were desired. He explained that the company had already equipped a laboratory and had proceeded to arrange for massive shipments of fresh pancreas with the sprawling commercial abattoirs of the Midwest. Its legal department could assist the university in protecting their discovery by securing a patent. Just exactly how many more diabetic lives was the University of Toronto willing to sacrifice in order to resist the help of a capable partner and a potential solution?

While Clowes worked on Macleod, Falconer, and FitzGerald in Toronto, Brown spent several weeks in his car traversing the Midwest in a single-minded effort to make the very arrangements that Clowes was describing. Meatpackers, it seemed, habitually discarded the pancreas glands. The procedure for the slaughter and processing of livestock in the slaughterhouse was a well-choreographed system of highly interdependent steps, timed to the second. To introduce an intermediate task into this intricate scheme was obviously to invite disaster, tantamount to throwing the proverbial monkey wrench. It would not only require the complete reworking of the established procedures, but also decrease the critical efficiency of the process and put the accommodating meat-packing plant at a disadvantage to its competitors.

Brown saw he would have to perform some near miraculous salesmanship to persuade them to preserve the glands for immediate shipment to Lilly. First he told them that there would be a high and steadily increasing demand for the glands. Then he said that every pound that the packers shipped to Lilly could potentially save a child's life. He began locally with Kingan and Company, and went on to visit Swift and Armour in Chicago and Cudahy in Omaha. He often took his petition right to the top man and sometimes enlisted Mr. J. K. Lilly to accompany him to these meetings. Slowly, the meatpackers began to agree, at least on a trial basis.

During Toronto's agonizing two-month-long insulin famine, the group prepared the most comprehensive paper on the subject to date. "The Effect Produced on Diabetes by Extracts of Pancreas" was written by Banting, Best, Collip, Campbell, Fletcher, Macleod, and Noble. This paper described all of the work to date, from Banting's initial inspiration to the hypoglycemic shock that resulted from an insulin overdose to the extreme difficulty of establishing a standard unit to the respiratory quotients and the liver-glycogen findings. In this paper the extract was officially named insulin, in accordance with Macleod's insistent reasoning.

The group agreed that Macleod would present this paper at the meeting of the Association of American Physicians. This was to be the official announcement of the discovery of insulin. The presentation was scheduled for noon on May 3, 1922. Clowes made arrangements to attend the meeting also. When Macleod finished speaking, the room erupted in a thunderous standing ovation. Joslin would later say that in twenty years of attending AAP meetings he had never experienced anything like it. The news made headlines around the world. Collip had been present to witness the glorious event, but Banting and Best were not. At the last minute they had decided not to attend, claiming that the trip to Washington, D.C., was too expensive.

Within days of the conference Clowes wrote to Macleod that he had consulted Lilly's patent experts on the best form of protective patent to take out in the United States and that he was more convinced than ever of the necessity of starting work on the problem of large-scale production right away. Clowes warned that if insulin were not protected by a patent there would be nothing to stop unscrupulous vendors from advertising ineffective anti-diabetic preparations as insulin.

Finally, in mid-May the University of Toronto invited Clowes to make a presentation to the Board of Governors about Lilly's offer of assistance. Mass production had proved to be a bigger challenge than Toronto had anticipated and the discovery team reluctantly admitted that they needed help to bring insulin to the world. For the first time, the Board of Governors agreed to listen to what Lilly had to say about protective patents and international distribution of insulin.

Working tirelessly at Connaught, Charley Best recovered his ability to make insulin in mid-May while Collip continued to struggle. The reasons for the failure have never been conclusively determined but were likely related to variations in temperature during the evaporation of the alcohol.

Unlike Collip, who had always surrendered his insulin to Toronto General Hospital, Charley gave his insulin directly to Banting, apparently without discussing this with FitzGerald or Macleod. On May 15 Banting's friend Joe Gilchrist, who had merrily dubbed himself "Toronto's human rabbit," became the first recipient of the new batch of insulin. It was effective. With Best in charge of insulin manufacturing at Connaught and Banting in charge of the best available clinical facilities at Christie Street, an agreement was reached with Connaught that one-third of all insulin produced would go to Banting for his private practice, one-third would go to Banting for Christie Street, and one-third would go to Toronto General Hospital or the Hospital for Sick Children.

Following Gilchrist's successful test, insulin was provided to an American doctor named John R. Williams in Rochester, New York, just across Lake Ontario from Toronto. Williams had been promised insulin for the desperately ill son of a vice president of Eastman Kodak. James Havens, a skeletal twenty-two-year-old, had been maintaining the Allen diet since his diagnosis *seven years previously*, at the age of fifteen. In the fall of 1919 he had spent more than a month at the Physiatric Institute and remained stable on Allen's starvation diet until May 1920, when his precarious metabolic equilibrium was upset. He was put on a diet of two hundred calories per day for three weeks and was subjected to daily visits to the doctor and weekly blood tests. His decline continued despite all efforts to help him. By the spring of 1922 he weighed seventy-three and a half pounds, was too weak to sit up in bed and cried most of the time.

On May 21, 1922, when it appeared that Havens had only a week to live, he became the first American to receive insulin. Banting spent two days with him in Rochester. At first the miracle cure seemed ineffective, but after the dose was tripled according to Banting's instruction, Havens began to show improvement. Banting promised to keep Williams supplied with insulin so long as there would be no publicity.

In 1922, the separation of university research from commercial enterprise was roughly equivalent to that between church and state. It was thought that the objectives of research and industry were simply too disparate to allow productive collaboration. And yet, the University of Toronto now found itself in a position where to hold to the moral high ground was to cause the deaths of children—a morally indefensible position. Clowes was uniquely suited to facilitate such an unlikely collaboration. Although he was embedded in commercial industry, he was a researcher and could "speak the language" that the members of the Insulin Committee could understand and, more importantly, trust.

Eli Lilly and Company had been poised for this opportunity for nearly five months. On May 22, Clowes arrived in Toronto with chemist Harley W. Rhodehamel, patent attorney George B. Schley, and Vice President Eli Lilly. They met Banting, Best, Collip, and a patent attorney representing the university named Mr. C. H. Riches at the King Edward Hotel in Toronto. During the next three days the masterful diplomatic skills of George Henry Alexander Clowes were put to the test.

Banting still refused to have anything to do with the patent, so the group prepared and submitted a patent application for the *process* of producing insulin under the names of Best and Collip. Two months later, on the advice of Lilly, a patent application was submitted for the *product* of insulin under the name of Best alone. These efforts were necessary, Clowes explained, to protect diabetics. Now that the discovery was public, attempts at independent manufacture began but, for once, the vexing difficulty of making insulin worked in Toronto's favor. Still, if the university wished to maintain control over the development for the sake of safety, it was imperative that they protect their process and prevent unregulated development.

An advisory group was formed in Toronto to assist in the administration of product development, testing, and clinical distribution. The Insulin Committee would be the guiding force overseeing all critical decisions related to insulin. It was led by Professor Macleod and included the following members: Dr. Banting; Mr. Best; Dr. R. D. DeFries, director of Connaught Antitoxin Laboratories; Professor Duncan Graham, head of the university's Department of Medicine; Professor J. G. FitzGerald, head of the university's Department of Hygiene; Colonel Albert Gooderham, university board of governors; Sir Robert Falconer, president of the university; Mr. C. H. Riches, legal advisor; and others.

The Insulin Committee alone approved a list of clinicians to whom insulin could be distributed by Lilly for human testing. The initial list was Dr. Frederick Allen of Morristown, New Jersey, Dr. Elliott P. Joslin of Boston, Massachusetts, and Dr. Rollin T. Woodyatt of Chicago. Within a month seven more doctors were added to the list, including Dr. John A. MacDonald, who would administer the human clinical trials at the Methodist Hospital in Indianapolis on behalf of Lilly. Dr. John R. Williams (Jim Havens's doctor) of Rochester and Dr. H. Rawle Geyelin continued to be supplied through Toronto's allotment from Lilly.

Eli Lilly and Company called itself an ethical drug company, distributing its products only and always through licensed medical doctors and pharmacists and never directly to the public (as distinct from the makers of patent medicine, whose products were advertised and distributed directly to patients). Lilly agreed to submit each batch of insulin it made to Toronto for approval and then to provide 28 percent of each approved lot to the university gratis. In addition, Lilly would supply insulin to university-approved physicians and institutions for testing purposes.

Clowes estimated that the effort to develop insulin would take at least a year and that the costs of the effort would be great. Mr. Lilly stated that he was prepared to invest two hundred thousand dollars (equivalent to roughly two million dollars in 2010 dollars) to help Connaught and the insulin discoverers realize practicable large-scale production methods. This was an especially brave commitment given that the United States was struggling to regain economic equilibrium in the throes of a post-war recession. Eli Lilly and Company itself had just barely emerged from a profound slump that had begun in October 1920 and extended through most of 1921. In an effort to avoid layoffs and excess inventory, the company had been forced into a four-day workweek for several months, but it had not reduced wages. The pledge made to the University of Toronto was a measure of the company's founding belief in science in general and in the idea of insulin specifically.

In exchange for undertaking these financial and manufacturing challenges, the University of Toronto would allow Eli Lilly and Company a one-year exclusive contract to make, use, and sell the extract in the United States, Mexico, Cuba, and Central and South America. During this time the university would not release the formula for making insulin to any other commercial enterprise. There was to be full collaboration between the two parties, and if in the course of the year Lilly developed patentable methods of production, it agreed to assign the U.S. patents to the university.

One of Mr. Lilly's own requirements was that his company be permitted to assign a brand name to the insulin they produced. The Lilly brand would help druggists and physicians safeguard against substitutions and inferior preparations that would inevitably flood the market. The name would help to compensate Eli Lilly and Company for their investment by giving them an advantage over competitors after the one-year exclusivity had expired. Eventually, Mr. Lilly would choose the brand name Iletin, in part because it echoed the name that Banting had originally assigned—isletin.

Within three days of discussion at the King Edward Hotel the negotiators had drafted an agreement, which would be referred to as an "indenture" and was officially dated May 30, 1922. Toronto was to prepare a final version of the indenture, sign it, and send it to Indianapolis for signatures. The team in Indianapolis did not wait for signatures but launched into action immediately. George B. Walden was put in charge of the program, to be assisted by Harley W. Rhodehamel and Jasper P. Scott. George Walden was a twenty-eight-year old chemist who had joined Eli Lilly and Company in 1917 with a salary of $85 per month.

Collip's appointment at Toronto expired on May 31, 1922. On June 2 and 3, he and Best went to Indianapolis and told the Eli Lilly chemists everything they knew about making insulin. They walked the Lilly chemists through the process. From Indianapolis Collip went directly to Alberta. Best returned to Toronto. The discovery team was abruptly and unceremoniously dissolved.

Seventeen days later, Lilly had yet to receive the signed indenture from Toronto. Still the Indianapolis team hurled themselves into the work of making insulin. On June 17, 1922, Mr. Eli Lilly wrote to Macleod. "Our chemists here have been working very intently on the production of insulin, and have gotten a good deal of experience, and at last have turned out about twenty doses of something that approximates very closely the material made in Toronto." He asked Macleod to send ten doses of their product so that the team at Lilly could compare the preparations. Macleod forwarded the request to Charles Best at Connaught.

In Indianapolis, Billy Sylvester, custodian of the Science Building at Eli Lilly and Company, was assigned the task of traveling by taxicab to Kingan twice a day with several white enamel twelve-gallon stock pots as containers to retrieve the fresh glands. Experimental runs were made almost daily beginning on June 2, and on June 19 Lilly sent Banting its first insulin, a shipment of fifty units. But it was not enough to supply clinicians who had patients with legitimate need, and so on June 21 Macleod sent the insulin formula to Dr. W. D. Sansum in Santa Barbara, California, and to Dr. Rollin T. Woodyatt in Chicago. (Sansum had already begun experimenting with making insulin.) Both doctors began small-scale production of insulin for clinical and experimental uses. These independent efforts annoyed both Banting and Clowes and placed even more pressure on Lilly and Connaught to produce large volumes of potent, stable extract. As is often the case in graduating from small- to large-scale production, great difficulties persisted in both Indianapolis and Toronto.

Macleod sent three copies of the signed indenture agreement to Eli Lilly on June 29, 1922, less than a week before Elizabeth Hughes was to totter down the gangplank of the Fort Hamilton. On July 10, the same date that Banting replied to Antoinette Hughes to discourage her from bringing Elizabeth to Toronto, Eli Lilly returned the agreement to

Toronto, signed by President J. K. Lilly and General Manager Charles J. Lynn. It was official.

Around this time Banting was approached by several American institutions with attractive offers to leave Toronto. The University of Buffalo offered him a faculty position. George Eastman of Eastman-Kodak pressed him to accept a role at the new medical school at the University of Rochester. And Harvey Kellogg, inventor of cornflakes and peanut butter, offered to build Banting his own wing at the Battle Creek Sanitarium and pay him an annual salary of ten thousand dollars to join the staff. Were Banting to move to the United States, Toronto would lose insulin for the university, for Toronto, and for Canada.

Although Duncan Graham objected to giving Banting anything, the University of Toronto persuaded him to offer Banting an appointment under his direction. With Doctors Campbell and Fletcher, Banting was to oversee a thirty-two bed diabetic clinic at Toronto General Hospital. For this Banting would receive a salary of $6,000 a year and a university appointment in the Department of Medicine. As part of the new arrangement he agreed to close his private practice to new patients. Banting's friend from the Hospital for Sick Children, Dr. D. E. Robertson, was instrumental in persuading Graham to accept the arrangement, although their heated arguments over the subject of Frederick Banting nearly destroyed their friendship.

In mid-June Macleod left Toronto for the Marine Biological Station at St. Andrews, New Brunswick. He had been granted $8,000 by the Carnegie Corporation, some of which he used to fund the research project to explore the manufacture of insulin from teleost. Macleod was certain that fish pancreas held the solution to the difficulties Connaught had experienced in producing insulin and was determined to prove it. Dr. N. A. McCormack and Clark Noble worked with Macleod through the summer of 1922 at the Marine Biological Station and documented some encouraging results from several fish, especially cod.

Unfortunately, Macleod discovered that commercial fishermen were far more resistant than were the meatpackers to the idea of saving pancreatic glands, or perhaps he was less persuasive in selling the idea.

The first factory-scale run was made at Eli Lilly and Company on June 26 and the second on July 5. The July 5 yield was about thirty units of insulin from about thirty-four kilos of fresh hog pancreas. Through tireless experiments with alcohol concentrations, temperatures, and adjustments to the extraction process, Lilly gradually increased the yield over the summer months, but the ability to make truly large amounts of insulin eluded them.

TWENTY-FIVE

Fame and Famine, Summer 1922

Ever since the AAP meeting in May newspapers around the world heralded insulin as a miracle cure, saying that it would do for diabetics what antitoxin had done for those with diphtheria at the turn of the century. The inevitable result was that in July, the Toronto train stations teemed with emaciated children and their distraught families, drawn by the stories in the press. Best went to Maine for a vacation, and once again Banting found himself alone in Toronto's sweltering summer climate. Each day's mail contained a deluge of desperate entreaties. One envelope was simply addressed: "To the Dr. who cures Diabetes, Toronto, Ont." A daily pageantry of illness filed up Bloor Street West to the tiny waiting room of his clinical office. Each child's distended stomach and huge staring eyes were more heartrending than the last, but there *was* no stable, nontoxic insulin. It was an excruciating conflict: He had agreed not to accept any new patients in his private practice once the diabetic ward at Toronto General Hospital was open, but it wasn't yet open. In the meantime, didn't the Hippocratic oath require him to do what he could to help these children? That month Antoinette Hughes's letter was one of dozens of desperate entreaties that arrived at Banting's Bloor Street office, either directly or via Macleod. Some came from family members and others from physicians. A typical exchange, as terse as it was tragic, was this one, via telegram, with a doctor in Atlanta:

Dr. J. R. Macleod — Is there any possible chance for you to take Graves Smith the patient about whom Joslin wrote you some weeks ago any time soon[?] His father is anxious to bring him to you if there is any hope of getting him under Banting[.] The boy is in a very serious condition and unless something is done soon it will be too late please wire at my expense.—Dr. J. E. Paullin

Dr. J. E. Paullin — No insulin available at present. Will wire you whenever supply is obtained.—F. G. Banting

Dr. Morton Ryder, uncle of the twenty-six-pound Teddy, was another whom Banting initially turned away. Trying to offer some hope, Banting suggested that he write to him again in September when there might be some insulin. Ryder replied, "Teddy won't be alive in September."

In 1922 there was a fine line between help and harm. Even laying aside the problem of purity, until they were able to achieve a stable potency in the insulin they produced, it was almost impossible to prescribe the right dosage. At Christie Street, several diabetics had suffered hypoglycemic shock as a result of an overdose and had to be revived with glucose. The lack of supply placed diabetic specialists in both countries in grueling dilemmas about which patients would receive insulin, and these decisions had life-and-death consequences. Most doctors agreed that during the experimental stage, only the most severe diabetics should receive insulin. But others argued that if these cases were so frail that the patient would not survive the experiment, shouldn't they be turned away so that a less desperate case might be given the chance to recover?

Banting turned nearly every case away, yielding only when he was sure that the child was so close to death that the risk of using unstable or impure insulin was justified. He finally accepted three new private patients, three living skeletons from the United States: Myra Blaustein, age eleven, forty pounds; Ruth Whitehill, age seven, forty-three pounds; and Teddy Ryder, age five, twenty-six pounds.

When Mildred Ryder left New York with Teddy for Toronto in early July, a friend helped Mildred with their luggage and waved them off at the station. As the train pulled away, the friend recalled feeling sure that Mildred would never bring Teddy back alive. Mother and son arrived in Toronto on the sleeper on Saturday morning, July 8. They went directly to 160 Bloor Street West. There was no insulin: The last batch had gone inexplicably bad. While Connaught struggled to recover the ability to make effective, nontoxic insulin, the discoverers were dependent upon the Americans for insulin to supply to their own patients. There was nothing to do but wait until Monday when the Lilly shipment would arrive. That Teddy might die within reach of the cure was almost more than Mildred Ryder could bear. To make matters worse, the diabetic clinic at Toronto General Hospital was still a month from opening, and the regular hospital kitchen could not accommodate the diabetic diet, so Mildred Ryder carried poor Teddy through the blistering heat to find a room to rent. She found a suitable situation on Grenville Street, with kitchen privileges so that she could prepare Teddy's exacting meals herself.

On Sunday Banting took delivery of the first new car he had ever owned. He came by Grenville Street and took Teddy and his mother for a drive in it to lift their spirits. On Monday the shipment from Indianapolis arrived, and Teddy's recovery began.

Mildred and Teddy liked Banting right away. He was not at all the intimidating celebrity they had expected him to be. He was a plainspoken man who loved children and had struggled with romance. Often, after giving Teddy his injection, he would linger at the Ryders' room to confide his troubles to Mrs. Ryder.

Until the diabetic clinic at Toronto General Hospital opened in late August, Banting had been squirreling away his private patients in rented rooms. Several were living at the Athelma Apartments at 78 Grosvenor Street, about a half mile from Banting's Bloor Street office. In this way he made his daily rounds, walking around the neighborhood from room to room and floor to floor and building to building. Some of these patients and their families became quite friendly with one another. While there was certainly a great deal of hand-wringing, there were occasional light moments too.

Teddy Ryder made a wonderful recovery, but he required up to four insulin injections a day. When he turned six that summer, the Whitehills threw him a costume party at their apartment at the Athelma. Teddy came dressed as an Indian chief with a feather bonnet so long it dusted the floor behind him as he walked around the room greeting everyone.

The last guest to arrive was a tall, mysterious woman in a large white hat, elbow-length white gloves, and a long pink dress. No one knew who she was. When she went to greet the birthday boy, she revealed herself to be none other than Dr. Banting! The room dissolved in torrents of laughter. Teddy Ryder never forgot it.

That summer Banting's old medical officer from Cambrai called him. Former captain L. C. Palmer asked Banting to see one of his patients—a fifty-seven-year-old woman named Charlotte Clarke. She was a severe diabetic with a badly infected, gangrenous leg whose condition was so poor that she was nearly comatose. At that time, no one had ever survived a diabetic coma. Unable to refuse his old military friend, Banting agreed to see her. The leg had to be amputated, but no one had ever performed surgery on a diabetic, and certainly not one nearly comatose. On the other hand, she was so near death that there was little risk in trying.

Clarke was admitted to Toronto General Hospital, but there was no insulin for her, so five diabetic patients were deprived of their insulin to provide enough to stabilize Clarke. She received her first injection on July 10. Next day, she was wheeled into the operating room and Palmer removed her right leg above the knee. After the surgery her metabolism was kept stable with insulin. Much to everyone's amazement she began a completely normal recovery. It was the first time that major surgery had been performed on a severe diabetic. Without insulin she would not even have survived the anesthesia.

After about a week, Palmer removed her stitches to reveal an incision that appeared to have healed perfectly. Believing that the insulin had done its work, Clarke received no more insulin after seven days. On July 25, Clarke's leg became swollen and discolored, and the wound split open to reveal an infection so deep and virulent that Palmer doubted anything could be done to save her, with or without insulin.

Just then, the Connaught insulin production failed again.

Fed up with Connaught's erratic production, and unable to get a satisfactory explanation from the Toronto chemists, Banting made a frantic trip to Indianapolis to see for himself why the Indianapolis production was working while the Connaught production was failing. He hoped, too, to carry enough insulin back to Toronto to save Charlotte Clarke.

During the journey he fell prey to his old paranoia and began to question why it was that Indianapolis had not experienced nearly so many difficulties as Connaught. Although it was true that Connaught was inexperienced with large stills and equipment to concentrate large volumes, he wondered if the Indianapolis team could have withheld some crucial secret of their process. By the time he arrived in Indianapolis, he was sure he had been betrayed. He determined to demand a complete tour of their facilities and a thorough explanation of their process and refuse to leave until he was satisfied that he had gotten the real story.

He charged off the train in an angry lather, ready to do battle. He was met on the platform by J. K. Lilly, Alec Clowes—and 150 units of insulin. When he was told that he could take it all back with him, Banting was so overcome that he fell onto Lilly's shoulder and wept. Whether the Toronto team had been too proud or too busy to communicate the dire circumstances in that city, the critical nature of the situation came as a surprise to the Indianapolis team. (It later came to light that Best *had* communicated the difficulty with the Toronto process to Rhodehamel in Indianapolis, but Clowes had been in Woods Hole and had not seen the correspondence.)

Eli Lilly and Company agreed to delay its own clinical work at Methodist Hospital in Indianapolis in order to supply extra insulin to Toronto until Connaught could recover the ability to make its own. Banting got his tour of the insulin manufacturing plant and process and was dumbfounded by the operations he saw there. He was particularly impressed with the large vacuum still, which was far superior to the antiquated tunnel process that they were using in the basement of the Medical Building, which relied upon evaporation. It was during this trip that Banting confided to Clowes his tribulations with Macleod and his suspicion that he intended to corner the credit for the discovery. Clowes pledged to do whatever he could to protect and assist Banting.

Upon his return to Toronto with the insulin, Banting stopped first at Toronto General Hospital to see Charlotte Clarke. As soon as her injections resumed, Charlotte Clarke's wound began to heal again. She made a full recovery and lived for many years afterward using a prosthetic leg.

Banting went next to the downtown office of Sir Edmund Walker, chair of the university's board of governors to procure the money to buy a vacuum still and other equipment necessary to bring Connaught up to the manufacturing standard he had seen in Indianapolis. In his typical combative fashion, Banting marched in and demanded ten thousand dollars immediately. Walker coolly assured Banting that he would raise the issue at the next board of governors meeting in the fall. Knowing that such a delay would cost lives, Banting was outraged by what he saw as a smug bureaucratic attitude. He asked Walker if the board of governors would accept the money if Banting could get it for them. Walker agreed. Banting stormed out.

Next day he was in New York with Dr. Rawle Geyelin, one of the original recipients of insulin and a member of Toronto's Insulin Committee. Banting watched in awe as Geyelin picked up the phone and called Robert Bacon, the wealthy parent of a diabetic child. Geyelin briefly explained the situation, then turned to Banting and asked how the check should be made out. Banting had a check for the full amount that day, and Toronto got its vacuum still.

Geyelin was appalled to see the discoverer of insulin begging for money. He told Banting that if he moved to New York he could make one hundred thousand dollars a year without any difficulty. Geyelin was amazed to learn that Banting had charged only a hundred dollars to Charlotte Clarke and twenty-five dollars a week to his insulin-dependent patients in Toronto. That summer Frederick Allen offered him a job at the Physiatric Institute, and according to Banting, an American investor offered him a million dollars for the rights to insulin.

On July 26, J. K. Lilly wrote directly to Banting.

> We were sorry that you found it necessary to hurry off so quickly after our very pleasant visit from you, yet we appreciate the necessity of your returning, and were very happy indeed that we were able to have you return with 150 units of insulin. Appreciating, Doctor, that Mr. Scott may not get into production until well into August, we have arranged a program that will enable us to increase our production in such a manner that we believe that we can supply you 500 units per week during the month of August. We sent another 150 units by Mr. Scott, and will use our utmost to get to you promptly each week in probably two or three shipments 500 cc's. We trust this will be of substantial assistance to you. We are having apparatus constructed

to enable the large scale production. . . . Working as quickly as possible.

On July 29, Lilly sent 200 units of insulin to Toronto. On August 8 they sent 500 units and pledged to try to continue to send 500 units per week. Canada's entire production of insulin depended on Connaught, and Connaught depended on Charley Best. At twenty-three years of age, Charley Best was now responsible not only for directing Connaught's insulin production but also for working with Lilly on standardization and stabilization.

The question of who should be the first American given the first injection of Lilly insulin was resolved by J. K. Lilly Sr. He decided that Dr. Elliott Joslin, who had devoted so much of his life to the care and study of diabetics, should have the honor of giving the first American preparation of insulin in an American institution by an American doctor to an American patient. (Dr. Woodyatt in Chicago was the first American physician to use insulin on a human patient, but the extract came from Toronto.) Miss Elizabeth Mudge, a nurse with (Type 1) diabetes, was forty-one years old and had no hope of seeing forty-two when Joslin chose her as the most desperate case to receive insulin. She weighed 69 pounds on August 7, 1922, and was in a near coma when she arrived at Boston's Deaconness Hospital by ambulance. So dire was her condition that Dr. Howard Root, a colleague of Dr. Joslin who happened to meet the ambulance, recognized immediately that there was no time to lose. With the ambulance still idling in the street outside the hospital, Root injected Mudge with two units of insulin while she lay moribund on the stretcher, pushing the needle through the blanket in which she was wrapped. She made a full recovery.

Hearing this news, Charley Best could not help but think of his favorite aunt. Among the thousand or so names recorded in Dr. Joslin's registry was the name of Helen Best. She was a nurse in her thirties when she went to see Dr. Joslin in February 1915 to seek help for her diabetes. At the time all Joslin could do for her was to prescribe the Allen diet. As a nurse, Helen well understood the seriousness of her disease and the importance of absolute compliance with the dietary regimen. Despite her strict observance, she died in a diabetic coma in May 1917.

★ ★ ★

In early August, Dr. Allen traveled to Toronto. There he met Teddy Ryder—not the Teddy Ryder he had treated at the Physiatric Institute, but an entirely different boy with the same name. The new Teddy was a vigorously healthy, happy boy with a round face and a thick mop of brown hair. For the first time in his life the voluble Dr. Allen was struck dumb. When he returned to the institute in Morristown, he stood humbly before his gaunt charges and said quietly, "I think I may have something for you."

Throughout the summer of 1922, the insulin plant at Lilly had been running three shifts. The lights never went out in the Science Building. Over one hundred workers focused solely on the problem of large-scale production of insulin. By August, Walden and his team had been able to increase the yield to roughly one hundred units per pound of pancreas. Kingan (and Billy Sylvester) could not meet the demand at Lilly. The first shipment of frozen pancreas glands by refrigerated railroad car was arranged with Swift and Company of Chicago.

Now Indianapolis began to experience the problems with potency that Connaught had experienced. Although Lilly had succeeded in increasing scale and yield, the potency of the final product decreased by as much as half. Thus in order to meet the agreed-upon shipments of insulin to Toronto and to the sixteen clinicians, production had to be doubled. The stress on George Walden, Harley Rhodehamel, and Jasper Scott was overwhelming. While Lilly was making every effort to help Toronto with their crisis, the unintended result was to create a second crisis in Indianapolis.

In August 1922 Walden was near nervous collapse. In order to forestall a complete breakdown, Clowes insisted that he join him in Woods Hole for a two-week rest. However, while Clowes had narrowly averted one nervous breakdown, Jasper Scott, who had been assigned Walden's responsibilities in his absence, did suffer a breakdown. This required his taking a rehabilitative rest of three weeks.

Clowes now received a telegram from Lilly in Indianapolis informing him that production had fallen below expectations, and if they were to continue to send Banting five hundred units per week, they would be unable to supply Woodyatt, Geyelin, or Wilder at the Mayo group. On

August 8, he sent a telegram to Banting, asking if he could reduce dosages and work with three hundred to four hundred units per week instead of the usual five hundred.

In August 1922, the quality, quantity, and potency of each batch were utterly unpredictable, and deterioration and sensitization reactions continued to present problems for clinical use. Clinical data from all of the participating physicians accrued and was analyzed in Toronto: There was a frustrating mixture of miraculous recoveries and baffling failures. Both Williams of Rochester and Woodyatt of Chicago had patients who died of hypoglycemic shock after receiving an overdose of insulin. Some parents of children who had endured the Allen treatment were desperate enough to be fearless. One eight-year-old boy, too weak to stand, was carried in to Joslin's office by his parents, who reportedly told the doctor, "Do anything you want with Frederick, you can't make him any worse." The human trials at Banting's clinic at the Christie Street Military Hospital had been discouraging. Stories about painful abscesses and hypoglycemic reactions deterred many diabetic veterans from participating in the program. Even Joe Gilchrist, who was promoting the program, suffered a dramatic hypoglycemic reaction. But then Banting decided to teach participants to administer insulin themselves so that they could take leave of the hospital on the weekend, and interest picked up. Interest increased even more when the first few men returned from weekend leave to report that insulin had a restorative effect on both their libido and their performance.

On August 10 Allen injected six patients with Lilly's insulin. Had Elizabeth been in Morristown she certainly would have been among them. In order to distribute the supply to the most recipients—and for fear of hypoglycemic reaction—he gave each less than one unit. The results were dramatic. Patients were restored to vigor so quickly that the results were sometimes referred to as resurrections. Blanche took Elizabeth to Morristown to await the next shipment of insulin. Antoinette wrote another letter to Dr. Banting, again urging him to accept Elizabeth as his private patient. And then she did something she had never done before, something that she had sworn she would never, ever do. She asked her husband to intervene.

TWENTY-SIX

Four Trunks, Washington, D.C., August 1922

Intervene? How exactly?" Charles asked, because he could see from the subtle pucker between Antoinette's eyebrows that she had a very specific idea in mind.

"Is there no one you can call?" Antoinette asked. "Mackenzie King. Or President Harding. Or better yet, ask Harding to call Mackenzie King."

Charles was startled by his wife's suggestion that he use his political influence to achieve such a deeply personal objective. But this was Antoinette asking, his own conscience, his trusted and intimate soul mate, and so he paused to consider the ramifications.

"This is not really a state matter."

"I'm not sure that's true," she replied with an unfamiliar tightness in her voice. "If you don't get Elizabeth to Banting, I can't get on the boat to Brazil with you."

In their thirty-four years of married life the longest time they had been apart was in the summer when Helen was dying. That was only for five days at a time and, had they needed to, they could have gotten to each other within hours. He could not seriously consider leaving for a month or more to sail to South America alone. She knew this. The starkness of her ultimatum took them both aback.

When he had taken the oath of office as secretary of state in the wake of the worst war in history, his biggest fear was that he would not be up to the task. He set a high standard for himself and for how he would serve, but it was Antoinette's support that allowed him to uphold that standard. Antoinette managed their home and family to perfection so that he could undertake the enormous workload that the office had required of him, beginning with developing a plan for world disarmament. She protected him from distraction and worry, safeguarded his social calendar, kept him fed, and saw to it that his wardrobe was clean and complete. She had always spared him from having to choose between his commitment to his family and affairs of state, even when Helen was dying. Now she was asking him to return the favor.

"If you had seen her come off that ship—," Antoinette choked back a sob. They both knew that time was running out for their youngest child. A cold, an ear infection, a skinned knee—virtually anything could send her into her final descent now. She weighed forty-eight pounds. That was twenty-seven pounds less than she weighed three years ago.

"Still, I can't call a president or a prime minister."

"Why not?"

Hughes knew that if he were to call Harding, he would intercede. Harding was virtually incapable of saying no to his friends. When he was a boy, his own father once told him that it was good that he had not been born "a gal," or else he would have been "in the family way all the time."

"Well, let us say that I do call President Harding. Harding would call Mackenzie King and King would call Sir Robert Falconer. Falconer would call Banting, and Banting would see Elizabeth. But Banting has already told you there is no insulin to give her."

"All I ask is that a meeting be arranged between Dr. Banting and Elizabeth. *Then* I will leave the matter to God. Whether Dr. Banting gives Elizabeth insulin or not is out of our hands, but we must arrange the meeting. That much we can and must do."

"But the problem is one of shortage, is it not? If so, then if Elizabeth receives insulin it may be at the cost of another child's life." Antoinette stared back in silence.

Throughout his professional and personal activities, Hughes had been guided by integrity and impartial commitment to the public weal.

He was universally recognized by both the powerful and the powerless as being someone who could be counted on to do the right thing regardless of any circumstances or personal stakes that might lead him to do otherwise. He keenly felt the gravity of the public trust and held it sacred and himself a servant to it. He knew that Antoinette felt the same way.

"Are you asking me to allow my heart to direct affairs of state? Are you asking me to use political power to achieve a personal objective? Didn't you marry me because I am the kind of man who has not and would not make such an error?"

Antoinette stared back in silence. A hundred thoughts raced through her tormented mind. Was it an error to do everything, everything possible to save your child's life? She was not sure she could live through the pain of losing another child. She wondered if she could love Charles if he didn't do everything he could to spare her from this.

"If you are asking me to do this, I will consider it." He held her gaze for a long time, watching her carefully. "Are you asking?"

"I am asking," she said in a barely audible voice. And then she went to bed.

A stillness settled over the house, like the eerie hush in the eye of a storm. Charles sat alone in the dark. He tried to imagine himself calling President Harding. Was this a public official pulling the strings of privilege or was it a father doing all that he could on behalf of his daughter? Was his responsibility to the principles he had sworn to abide by greater than his responsibility to his daughter? One was broad, the other deep. Which was the greater good? What exactly would he say to the president? Even if he did place the phone call, would there be time to arrange for Elizabeth to be placed in the care of the Toronto doctor before the SS *Pan America* sailed for Brazil on August 24?

Three hours later Antoinette came downstairs to find Charles sitting in his study staring at a five-by-seven-inch hand-colored photograph. She had the sense that he had not moved since she left him to go to bed. The photograph was of the house where he was born. It was a modest, one-story home with green shutters and three steps leading up to a front porch that wrapped narrowly around one side. He stared into the image of his childhood home and sounded the depths of his soul for the familiar certainty of his father's voice. He was looking for something that wasn't actually contained in the image at all: an answer. What would his father say to Antoinette's request?

If only there were a way to stroll up Maple Street, over the freeze-crazed cement of that familiar sidewalk, under the leaf-flocked, nodding boughs of maples and elms, and up the three steps to the porch. There his father would be slumped in the rocking chair, half asleep, chin turned to the side as if muttering a secret to his shoulder, a copy of Maimonides's *Guide for the Perplexed* open on his chest. Ironically, this was one of his favorite books, and yet David Charles Hughes never seemed in the least bit perplexed.

The elder Hughes had undertaken his own intellectual education; he was studious, well read, and self-taught. He took a special interest in Latin and Greek. In his later years, he studied Hebrew with a rabbi. Charles often heard him quote a favorite line from the Talmud: "Save one life, and save the world."

Antoinette had not been sleeping these last hours. She had not even changed into her nightclothes. She had been busy preparing four lists of clothing, toiletries, and sundries. In the morning she would ask the maids to ready four trunks. The first would furnish Charles with all that would be necessary for the two-week trip to Brazil to attend the Brazilian centennial. This trunk would include formal attire for shipboard dinners and centennial festivities, summer-weight touring clothes for sightseeing and business attire for state meetings. The second trunk was to be for Elizabeth, to supply her with all that she would need for her experimental treatment in Toronto, including the cornflower blue sweater that she had knitted while in Bermuda, film for her camera, stationery and her ever-expanding collection of books and scrapbooks. The third and fourth trunks would both be for her. One would prepare her to join her husband aboard the *Pan America;* the other would prepare her to accompany Elizabeth and Blanche to Toronto.

Antoinette stood at the door to her husband's study. "You say you cannot call a president or a prime minister. Well, I have another proposal."

Charles nodded. Antoinette took a deep breath.

"Insulin has been discovered by Dr. Frederick Banting at The University of Toronto," she began. "The University of Toronto received a million-dollar grant from the Rockefeller Foundation," she continued, studying her husband's impassive expression. "We attended the same church as the Rockefellers. You served on the board of trustees of the church with both John D. Rockefeller and John D. Rockefeller Jr. You started the Sunday school class that John D. Rockefeller Jr. now teaches."

"What of the impact on Elizabeth, years from now, knowing that her life had been spared at the expense of the life of another child?"

"Let Elizabeth live to grapple with that conflict." She argued. "Let Elizabeth choose." He shook his head. "God placed you in a position of influence." She persisted.

"Because God trusted me not to abuse it."

"God gave you legs, is using them unfair to the lame? Think of the parable of the talents. It's a sin *not* to use the gifts God provides. Please think about it."

"I will do nothing else *but* think about it."

Antoinette went back upstairs to the bedroom. It was now nearly dawn. She might still get an hour or two of sleep.

Apparently Charles had meant what he said quite literally. When she dressed and came down the stairs the next morning, he was still staring into the photographic image, where the rocking chair remained motionless and empty on the front porch, locked in silvery emulsion. In busy-ness was salvation, at least that had always been his credo. It unnerved her to see him so still for so long, lost in the deep whorls of his bright and terrible mind.

"Good morning," she said.

"Good morning," he said. "Aside from the meeting with Banting, do you have any other requirements that must be met before you are free to accompany me to Brazil on the twenty-fourth?"

"Yes," she said. "There must be some kind of two-way communication with Elizabeth while we are at sea. Morse code, radio telephone, wireless, carrier pigeon . . . something."

This seemed to him completely outlandish. Even the secretary of state could not speed the pace of technological advance. But he only bowed his head.

"Is there anything else?"

"No."

Charles Evans Hughes could not bring himself to call Rockefeller or

Harding or Mackenzie King. But that day he did call President Falconer. They had corresponded a few times after Falconer had tried to arrange for Hughes to speak at Toronto. Hughes sat and stared at the telephone for an entire hour before lifting the receiver. In one sense, it was a phone call. In another, it was a shattering breach of moral code, an act the person he was could not possibly, would not ever perform. Except for one thing: Antoinette had asked him to.

TWENTY-SEVEN

Escape from Morristown, August 1922

PRESIDENT FALCONER WAS IN A MEETING WITH COLONEL ALBERT Gooderham when the phone rang in the outer office. Gooderham was an intimidating character, with a dramatic mustache and a commanding voice, and heir to a family fortune. The Gooderham and Worts distillery, founded in 1832, was the largest distillery in the world, providing over two million gallons of Canadian whisky to the world market. One of Toronto's proudest architectural accomplishments bore the name Gooderham—the red-brick flatiron building built in 1892, ten years before the famous New York City landmark. It had been Gooderham who had donated the land on which the Connaught Antitoxin Laboratories were founded in 1915. He was a longstanding member of the board of governors of the University of Toronto, and throughout the city, the mere mention of his name was sufficient to capture attention.

So it was with grave trepidation that President Falconer's secretary dared to interrupt the meeting with Gooderham. The initial expressions on the faces of both Falconer and Gooderham confirmed that she had cause for hesitation. But when she said the words, "Secretary of State Charles Evans Hughes is on the phone for you, sir," the look of indignation that caused Gooderham's elaborately waxed mustache to quiver melted away. Falconer excused himself.

Hughes stated his request. Falconer was gracious and promised to do what he could to help. But it would prove trickier than he anticipated. First, Falconer started to call Macleod but realized that the last thing Macleod would want to do is help the secretary of state of the United States of America. Further, Banting would be unlikely to comply with any request made by Macleod. The same reason stilled his hand from phoning Duncan Graham. He did not relish making the request directly to Banting, imagining that Banting might go to the press with the story that the president of the University of Toronto was trying to tell him how to run his private practice after denying him one under the aegis of the university's teaching hospital.

So, he called Banting's political champion, Dr. Billy Ross, who was only too delighted to talk to Banting.

Banting was at first reluctant to bring in another American. After all, he had three American children as patients already. Further, he was naturally resistant to the idea of anyone using power to skip to the front of the line. He had already turned down Mrs. Hughes twice.

Ross reminded him of his new commitment to beat Macleod at his own game. For this he would need all the highly-placed allies he could get. Banting objected, saying that treating the secretary of state's daughter was only an advantage if he was successful, and that was hardly guaranteed. Neither was it guaranteed that once she began on insulin she would be able to continue. The insulin supply was erratic, and even when they could get it, the potency varied so much from batch to batch that it was hard to find the right dosage. There had already been one death at Toronto General Hospital for lack of insulin and plenty of accidental overdoses at the Christie Street Military Hospital. But Ross persisted. He asked Banting to consider what a Nobel Prize would mean to Canadians—*our first!*

Banting agreed to see Elizabeth, but only to examine her. He would make no promises to treat her or to supply insulin. Billy Ross helped him compose the letter to Antoinette in which he made it plain that he would see Elizabeth, but that she should not expect to receive insulin. On August 8, Ross took the letter with him when he left Bloor Street. He wanted to post it himself so that there would be no chance for Banting to have second thoughts.

A few days later, at two o'clock in the afternoon, Antoinette received Banting's letter.

★ ★ ★

Charles that day was at the State Department talking with Admiral Carl T. Vogelgesang, commander of the Third Naval District and the Brooklyn Navy Yard, who was scheduled to accompany him on the *Pan America*. Vogelgesang reported to Hughes that arrangements for two-way radio communication during the trip to Brazil had begun. Naval radio stations along the coast and in the West Indies had been notified to be on the alert for messages *from* the vessels. Messages *to* the vessels could be sent at certain hours through the navy's high-powered radio stations at Sayville, Long Island; Cayey, Porto Rico; and Balboa, Canal Zone. The battleships *Maryland* and *Nevada,* which would accompany the *Pan America,* would also copy the messages and relay them if necessary.

American press messages would be received direct aboard the ships each day of the trip, and special arrangements would be made with the navy for the newspaper correspondents on board to report to the world interesting bits of information about events aboard the ships.

Charles could hardly wait to report the good news to Antoinette that evening. Unfortunately, he would not have the chance. When he returned home after work, Antoinette was gone. Shortly after receiving the letter that Banting would see Elizabeth, she was on her way to New Jersey. She left a message for him at his office and asked him to send a telegram to Dr. Allen to let him know that Banting had agreed to see Elizabeth. The telegram failed to mention that Antoinette was on her way to New Jersey.

Not understanding the immediacy, Allen drafted a letter to Dr. Banting in support of his decision and considered how to arrange Elizabeth's transfer with the least disruption to her emotional and dietary well-being. On the following day, he would prepare a dossier of information for Dr. Banting about Elizabeth's medical history to accompany her to Toronto. Then he went to bed.

By the time Antoinette arrived at the Physiatric Institute, it was nearly midnight. As the taxi pulled into the driveway, the windows of the great mansion were dark. Antoinette gave the driver a twenty-dollar bill and asked him to wait and to keep the engine running. Then, not waiting to hear his reply, she bounded from the car and hurried up the broad alabaster steps. She pushed through the massive bronze door and walked briskly past the startled night guard, continuing through the silent halls and up the stairs. As Antoinette rounded the corner to Elizabeth's suite, she nearly tumbled into a nurse.

"Excuse me, madam!" the nurse began, but Antoinette entered the room where Elizabeth and Blanche were sleeping and turned on the light. The nurse followed her in.

"Visiting hours are over!"

"Mrs. Hughes?" Blanche squinted and sat up in bed.

"Mumsey!" Elizabeth chirped.

"Wake up, darling. Get dressed. It's time to go."

"Is everything all right?" Elizabeth asked.

"Yes, dear. Everything's fine. We're going on a trip."

"Do you have Dr. Allen's permission to take this patient off campus?"

"Chop-chop! There's a car waiting outside!"

The nurse hurried out of the room to summon Dr. Allen. Blanche pulled on the dress that was draped over the chair in the corner. Then she turned to help Elizabeth into her clothes.

"Where are we going?" Elizabeth asked brightly as Blanche pulled her arm through a sleeve.

Antoinette had found the suitcase under the bed and was moving clothes from the dresser to the suitcase.

"Where are we going, Mumsey?"

"Toronto, darling."

Just then Dr. Allen entered.

"What is the meaning of this?" he thundered.

"Good evening, Doctor," Antoinette replied, spinning to face him.

Blanche quickly finished packing the suitcase and snapped the latches shut. Then, quietly pulling the suitcase from the bed, she slipped as inconspicuously as possible out the door.

"Mrs. Hughes, I'm afraid I cannot allow you to take Elizabeth from this room—not like this, not in the middle of the night!" Allen positioned himself in front of the door.

"Excuse us." Antoinette interrupted the doctor as she guided Elizabeth toward the door. "We've a long trip ahead and no time to spare."

Antoinette now stood nose to nose with Allen.

"This is my institute!" he snapped.

"This is my daughter!" she rejoined.

"Do you think that being Mrs. Charles Evans Hughes gives you any authority in my hospital?"

"I am her mother! Now please, step aside!"

In that moment, Dr. Allen realized that he could no more stand in the way of Antoinette Hughes than he could stand in the way of progress. It was only a matter of time before insulin would take all of his patients from the institute. The magnificent breakthrough that he had so long predicted would come *had* come. It would be his ruin.

Allen stepped aside.

Antoinette swept past him and hurried Elizabeth around the corner, through the corridor and down the stairs. Outside, the night air was charged with an exultant chorus of crickets and peepers. The engine of the waiting taxi purred in the darkness. The driver slammed the trunk on Elizabeth's suitcase and settled behind the wheel. Antoinette ordered the driver to take them to Grand Central Terminal in Manhattan. Blanche was already seated in the front seat; Antoinette and Elizabeth snuggled into the backseat together. As the car pulled around the curve of the driveway, Blanche, Elizabeth, and Antoinette looked back at the behemoth structure, as if they sensed somehow that they would never return—or hoped so anyway.

In the back of the taxi, Antoinette was quietly trembling at what she had just done. But just as she thought she might lose her ironclad composure, something outside the car window caught her eye. It was a light in the deep and distant darkness beside the mansion, like a single glowing ember in the ashes of a spent fire.

"What is that light?" she asked.

"That's the groundskeeper's cottage," Elizabeth answered.

She thought of the old man's kindness and his remarkable ability to fix anything mechanical or wooden just by turning it in his gnarled hands. She remembered how he fixed up the birdcage for Eddie's canary and was sorry not to have said goodbye to him. But Elizabeth had no time for sad thoughts now. She was on her way to a city she had not visited, to a facility she knew nothing about, to be treated by a doctor she had never met.

TWENTY-EIGHT

The Transformation Begins, Toronto, August to November 1922

ON AUGUST 15, 1922, ANTOINETTE, ELIZABETH, AND BLANCHE arrived in Toronto and rented a large apartment in the Athelma Apartments on Grosvenor Street. The next morning, the trio left the apartment by taxi to go to Banting's office on Bloor Street West, where he would examine her. There had been quite a bit of talk about Dr. Banting and his amazing discovery among the staff at the Physiatric Institute and, of course, Elizabeth and Blanche had read the news articles, so on this morning Elizabeth's spirits were high. She had always harbored a special fascination with meeting people of note and she was eager to meet a bona fide scientific genius. But despite her optimism Elizabeth was so weak she could hardly walk. Still, she was determined to greet Dr. Banting on her own two feet. Supported by Blanche, she shuffled from the door of the taxi, up the stoop steps to the door of the office, a laborious process closely watched from the windows of 160 Bloor Street West by several patients in the waiting room and by Dr. Fred Hipwell, Banting's cousin and classmate, who now shared the office with him.

Banting invited Elizabeth, Antoinette, and Blanche into the examination room. He was quite a bit younger and rougher than Antoinette expected. His hair was badly cut (she thought perhaps he'd done it himself). He was wearing a poorly made suit that appeared to have never encountered an iron in its long, adventurous life. When Banting extended his large bear paw of a hand to Antoinette, she was surprised to find it curiously rough for someone in his profession. She could not help but wonder if the whole desperate endeavor was for naught. Could this disheveled character possibly save Elizabeth's life? Could she actually leave her daughter in his care?

Elizabeth's first impression of Banting was entirely different from that of her mother. What Elizabeth saw and heard was the walking, talking opposite of everything that was Dr. Allen. She couldn't have been more delighted by or more curious about him if he had had a tail and spoke in rhyme.

Banting left while Elizabeth changed into a hospital smock for the examination. Returning, he weighed and measured her. He looked into her eyes, nose, ears, and mouth. He examined her fingers and toes. He checked her reflexes by tapping on her knees and ankles with a triangular rubber hammer. He palpated the glands in her neck and armpits. He took the following notes: "Height five feet. Weight forty-five pounds. Emaciated. Skin dry. Slight edema of ankles. Hair brittle and thin. Abdomen prominent. Marked weakness."

"Does it hurt when I press here?" he asked.

"No," she replied.

"Here?"

"No. Do you mind if I ask you how old you are, Dr. Banting?"

"I'm thirty."

"That's exactly twice my age, or it will be in four days when I turn fifteen. Are you married?"

"No. Are you?"

"Oh yes," she replied, trying to sound nonchalant. "I've been married several times."

He looked at her. She looked at him. They both broke out into identical, simultaneous grins. Antoinette shook her head and Blanche tried to hide a smile by looking into her lap.

"Do you like animals?"

"Very much. I grew up on a farm."

"Is that your farm?" Elizabeth indicated a partly finished oil painting on the desk.

"Why, yes, as a matter of fact it is."

"Did you paint it?"

"This is the first examination I've ever conducted where the patient asks more questions about me than I ask about the patient!" Banting turned away to prepare a syringe. "Okay with you if I draw some blood?"

Elizabeth held out her arms, allowing him to choose. In 1922 blood sugar analysis was time consuming and inaccurate. It also required up to 20 mL of blood.

"Aren't you going to say, 'This might pinch a little bit'? I thought they teach you to say that in medical school."

"Not in Canadian medical school." Banting smirked. He was charmed.

"What's your favorite animal?" she asked, trying to distract herself from the sight of her blood filling the syringe.

"The dog, I guess. Sometimes I think I get along better with animals than I do with people."

"Well, I like you pretty well so far."

"Well, I like you, too. So far."

Banting dragged the chair from the desk over to the examination table. He turned it around and sat on it backward, resting his arms over the back. He looked seriously at Elizabeth.

"How do you feel generally?"

"Hungry."

"Besides that."

"Thirsty."

"How long have you felt this way?"

"Three years and nine months." Elizabeth turned serious for the first time during the examination.

"You look sick but you don't act sick. Why is that?"

Elizabeth took a deep breath and leveled her gaze at the young doctor.

"Dr. Banting, have you ever known something, just known it in your bones? And even though everything may seem to point to the opposite, you still know it's true?"

"As a matter of fact I have."

"Really?"

"Truly."

"Well, I know that I'm going to get better. Do you believe me?"

"Yes, I do."

"Really?"

Banting nodded solemnly.

"Then you're the first one ever."

"The only question I have is when would you like to start getting better," he said.

"Of all the questions of all the doctors I've seen, no one has ever asked me that."

He stood up and returned the chair to the desk. "How do you feel about shots?"

"Will they make me well?"

"Yes, I think they will."

"Then I'm crazy about them."

Banting pulled a string from around his neck on which there was a key. He bent to a locked cabinet in the corner of the room and opened the cabinet door. Elizabeth could see now that it was a kind of icebox and that there was nothing inside but two small brown glass vials. She watched him closely.

"Is that insulin?" she whispered.

"Yes," he whispered back. He swabbed her thigh with alcohol.

She watched him fill the syringe.

Just before he injected her he asked, "Will you promise me one thing, Miss Elizabeth Hughes? Will you promise me that if you get well—when you get well—you will grow up to be whoever and whatever you want to be and you won't let anyone persuade you to do or be something or someone else?"

Elizabeth must have sensed what it had cost Banting to become who he was, what it had cost him to carry the idea of insulin against seemingly impossible odds, repeated failure, and constant debt and doubt, all the way to the office in which they sat now. Or perhaps she had caught a glimpse of a profound loneliness behind his eyes. In any case, she nodded solemnly, just before the needle pierced her meager hip. She flinched but did not look away as Banting squeezed the plunger, pressing the murky beige extract into her flesh. Neither Banting nor Elizabeth spoke. Then Banting turned away to discard the empty vial.

"Wait!" Elizabeth's voice broke the silence. "May I keep it?"

"The vial?"

"Yes."

That, too, was a first for Banting. He placed the vial gently in her palm. She closed her fingers around it.

★ ★ ★

That same day, Dr. Allen wrote a letter to Banting.

> *I take pleasure in informing you that our first results with your pancre-atic extract have been marvelously good. We have cleared up both sugar and acetone in some of the most hopelessly severe cases of diabetes that I have ever seen. No bad results have been encountered either generally or locally. We have been able to increase diets, and already an effect seems evident in the form of increased strength. I am making all observations on an experimental as well as therapeutic basis, and only wish that we could have several times as much extract as is available just now. You deserve all congratulations, but as you will receive them so abundantly, I need not express myself at length now. Unless notified by you to the contrary, I shall include your name in the list of editors in the next issue of* The Journal of Metabolic Research, *to appear probably within two or three weeks from date.*

That afternoon Banting had lunch with D. E. Robertson at the university's faculty club. When Banting told him about the happy events of the morning, Robertson blanched and asked Banting if the suit he was wearing was the same suit he had worn to meet Mrs. Hughes.

"I only own one," Banting replied.

"What are you doing after lunch?"

"Nothing right away," Banting shrugged. "I have patients later this afternoon. Why?"

After lunch, Robertson took Banting to the most exclusive tailor in Toronto to be fitted for a suit and overcoat. Banting complained about the expense and protested that "no one ever had a good idea in a dress suit," but Robertson prevailed. He could see that Banting would soon be meeting with dignitaries and representing Canada to the world. The elder man took it upon himself to provide Banting with a good suit and some basic manners.

Elizabeth responded well to the insulin; no reactions developed either at the injection site or elsewhere. Banting had assumed that Antoinette would remain in Toronto for a while, as had been the case with all of his other patients. But after just a few days, Antoinette informed him that both she and her husband would be at sea for most of the next four weeks. Antoinette left Blanche a considerable sum of money for "expenses," which presumably might include the transportation and burial of Elizabeth's body in the Hughes family plot at Woodlawn Cemetery.

On August 18, 1922, George B. Schley, the patent attorney for Eli Lilly and Company, happened to see a short newspaper article reporting that the daughter of the U.S. secretary of state was in Toronto taking insulin for diabetes. It described Dr. Frederick G. Banting as the *original inventor* of insulin. This detail alarmed Mr. Schley, who was aware that the Toronto team had drafted two patent applications: the first, a process application, by Best and Collip, and second, a product application, by Best alone. In neither of these applications did the name of Banting appear as inventor.

On August 22, 1922, Schley wrote a very stern letter to Clowes informing him that the law required that a patent application be filed by the actual inventor or inventors. If the patent is applied for by one who is not the inventor, the patent is absolutely void if that fact is found by a court. Furthermore, there was a real danger of criminal prosecution for perjury should it be shown that Best or Collip had misrepresented himself as the sole inventor(s) of the product and process when in fact both knew that Banting was the original inventor, or at least a coinventor.

At first, Banting dismissed the matter, but when he heard about the possibility of criminal charges against Best, he changed his mind. The name Banting was added to the two U.S. patent applications and to those for the United Kingdom, Europe, and the rest of the world.

On August 21, 1922, the diabetic clinic at Toronto General Hospital finally opened. Through the summer and fall of 1922 its patients were sustained largely with Lilly's help because of Connaught's sporadic output. The insulin directed to Banting's patients in Toronto, including those at Toronto General Hospital under Banting's care, was provided at no cost to patients.

Elizabeth took insulin twice daily, fifteen to thirty minutes before her morning and evening meals. Each specimen of her urine was tested, and when sugar appeared, her dosage was slightly increased. Banting visited her at the Athelma Apartments each day at 5:30 in the afternoon, bringing with him her evening dose of insulin. During this period of dose testing and regulation, her caloric intake was also steadily increased, and so there ensued a precarious simultaneous balancing of an increased insulin dose to match the increased calories. A failure to balance these produced two risks, either potentially fatal.

Before 1922, hyperglycemic coma, induced by total lack of or insufficient insulin, accounted for 86 percent of the mortality of diabetic children; after insulin, from 1922 to 1936 the mortality rate of diabetic children from hyperglycemic coma declined, but was still 56 percent. The first diabetic "resurrected" from a hyperglycemic coma by the injection of insulin was eleven-year-old Elsie Needham, at the Hospital for Sick Children in Toronto in October 1922.

The introduction of insulin saved diabetics from hyperglycemic coma, but it also introduced a second type of coma—*hypo*glycemic coma. Diabetic children were more susceptible than diabetic adults to hypoglycemic coma. Soon after the discovery of insulin, the need to control the dosage became apparent.

Too much insulin drives the blood sugar down to dangerous levels; hypoglycemia occurs when it falls below 60 milligrams of sugar per deciliter. (An average person's blood sugar is 80 to 120 milligrams of sugar per deciliter of blood.) The symptoms of too little sugar in the blood, which involve the autonomic and central nervous systems, include numbness and tingling, rapid heartbeat, trembling, weakness, sweating, pallor, and nausea. These symptoms are often accompanied by confusion or stupor, which can prevent the diabetic from taking the simple steps necessary to save himself—most important, a quick dose of sugar. If not treated, hypoglycemia can lead to seizures and coma.

Elizabeth called these hypoglycemic episodes "the feels," and she often had them, sometimes three episodes a day. To prevent Elizabeth from lapsing into shock during the night while she was asleep, Blanche and Elizabeth shared a bed in hope that Blanche could better detect and respond to a nighttime attack of "the feels." In those early months of experimental insulin, Blanche saved Elizabeth's life dozens of times by reviving her with orange juice or a molasses kiss during the night.

And there arose other problems with the miracle cure. Protein impurities caused abscesses in many patients and salts in the solution made injections painful. Elizabeth's hips and thighs were soon upholstered with egg-shaped welts. The new ones were purple, the older ones were green fading to yellow. Banting had taught Blanche to administer the injections using this color-coded pattern of wounds to guide where to place the next injection. When the insulin was weak, the injections were necessarily large. In October the only insulin available was so weak that Elizabeth had to take 5 cc at a time. Her syringe held only 2 cc. So Blanche filled the syringe and injected 2 cc, then unscrewed the glass barrel from the needle, which she left sticking into Elizabeth's hip, filled the syringe again and screwed it to the needle, and injected the insulin into Elizabeth, and then unscrewed the syringe one final time and repeated the process for the final cc. The whole procedure required about twenty minutes, and in this time Elizabeth's hip swelled and her whole leg became numb. It took about an hour of careful walking on it for the sensation to return, but it was worth the trouble if it allowed her to eat real food again.

Both Elizabeth and Blanche were compelled to acquire a thorough understanding of sterile injection and urinalysis procedure. For the rest of her life Elizabeth would need to have with her certain necessary equipment. For injection of insulin she would need two syringes, two rustless 3/8-inch, 25-gauge hypodermic needles, a supply of insulin, a small covered pan for sterilization, clean cotton and rubbing alcohol, and a sponge and cleanser for cleaning her needles. For urinalysis she would need a supply of Benedict's solution, two test tubes, one eyedropper, a teaspoon, an open-mouth bottle for urine, and an aluminum cup. All of this was in addition to the meticulous charts that detailed her caloric intake, exercise, insulin reactions, and urine readings, which she was still required to keep. As Frederick Allen said, insulin *improved* but did not *simplify* the treatment of diabetes.

Problems with the potency of the extract threatened her recovery. One shipment of insulin from Lilly had proved to be very unsatisfactory, and Banting had given doses as high as 15 cc a day to Joe Gilchrist with very little effect. If no effective insulin could be obtained Elizabeth and the other diabetics would be forced to return to fasting and the Allen diet. On August 21, Dr. Banting visited at his usual time of 5:30 P.M. to tell Elizabeth that Connaught was about to produce its first substantial batch of truly potent insulin. It was so potent that she would only have to take one cc at a time. He said that she would soon be on a diet of 2,240 calories, like a normal girl.

Banting was not nearly as cautious about the process of increasing the caloric intake of his patients as was Allen, and Elizabeth was soon experimenting with previously forbidden foodstuffs such as cereal, bread, potatoes, and rice. In this once forbidden domain of food, revelation followed revelation on a near daily basis. Elizabeth described it as "unspeakably wonderful."

On August 25, she ate a piece of white bread for the first time in three and a half years.

On August 29, she ate corn for the first time in three and a half years.

On September 7, she ate macaroni and cheese for the first time in three and a half years.

On September 13, she ate grapes for the first time in three and a half years.

On September 21, she ate bananas.

On September 22, she ate plums.

In Rochester, New York, James Havens had a similarly ecstatic reaction. He wrote to Banting: "A week ago last Thursday . . . marked an historical event as I then tasted my first egg on toast. Egg on toast is my idea of the only food necessary in heaven. Moreover if they don't pass out at least that much rations up there I guess I prefer the other place."

Banting encouraged Elizabeth to eat unreservedly. For breakfast she ate peaches, three-quarters of a shredded wheat biscuit with cream, an omelet with an ounce of butter, some bacon, some cream cheese, and a big slice of toast. For lunch she ate meat, a hot vegetable, celery or tomatoes, and a large serving of custard for dessert. For supper she might have cold roast beef and potato salad and eggplant, celery with lots of butter, cocoa, saltines with cream cheese, junket pudding with fruit, and a big bunch of grapes.

Although Elizabeth could not send letters to her mother in Brazil, she had promised Colonel Swalm that she would maintain the exercise of writing every day and so she continued to write to her mother and to her sister, Catherine, and brother, Charlie, too.

No body up here except Dr. Banting of course knows what a big diet I'm on and the foods I'm eating on it either, and I know if they did know

they'd nearly roll off their seats. It's our great big secret! [Her diet con-
sisted of 2512 calories.] I could use up pages just in innummerating [sic]
all the dishes I have nowadays and it seems to me that I eat something
everyday that I haven't tasted for over three years, and you don't know
how good it seems and how I appreciate every morsel I eat.

At this time there was happy, if slightly mysterious, news for Blanche
too. As Elizabeth wrote to her mother:

I suppose you've heard either from Catherine or Charlie of Dr. Mc-
Clintock's appearance and how he accompanys [sic] us on all our picnics
and comes up to see Blanche every night. . . . I'm simply positive they
must be engaged for they call each other "dear" and do other very signifi-
cant things, but Blanche won't vouchsafe anything to me as yet. Isn't it
queer? I'm glad I know him as well as I do though, for he really is wor-
thy of her in my opinion now, although what he does is beyond me. He
seems to have plenty of money so as not to have to work, yet if he has
why don't they get married. Well it's a mystery as I say, and yet it strikes
me very funny too, doesn't it you?

As Elizabeth gained strength, she and Blanche often spent afternoons in
Queen's Park reading and walking the lovely footpaths of the campus
and the city, always accompanied by the enigmatic Dr. McClintock. In
October, she wrote:

Yesterday afternoon I had an awfully good time going over to the library
here on College St. and reading while Blanche and the Dr. took a walk.
I love to do that and in that way I can almost read in one afternoon one
of the short books that really wouldn't be worthwhile to take out on my
card. Yesterday I read and almost finished Hudson's charming book of
tales of the Pampas land and it was great, the way all his books are. . . .
It certainly is one of the best librarys [sic] I've ever been to, and they
have the nicest, cleanest books as well as almost all the latest ones. I was
astounded the other day in looking up, to gaze on a book called, "Charles
E. Hughes." Jurist and Statesman [sic], which I had never seen or
heard of before, and which I immediately took down and perused. It's

very interesting being of his law cases and how he handled them on the Supreme Court. I suppose you know all about it but it was news to me.

And a few days later:

Blanche is going to let me tell just you and Catherine the exciting news she told me the other day in the most casual manner ever, which I have been expecting and waiting for, for months now, and that is that she really is engaged to Dr. McClintock. She is most secretive about it as usual, and all I can get out of her is that they will be married sometime in the near future and are going to live way out in California. I am so glad for her, for she will be simply adorable as a wife and mother, and I am sure now that he is worthy of her, after having seen him everyday for two months. Upon first meeting him I know you would not think it at all, but upon knowing him well and after drawing him out he's perfectly adorable and so full of fun. He has a great sense of humor just like us, and the games he thinks up for us to play evenings here are lots of fun. I really have enjoyed his being here every day a lot, and accompanying us on all our picnics, etc. He is leaving Monday evening on the seven P.M. train. I know you'll be very much interested in all this, and that's why I wanted to prepare you for it before you came up. I was positive of it all the time. She couldn't have had all the various symtons [sic] of it and not have the malady.

Newspapers reported on Elizabeth's miraculous recovery, and not always entirely accurately:

NEW TREATMENT AIDS MISS HUGHES
Daughter of Secretary of State Improves Under Canadian Specialist's Discovery
Gains Sixteen Pounds
After Transfusions Diabetic Sufferer is Now Permitted Nearly Normal Diet

PERMANENTLY CURED BY INSULIN TREATMENT
Mr. Hughes' Daughter Treated Here a Year Ago—Fear No Return of Diabetes

NEW YORK EXCITED OVER NEW CURE
FOR DIABETES

Discovery of Dr. Banting of Toronto is
Discussed in American Press

Public Interested

Treatment of Miss Hughes Focuses Attention of America
on Toronto Experiments

LITTLE DAUGHTER OF HUGHES SEEMINGLY
CURED OF DIABETES BY SERUM
TAKEN FROM FISH

Banting said that Elizabeth was his "record case." She was gaining roughly two pounds per week. "You'd think it was a fairy tale," she said. She could hardly wait for her parents to see the transformation in her appearance. But she was irritated at the publicity. "I hate to be written up like that all over the country and I think it's cheapening to the discovery. Poor Dr. Banting's even gotten to the place where doctors are beginning to kid him about advertising his discovery through me. Isn't that perfectly horrid, though?"

Elizabeth had begun to receive letters from desperate diabetics who had read about her. At first she tried to reply to them all, but she soon felt burdened by them. "With your letter this morning came two more letters from poor diabetics which I suppose I've got to answer. The poor things. I feel so sorry for them."

She had no interest whatsoever in becoming a poster child for insulin: In fact, she had already begun to think of herself as a *non*diabetic.

Yesterday morning we were called on the telephone by this lovely lady, Mrs. Ferris who had Diabetes and wanted to know about the effect of the treatment on me and something about it and she couldn't find Dr. Banting and had read of my case in the New York papers. She said she was only going to be here until the late afternoon as she was with a party who were leaving then. They had been touring the US and the other member of this party were Sir Charles and Lady Wakefield and Sir Arthur and Lady Halmsworth . . . she came up to see us for a while and we told her all we could for she seemed very nice. It seems that she's had this since 1914 very mildly, but through great carelessness in han-

dling her diet she has now become quite a severe case I guess. She has no idea at all how to take care of her diet not knowing even what calories and carbohydrates meant so I don't see how she can be getting along very well. And I don't see how she could manage this treatment at all. She must be showing sugar all the time and has two diabetic carbuncles on her hands. Now you only get those you know from showing sugar constantly so that's the reason why she had them. Well we did all we could for the poor ignorant lady and she left hoping to come in touch with Dr. Banting sometime during the day. Well the poor thing must've passed him going down in the elevator and not known it, for immediately after she left, Dr. Banting appeared. . . . Wasn't that the perversity of fate though. . . . We have had several poor people come here to ask about the treatment and they were eventually all turned away. Its [sic] makes you feel so sorry and yet you can't do a thing about it. I can't get over how fortunate I was to get in up here.

This was not at all her idea of what life would be after Toronto. Instead, she imagined herself returning to Washington and to school and leading a completely normal life, which she hoped would commence before the end of the year. She intended to put the past forty months so completely out of her consciousness that it would be as if they had never happened at all. The only thing that was stopping her was that she had promised Dr. Banting that she would not leave Toronto until a meeting of clinicians could be arranged. At this meeting, she would be the main attraction. The meeting was scheduled for November 25. Elizabeth and Blanche planned to leave Toronto on December 1—each to begin a new life. Blanche was to marry Dr. McClintock and move to California and Elizabeth would begin an ostensibly nondiabetic life in Washington. Only one of these scenarios would come to pass.

TWENTY-NINE

Crossing the Line Aboard the SS Pan America,
August to September 1922

On Monday, August 21, 1922, Hughes began to organize the affairs of the State Department in preparation for Under Secretary William Phillips to assume the role of acting secretary of state during the month that Hughes would be away. He canceled all but the most pressing engagements for Monday and Tuesday in order to devote himself fully to the transfer of responsibilities. He planned to leave with Antoinette for New York on Wednesday morning and the following day depart for Brazil.

Having cleared his calendar, he now set out to clear his desk of pressing business. As the hours ticked by and the need for efficiency pressed down upon him, Hughes found himself slowing down and distractedly staring out the window. He watched clouds sail through the rectangular panes of his office window like aerial brigantines bound for planets as yet undiscovered. His famously focused mind wandered.

He had asked his staff not to disturb him and, obligingly, they did not. But as Monday morning wore on into afternoon, they began to be concerned. They bustled about the outer office wondering why he had not summoned them. At last, Under Secretary Phillips tapped on Hughes's door to ask if there was anything he needed. There was Hughes, sitting at his desk wearing an inscrutable expression. His inbox was just as full as it had been that morning, his outbox empty.

When Antoinette returned from Toronto, she saw that something about Charles had changed. The haberdashery in which he was packaged was as trim and pressed as always, but some aspect of his psychological architecture had slumped inward. The man who Supreme Court Justice Robert H. Jackson said "looks like God and talks like God" appeared to Antoinette distinctly more mortal than the last time she had seen him. The cost of the intervention was considerable, as she knew it would be. There was a vagueness in his gaze that she had seldom seen before. He had lost an important compass point on the map of his selfhood. Now she must try to help him get it back.

On Thursday, August 24, 1922, shortly before four o'clock in the afternoon, Charles was to meet Admiral Carl T. Vogelgesang at the Twenty-third Street Ferry in Manhattan. From there they would make the brief crossing to Hoboken, where the *Pan America* would depart from Pier 1 for Rio de Janeiro. And so, at four o'clock, a great crowd of dignitaries, journalists, and interested citizens gathered to catch a glimpse of the inimitable Charles Evans Hughes and witness the historic departure of the *Pan America*.

Ambassador Allencar of Brazil, Consul General Lobo of New York, and the entire staff of the New York Brazilian consulate were at the pier awaiting the arrival of the secretary of state. On the deck of the ship, the members of the Brazilian centennial delegation gathered. Representative Stephen G. Porter, Major General Robert L. Bullard, and Justice Edward R. Finch of the Supreme Court of New York stood at the railing in their dress uniforms and their fine summer suits and accommodated reporters with waves and countless poses. Admiral Hilary P. Jones was so resplendent in his full-dress uniform that he resembled a richly upholstered chair. His belted double-breasted coat reached to his knees and was embellished with enormous, domed gold buttons, six inches of thick gold braid encircling each cuff, and richly fringed epaulettes on his shoulders.

An hour crept by. The *Pan America* sat at the dock in Hoboken. Hughes did not arrive.

At five o'clock the sky was still bright, but the heat had subsided as the summer shadows reached for the eastern horizon. The crowd grew restless, then indignant, then concerned.

In an attempt to quell the unrest, Captain George Rose stood up before the well-dressed crowd on the deck and asked if they might be interested in learning something about the *Pan America*. It was a new steamship, he said, launched just the previous February. She had initially been called the *Palmetto State*. This was to be her fourth voyage to South America. Her crew numbered 220 men, some of whom had been standing at attention on deck for the better part of two hours.

The voyage to Rio de Janeiro, Captain Rose continued, desperately trying to think of things to say, would take roughly eleven days. After that the *Pan America* would proceed to Montevideo and Buenos Aires and the Hughes delegation would return to New York aboard the battleship *Maryland*.

Several members of the delegation began to quietly speculate about what could be keeping the secretary. Some wondered if there had been bad news about the daughter whose precarious health had been described in the newspaper. And then, of course, it might well be that Hughes, like Wilson, had simply collapsed. In this last speculation, they were not far wrong.

At 5:25 Captain Rose directed the band on the deck to play "The Star-Spangled Banner" and the "Hino Nacional Brasileiro" (the Brazilian national anthem) for the third time. The crowd of spectators began to thin.

At 5:40 P.M., Charles Evans Hughes threaded his way through the knot of spectators on the pier and shuffled up the red carpet that had been laid over the gangplank. He was met by Admiral Vogelgesang, to whom he muttered something about being unable to dispose of the crushing "accumulation of business" in time for the scheduled departure. The ship finally left two hours late, at six o'clock. Tugboats, ferries, and small boats in the harbor whistled a cacophonous farewell salute. Hughes told reporters that he hoped to obtain as much rest as possible during the voyage. Then he and Antoinette excused themselves and retired to their cabin.

Secretary Hughes and his party occupied the entire promenade deck of the 518-foot-long, 72-foot beam steamer. Charles and Antoinette's suite consisted of a bedroom, dressing room and bath, dining room, and parlor. The other cabins were to be occupied by Representative Porter; General Bullard representing the army; Admiral Vogelgesang, several secretaries and aides, and Mrs. Jones, wife of Admiral Jones, who was in command of the *Maryland*, one of the two battleships accompanying the *Pan America* on its mission of peace. During the first day at sea neither Charles nor Antoinette left their suite once.

There were five thousand miles of reseda sea between New York and Rio de Janeiro. In Toronto, Elizabeth spread out the pages of *The New York Times* each day and followed every mile of her parents' journey.

Hughes had mastered the art of using the press to communicate with members of his family, particularly Elizabeth, whose condition required her to be away from home for long periods of time. He knew that wherever she was she would be reading the newspapers. Never was this system more in evidence than during August 1922.

During this journey, the printed word would not be the only form of communication. Even before the journey began, the Naval Communications Service had made "elaborate arrangements" to ensure radio communication with Secretary Hughes every single day of his voyage to and from South America. Although world peace continued to be precarious, it was not the radio dispatches related to official state business that the Hugheses awaited with dread; it was bad news from Toronto.

Two days after the *Pan America* set sail there was a knock at the cabin door at nine o'clock at night. Antoinette opened it to reveal a steward with a grim expression and a wireless message in his hand.

"For Secretary Hughes," he said. She reached for the envelope. "I'm afraid it's bad news."

Antoinette skittered away from the door and into the bedchamber. Hughes stepped forward and took the envelope from the steward and closed the door. He paused for a moment before reading the message, listening to the muffled sobs from behind the bedroom door. Charles read the words of the wireless message.

Albert W. Swalm, American consul at Bermuda, had died on August 24.

Charles showed the message to Antoinette, who stared at it uncomprehendingly. Supporting each other, they silently made their way to the upper deck and stood at the railing beneath the darkening dome of cobalt sky that stretched in all directions. The *Pan America* and her escort ships had been under sail for more than one thousand miles and had not seen a single ship since leaving New York. Everything seemed to be moving too fast and too slow at the same time. Antoinette turned to the old man beside her. He was not old yesterday. He patted her hand.

"I fear I am not the man you married, my dear."

Antoinette began to protest, but he silenced her with a queer expression that was both intimate and distant at the same time. His lips were pressed close in a tight little smile, but his eyes swam with profound sadness. Charles now understood something that Elizabeth had learned through her years of trial—that the purpose of living is not to *preserve* life but to *lose* it. Living is by necessity a process of continuous loss. As we live we lose time, we lose innocence, we lose family and friends, we lose memories, and the longer we live, the more we lose. Ultimately, we lose the process of losing itself. Accepting this, Charles was free. He was no longer a standard-bearer; he was a man. Antoinette's request on Elizabeth's behalf had released Charles to become more fully human than he had ever dared to be. In a sense, Elizabeth and Charles had saved each other's lives, and Antoinette was the catalyst.

He had crossed the line from his head to his heart, and through that trespass, Elizabeth crossed from dying to living. In all the remaining years of his life, he was never again referred to as a human icicle, a bearded iceberg, a mental machine. Elizabeth began transforming herself into a nondiabetic, a transformation that would last for sixty years.

On September 1, as the *Pan America* approached the equator, the crew busied themselves with preparing for the traditional ceremony of "crossing the line." This initiation rite began on naval ships to commemorate a sailor's first crossing of the equator. While the original military form resembled a two-day hazing, a much more polite version of the ceremony continued on cruise ships as a form of entertainment. Those passengers who had already crossed the equator were called Sons of Neptune.

A bulletin issued to members of the Hughes delegation explained that according to tradition, on the evening before the equatorial crossing, the uninitiated (the "Pollywogs") stage a "revolt" involving high jinks and revelry, often at the expense of the Sons of Neptune (the "Shellbacks"). After crossing the line, the uninitiated would be issued subpoenas and "tried" in the court of Neptune. King Neptune, it was rumored, had been eagerly awaiting the arrival of the American mission.

Hughes and members of his delegation were tried for numerous crimes and misdemeanors. Representative Porter was convicted of perjury for claiming to have previously crossed the equator. The charges against Hughes included "undermining the prestige of Neptune by scrapping battleships." The Associated Press headline on September 1 read "Hughes Pleads Guilty in Neptune's Court/Charged With Boisterous Conduct, Loud Laughter and Antique Jokes."

The secretary pleaded guilty to all counts against him. However, in his defense he pointed out that Neptune now ruled over a kingdom of peace rather than over a kingdom of war. The ceremony completed, each new initiate was declared to be a Son of Neptune.

While Hughes had previously hardly left the cabin, he now rarely entered it. He participated in deck sports. He entertained his fellow travelers with humorous stories and political commentary, staying up well into the night to do so. Even the reporters appeared flummoxed by his sudden transformation. One newspaper recounted his strange behavior as follows, "One never can judge all the possibilities of a man's nature by the way he appears in public and we see that Secretary Hughes had been acting like a regular cut-up on the way down to Brazil."

He had most certainly crossed a kind of personal equator and, once he had crossed, he could not or would not retreat. Once a Son of Neptune, always a Son of Neptune.

In Toronto, Banting continued to be besieged with letters very much like the one from Antoinette. Allen tried to help deflect some of the attention by sending a letter to all of his patients in September of 1922.

> *Every effort is being made by the discoverers and manufacturers to improve the process and increase the output. Dr. Banting in Toronto is overwhelmed with requests from patients whom he cannot treat or furnish with extract. He is devoting himself to experimental trials upon a few desperately severe cases and has generously shared the small supply with a few specialists who can aid in determining the value and the best method of use of the extract. . . . The small present supply of this Institute is being used for treatment of a few cases of the greatest severity.*

Nothing Allen could say could stem the storm of interest. By September 1922, one hundred or more units of insulin were distributed weekly to ten clinicians for human trial, and each of them could have easily made use of double the amount.

For her part, Elizabeth was canoeing in the little pond in Toronto's Hyde Park. She was tooling around town in Dr. Banting's new car. She was going to plays and concerts and exploring the city. But mostly she was eating. She gained so much weight that she had to add a link to her watchband. She was not the same girl Antoinette had left in Toronto a month before. Just as Elizabeth was returning, day by day, meal by meal, and pound by pound to the normal world, she knew from the newspaper that her parents had begun their journey back to the United States aboard the *Maryland*. She also knew that the Charles Evans Hughes who was returning was not the Charles Evans Hughes who had sailed to Brazil.

Among the items Elizabeth inherited from her father after his death were two medallions, each in a velvet-covered box. One was hexagonal, copper and 5-1/2 inches across. On its face was a bas-relief of an eagle surmounting a shield. The words "U.S.S. MARYLAND" were engraved above crossed anchors and "Rio de Janeiro to New York 9-12-22—9-23-22. Charles E. Hughes, Secretary of State U.S.A." The second medallion was round, gold and 2-3/8 inches across. It bore the inscription: "CENTENNIAL OF BRAZILIAN INDEPENDENCE." For Charles and Elizabeth these coins symbolized a much more metaphysical passage than that described by the words engraved in the metal. Unlike the obols that the ancient Greeks paid to Charon to cross from the land of the living to the land of the dead, these coins were symbols of new life for both father and daughter.

THIRTY

Fate, Fortune, and Forgetting, September to December 1922

IN THE SPRING OF 1922, FATE CONSPIRED TO ASSEMBLE A MOST UN-
likely team of four men in Toronto. For six uneasy months the four
collaborated and competed with one another. Shortly after these individual trajectories converged in Toronto to make medical history, another, broader convergence began. Hundreds of desperate and dying
diabetics flocked to the city from all over Canada and the United States.
And then, just as abruptly as these twin convergences began, they dissipated. By late September, many of the diabetic American children who
had made the near hopeless pilgrimage to Toronto to be treated started
to return home to begin the adventure of a normal childhood. Ruth
Whitehill, Myra Blaustein, and Teddy Ryder were among them.

Despite these remarkable stories, all was not well. The bitter dissension over who should receive credit for the discovery began to spread
beyond the immediate group to infect esteemed members of Toronto's
academic, political, and medical communities. Through their colleagues
and contacts, the rancor spread throughout the world. Sir William Bayliss of University College in London defended Macleod in *The Times*. In
Toronto, Billy Ross made sure that the name of Banting was at the top
of everyone's mind. Long-term friendships were sundered over the question of whom to support.

The University's patent attorney, C. H. Riches, pressed for an official, unified account of the discovery. The board of governors realized

that, sooner or later, the university would be asked for the official story of the discovery and, much to their embarrassment, they didn't have one. Their position thus far had been to ignore the problem and hope that it would be resolved among the participants. It was now clear that this had been an idle hope.

As the storm of controversy began to occupy column inches in international newspapers and journals, the publicity threatened to undermine what the university had hoped would be its moment of glory. To exacerbate the matter, several dignitaries from the European medical world were planning to visit Toronto that autumn to investigate the claims of discovery. These included the very influential Dr. August Krogh from Copenhagen, who had won the Nobel Prize for Physiology in 1920, and Dr. Henry Hallett Dale from Britain's Medical Research Council, who would be awarded the Nobel Prize for Physiology in 1936. Both men would certainly report their impressions to the Karolinska Institute in Stockholm, which decided the recipients of the Nobel Prize. If Toronto's nest of dysfunction and hostility were to be revealed, not only would the chance of a Canadian's winning a Nobel Prize be squandered, but it might relegate Canada to its pre–World War I status as a lesser player on the stage of world politics. And it wasn't just colleagues across the Atlantic that concerned the governors. Should Clowes learn the depth of the dissension among the insulin discovery team members, it could be used against Toronto in negotiations with Eli Lilly and Company.

In September 1922, Colonel Gooderham himself was asked to intervene to ameliorate the situation. With his barrel chest, his astonishing mustache and the awe inspired by his family name, he was exactly the lion tamer that Toronto needed and had not found in Macleod.

Under the elaborate script of his company stationery, "Gooderham & Worts, Limited, Distillers, Maltsters and Millers, Established 1832," Gooderham wrote a formal request to Macleod, Banting, and Best, asking each to submit a detailed, typewritten description of the development of insulin. Collip was not asked to contribute to the effort, but Gooderham asked each of the other three to include in his account an outline of those contributions made by Dr. Collip.

"I would then compare these statements and see wherein they differ," the letter said, "and ask you three gentlemen to meet at any early date with a view to harmonizing these statements with me. I feel that we should have as a result a connected account of the work from the very start, which would be available to anyone desiring information and which would be agreed upon by each member. This would, in my opinion, clear up all our misunderstandings and we would adjust this matter between ourselves before the gentlemen from England arrive. This understanding is urgent, as Mr. Riches requires me to give him such a statement in order that the question of the patents and amended patents which are now necessary may be proceeded with at once."

All three promptly complied.

Predictably, Banting's version reflected his view of his role as the overworked and underappreciated hero of the story and Macleod's role as the eloquent and arrogant disbeliever who had swooped in after the bulk of the work was done to claim a share of the glory. He described Macleod's lack of confidence in the project from the very first and went on to describe Macleod's continued lack of trust and cooperation throughout the discovery and development process. Banting reiterated that Macleod had sailed for Scotland in early June and did not return until late September—the exact period of critical work. His testimony described Macleod's subsequent refusal to grant Banting's requests for the most basic accommodations: a salary, a room to work in, a boy to look after the dogs, a decent operating room. He said that were it not for Professor Henderson's timely intervention, he would have gone to the Rockefeller or Mayo Institute.

Banting acknowledged that Collip had refined an extract originally made by Best, and that it was this extract that was sent to Toronto General Hospital for clinical tests. However, Banting accused Collip of reporting results to Macleod as his own that were not his own. Finally, Banting held Collip responsible for the desperate six-week-long insulin famine in early 1922.

Macleod's version granted Banting "complete credit" for the idea, but asserted that, given Banting's lack of familiarity with the subject, "he could certainly not have made such rapid progress without careful guidance and assistance." Macleod described his first meeting with Banting quite differently than Banting had. He stated that, based on that meeting, very few investigators would have given Banting the resources to pursue his idea. Macleod had been willing to take a chance on Banting. Moreover, Macleod felt unjustly criticized by Banting because, "in many, if not most, laboratories it is the custom for the 'chief' to have his name on the papers when the investigation is in a subject related to that in which he is engaged and if he stands responsible for the conclusions and had participated to the extent that I did in the planning of the research." Further, Macleod had declined to add his name to theirs in the first published report of their work, indicating, according to Macleod, that he made it "perfectly evident that I considered the full credit for this investigation to be Banting and Best's."

When Charley Best sat down to write his testimony, he was in a foul mood. He resented Gooderham's assignment. Further, he resented the abject negligence that the university had shown toward his education and the complete lack of appreciation for his precarious position. At the age of twenty-three he had found himself at the center of a major scientific breakthrough and a possible candidate for the Nobel Prize. It was an incredible stroke of luck for him, of course, because it could just as well have been Clark Noble who won the original coin toss. But if the members of discovery team were indeed the heroes that the press claimed they were, why were they being treated as naughty schoolboys by the University of Toronto?

If this was how the academic world worked, then they could have it. The idea that these men were supposed to be his mentors was laughable; he had hardly an ounce of respect left for the lot of them. Collip was selfish, Banting was crazy, and Macleod seemed completely ineffectual when you came down to it. Best was the only person on the discovery team that all of the other members were still speaking to. And now he was being asked to choose sides, the one thing he knew he could not do. All right, then. If Gooderham intended to corner him and insist that he take a side, he would: his own.

When Gooderham received and reviewed the three testimonies, he was utterly dismayed. There was very little commonality among the three versions. Neither was there any lack of conviction in any of them. Deeming the situation intractable, Colonel Gooderham abandoned his task of reconciling the versions. The lions had prevailed over the lion tamer.

* * *

In late November 1922, Danish biomedical scientist August Krogh arrived in Toronto. His visit was prompted not only by the disposition of the 1923 prize but also because Krogh's wife, Marie, was diabetic. He returned to Denmark with the formula for making insulin, courtesy of Macleod. H. H. Dale and Harold Dudley of Britain's Medical Research Council also visited Toronto and Indianapolis in the fall of 1922, and they, too, returned with the ability to make insulin for experimental use. In December 1922 clinical testing began in Britain, supervised by the Council. One of Dale's first juvenile diabetic patients was Paula Inge, the daughter of the noted theologian and dean of St. Paul's Cathedral, William Ralph Inge. Paula, like her American counterpart Elizabeth Hughes, had been diagnosed at the age of eleven.

In early November Charles and Antoinette traveled to Toronto to see Elizabeth. Banting put on his new suit to meet the secretary of state. Elizabeth weighed sixty-five-and-one-half pounds. For the first time in more than three and a half years, she was getting taller. She no longer recognized herself in the mirror. Blanche said that, with each day, she looked more like her father. For Elizabeth, the miraculous changes would not be complete until she could see them through her parents' eyes. As much as she longed to see her mother and father, she longed to be seen by them even more.

The day finally arrived. Much to her parents' amazement, the Elizabeth who opened the door of apartment number J-5 at the Athlema Apartments looked like the Elizabeth of four years ago, the Elizabeth who was not yet sick. Four years of fear and grief were dissolved in tears of joy. The three huddled together like survivors of three separate but simultaneous shipwrecks. Antoinette's desperate request for her husband's intervention was redeemed. Charles's journey away from himself and back again was justified. Elizabeth was saved.

News of her miraculous recovery spread fast. There was no telling what insulin could do. Some medical authorities even postulated that, with repeated use, insulin might restore the islets of Langerhans to their normal, functioning state. What Elizabeth craved more than anything was a normal life, a nurse-less life, an independent life. She had hardly spent five minutes alone since her diagnosis nearly four years ago. She recognized that self-care was the key to her freedom.

Shortly after her parents' visit she took the first bold steps toward a future as a secret diabetic. She wrote:

> Now I know I am going to shock you by what I am going to say next, but I seem to be always giving you surprises nowadays. . . . I will try to camouflage it in terms that I don't usually use for then you will get it more gradually and I'm sure you will be able to fathom it. . . . I decided that being captain of my own ship it would be very well for me to know how to manage the target practice every day. So yesterday I resolved to be bold and begin. Thus I cleared the decks for action, put the crew (including myself) on their mettle, boiled the gun (to make sure of the uttermost cleanliness on this ship) and finally gave the orders to pull up steam (or rather air), which I did. Everything then being at last ready I cleaned the target thoroughly, and I myself fired the first shot heard round the world (my world that is). I made a clean breast of it and hit the bulls-eye on the instant causing no ill effect whatever to my target. After shooting all the shells I had, and without the slightest leak whatever in the hold through the force of the concussion, I gave the order to heave to, (which I executed myself), and back went the gun and powder all cleaned and ready for further use the next day. I then immediately betook myself to the dining room saloon [sic], where I soon indulged myself into eating an enormous dinner, which under the impression that I had done a good job the first time, and with the effect of the first shot still upon me, I assimilated with no dire results whatever afterwards. . . . Compronez-vous? [sic] I certainly hope. If you don't I think I will have to tell you how I happened to start on this wild career of being Captain of my own affairs. Dr. Banting came in yesterday morning and he stated how he had gotten a letter from Mrs. Whitehill and how she had said that wonder of all wonders, little eight-year-old Ruth was giving herself her own injections. Well that was too much altogether for me. I was not going to be in any way outdone by a mere girl of eight, whereupon I made the bold resolve to give it to myself for the first time (doing absolutely everything) last night. So I did and thus you know the result. I can do it perfectly beautifully and it doesn't hurt me as much as anyone else giving it to me for I know just when it hurts and just when to give more and stop and so on. It really is

a wonderful thing to be able to do, and now I feel so absolutely indepen-
dent because I can do that. I can cook my food, and I can weigh and figure,
and so I don't see why I [wouldn't] be perfectly able to live alone. . . .
Listen Mother, I always know when I am having a reaction now because
I've had them so much and all I have to do is to reach on my table for a
[molasses] kiss and then in five minutes time I'm all right and ready to
turn over and go to sleep again, and if one candy didn't seem to be enough
for that time why all I'd do would be to eat another one and keep on
until I recovered. That's all there is to it, and there's nothing anybody
can do to help me but myself. Blanche always wakes up when I have one
here for she is sleeping in the bed with me and can't help herself, but truly
both Dr. Banting and Blanche think that I am entirely able to take care
of myself in every way.

In November, Toronto's insulin patent application was rejected by the United States Patent and Trademark Office, largely because of a prior American patent, U.S. Patent 1,027,790, which had been awarded on May 28, 1912, to Georg Zuelzer. In late November, patent attorney Charles Riches planned to appeal the rejection at a hearing before the chief American patent examiner. He charged the Toronto team to gather all of the evidence they could about the clinical results of their process. Affidavits were requisitioned from Doctors Joslin, Allen, and Woodyatt. Telegrams flew in all directions to rally support for the defense. Macleod raced to Washington to testify. Banting asked Charles Evans Hughes to help.

The new Charles Evans Hughes did not hesitate. On November 24, he wrote a letter to the Honorable Thomas E. Robertson, commissioner of patents. Although the letter was marked "personal" it was written on official State Department stationery. The letter explained that his youngest daughter, Elizabeth, had been diagnosed in 1919 and had been placed under the "best possible attention" in the care of Dr. Allen. It went on to explain that she had been placed under Dr. Banting's care in Toronto in August. "The results of the treatment are so important that I cannot forbear expressing the hope that, so far as is consistent with the exigencies of the Patent Office, there may be the utmost expedition in dealing with the application."

On January 23, 1923, two months after he wrote to the commissioner of the Patent Office, an American patent on both process and product was awarded to the applicants—Banting, Best, and Collip.

In the years to come, Charles Evans Hughes would become the friend to Banting that his daughter could not be. In 1923, he helped to fund the Banting Research Foundation and persuaded former president Taft, President Wilson, and Secretary of the Treasury Andrew W. Mellon, among others, to do the same. In 1926, Hughes served as an honorary vice president of the American Association for Medical Progress, a lobbying group that sought to block legislation prohibiting medical experimentation on living dogs. *Once a Son of Neptune, always a Son of Neptune.*

On Saturday November 25, 1922, the season's first snow fell in Toronto. Elizabeth longed to go out in it but had to stay in and await the arrival of the clinicians who were to visit sometime that afternoon. Her old life already seemed so long ago. "We've got to stay in all day Saturday waiting for those blessed Dr. Allens and Dr. Joslins to appear. I am simply scared to death to face the former."

Just as she and Blanche were sitting down to lunch, the bell rang and Dr. Banting ushered in the clinicians. It was an astonishing assembly of authorities on diabetes, all of whom had come to Toronto to see Banting's famously successful case. One by one they crowded around the girl at the table, who appeared to be about to eat a very generous midday meal. Some of the men were familiar to her, others were not. Along with Dr. Banting were John R. Williams, J. J. R. Macleod, W. R. Campbell, Elliott Joslin, R. J. Woodyatt, G. H. A. Clowes, Irvine H. Page, Russel W. Wilder, H. Rawle Geyelin, Duncan Graham, Arthur Walters, John A. MacDonald, A. A. Fletcher, Charles Best, Joseph Gilchrist, and, last but not least, "Dr. Goddlemidey" himself—Frederick M. Allen.

At first they said nothing, but stood there with expressions of bewildered joy on their faces. Then all at once they began a torrent of questions. Allen remained across the room near the door. He listened to Elizabeth discuss her experience with the other doctors, blinking and swallowing to contain his emotion. If Banting had not introduced Elizabeth, Allen would not have recognized her as the girl who had been under his care for more than three years.

* * *

Between August and January 1922 Elizabeth would gain nearly fifty pounds and three-quarters of an inch in height. Still, she had to guard against exciting her metabolism. A setback now would derail her plans to embark on a new and normal life at last.

> Mrs. (rather) Lady van Hoofenbhouck Tulleken called me up yesterday and I am going up to spend the afternoon with her daughter next Tuesday. She is going to send for me and bring me back in her car so that will be very nice as it's a kind of an out-of-the-way place to get to as you remember. This afternoon we are going to see Frances Hodgson Burnett's story played, up at the Yonge St. Theatre on Bloor St., "The Dawn of Tomorrow", and I think it will be awfully good. I am glad these last days up here I am going to have something definite to do, for otherwise I'm sure I would get all excited [sic] thinking about coming home so soon. Now I will be busy doing nice things and won't have time for many such thoughts. While Blanche is busy packing I am going to [go] over to the library to read if I have nothing else more thrilling to do and that will keep my thoughts busy too.

In March of 1923 Billy Ross and Sir William Mulock, then chancellor of the University of Toronto, mounted a campaign to secure government support for Banting and asked Hughes to provide a testimonial, and he did so. He wrote to Prime Minister Mackenzie King. Banting was awarded an annual lifetime financial stipend of $10,000 from the provincial government and $7,500 from the federal government. In June 1923 the Rockefeller Foundation gave $150,000 to fifteen hospitals in the United States and Canada to promote the use of insulin in the treatment of diabetes (equivalent to roughly $15 million today). A gift of $10,000 went to each recipient, with the exception of the newly established Banting-Best fund, which received $5,000, and the Presbyterian Hospital of New York, which received $15,000. Quite unexpectedly, Banting found himself a wealthy and influential man.

As Elizabeth prepared to leave Toronto to begin life as a completely different Elizabeth, Dr. Banting arranged to send her insulin from Toronto through the State Department on a regular schedule. This way it would not have to go through customs, and Elizabeth would not be obliged to divulge her diabetes to a doctor in Washington in order to get her supply; the fewer people who knew of her condition, the better. She hoped that as more stories of resurrected children appeared in the press, her own name might be forgotten, at least its association with the word that she and her family rarely, if ever, said aloud—diabetes.

Privilege contributed to both Elizabeth Hughes and her British counterpart, Paula Inge, receiving the insulin that so many other children desperately needed. But even after the wide availability of pharmaceutical insulin, complications of dosage, diet, and administration were such that long-term recovery was hardly guaranteed. In the early insulin era, from 1922 to 1930, juvenile diabetics who died did so relatively quickly, often within two years of their diagnosis. Such was the challenge of safe self-administration of insulin therapy in those early years. Only three of Dr. Allen's original one hundred patients survived to receive insulin. One of the three, a particularly dedicated and trustworthy disciple of Dr. Allen's diet, died in Dr. Allen's care in 1923, despite having made such a dramatic recovery with insulin that he could walk ten miles a day. Dr. Joslin also lost at least one early patient whom he treated with insulin, as did Williams and Woodyatt. Paula Inge died in a diabetic coma in March of 1923.

On December 1, 1922, Elizabeth left Toronto—alone. It was the first time she had traveled without a nurse in years.

She never looked back. At the age of fifteen, she set herself to completing high school and applying to college. During the summers in Washington, she might join her parents and president and Mrs. Coolidge for a weekend cruise of Chesapeake Bay. She and her parents agreed to forget about diabetes. And this was the most extraordinary feat of Elizabeth Hughes's life. More extraordinary even than her remarkable recovery from juvenile diabetes in August 1922 was the astounding disappearing act that began in December of that same year. Within months of her departure from Toronto, the Elizabeth Hughes who has been described in these pages was entirely eclipsed by an Elizabeth Hughes who had never been sick.

THIRTY-ONE

The Nobel Prize and Beyond

THROUGHOUT 1923, NOBEL PRIZE NOMINATIONS ARRIVED IN STOCK-holm. Banting was nominated by Dr. George Washington Crile of Cleveland and by Francis G. Benedict, a leading researcher who had worked with Elliott Joslin. Macleod was nominated by a former colleague from Western Reserve University, Professor G. N. Stewart. August Krogh, the Danish Nobel laureate, nominated both Banting and Macleod. To address the conflicting views about who should receive credit for the discovery of insulin, the Nobel Committee solicited two independent appraisals of the discovery. On October 25, 1923, nineteen professors of the world-renowned Karolinska Institute voted by secret ballot. The result was that Banting and Macleod were to be corecipients of the 1923 Nobel Prize in Physiology.

It was Canada's first Nobel Prize. As the news spread, spontaneous celebrations erupted throughout Toronto. Banting was an instant celebrity—a local Ontario boy, a veteran, and a Nobel laureate. Toronto's leading medical and political men congratulated each other. It was a great day for all of Canada.

Banting reacted to the news not with gratitude but with fury that Macleod had been included and Best overlooked. When Gooderham went to Banting's office to congratulate him, Banting threatened to refuse the prize. Gooderham told him to book a passage to Stockholm immediately, and that the University would pay for it. While Banting ultimately accepted the prize he made public his disagreement and announced that he would share his half of the financial award with Best. This left Macleod with no choice but to announce that he would share his half of the prize with Collip. The prize totaled $24,000, which was split between Banting and Macleod, and further split to $6,000 for each of the four members of the discovery team. Privately, Macleod grumbled that Banting's sudden prosperity made sharing the prize money an easy matter for him.

The 1923 Nobel Prize for Literature was awarded to William Butler Yeats, who had written the poem "The Second Coming," which was published the month that Banting first met Macleod.

Neither Banting nor Macleod attended the ceremony in Stockholm, largely because Banting refused to share the stage with Macleod and Macleod didn't dare accept the prize on Banting's behalf for fear of being accused of grandstanding. In 1923, Macleod, who had wanted to be elected to the Royal Society, got his wish. Banting finally delivered his Nobel lecture in 1925.

In November 1923, the University of Toronto held a celebratory banquet for four hundred guests in the Great Hall of the elegant Hart House. It was a lavish affair with some guests traveling many miles to attend. There was a jazz orchestra and after-dinner speeches. An official photographer documented the great event for posterity, but Banting refused to pose for a photograph sitting next to Macleod. To this day there exists not a single photograph of the four members of the discovery team in a single frame.

A Nobel Prize in Physiology (Medicine) would not be awarded to another Canadian for nearly fifty years.

After the Nobel Prize announcement, a number of bona fide researchers came forward with claims of having discovered insulin prior to Banting. Georg Zuelzer and Nicolas Paulesco appealed directly to the Nobel Committee. E. L. Scott published a claim to priority in the isolation of the active principle in the pancreas. Paulesco had applied for a Hungarian patent in 1922. Murlin applied for a patent for an antidiabetic pancreatic extract in 1923. Even Collip published a paper stating that he had succeeded in keeping a depancreatized dog alive for sixty-six days with injections of an extract he named "glucokinin," derived from plants such as lettuce and onion greens. But the insulin patent that had been secured (with help from Hughes) for Toronto and assigned to Toronto's board of governors held fast.

Now discussions began about the disposition of royalties. It was agreed that half of the insulin royalties would go to the University of Toronto and half would be split among the patent signatories, Banting, Best, and Collip. This income supplied these three scientists with many years of steady funding for their research. From 1923 to 1967 the University of Toronto's royalties from insulin totaled $8 million. By separate arrangement with Lilly, Clowes received a generous percentage of the insulin profits for his lifetime. Macleod never received any remuneration from the patents.

The year 1923 would prove to be both the most profitable year, to that point, in the history of Eli Lilly and Company and the year of its greatest growth. This was in large part due to the tremendous success of Lilly's insulin product, trademarked "Iletin® (Insulin, Lilly)." In January 1923 Eli Lilly and Company began to sell limited quantities of insulin to physicians through retail druggists. In October 1923, Iletin was released for distribution directly through physician prescription. At that time it was estimated that 7,500 physicians were treating 25,000 diabetic patients with Iletin. The first-year sales of Lilly's insulin came to $1,110,000—three times as much as any specialty drug had brought in for Lilly before in a single year. By the end of 1923, Lilly had sold almost sixty million units. Frozen glands now arrived at the Lilly plant by the refrigerated train car load.

In an address to an annual meeting of life insurance professionals in December 1923, Dr. Clowes said:

> *To give you some conception of the speed with which this valuable remedy has been applied to the treatment of diabetics, I can state that a year and a half ago there were less than ten cases under treatment; a year ago not more than five hundred, while today there are probably not less than sixty thousand cases under treatment of which more than forty thousand are in the United States.*

This rapid delivery of an effective extract would not have been possible were it not for the isoelectric and organoprecipitation methods—both of them George Walden's inventions on behalf of Eli Lilly and Company—which resulted in a purer and more stable product. According to the original indenture, the patents for the isoelectric and organo-precipitation methods were turned over to the University of Toronto.

Insulin was now not only readily available, but also affordable. George Walden's improved methodology also allowed Eli Lilly and Company to reduce the price per unit several times after its introduction. Although Eli Lilly held the exclusive franchise of insulin production in the United States, the company was committed to keeping the price as low as possible so that it would be available to all diabetics. A local newspaper reported:

> Many persons have the idea that insulin is as rare as radium and as hard to obtain. Those who have that opinion are in error. The enemy of diabetes is now being produced in quantities sufficient to meet the world's needs. Its cost is so nominal that, as Mr. Lilly said, it is available to the consumer at a price below what the average man spends daily for his cigars or a supply of gasoline for his pleasure automobile. Iletin costs less than three cents a unit, thus proving that the humblest man or woman may enjoy its benefits.

By the end of 1923 the cost of treatment per patient was frequently less than one dollar per week and seldom more than two dollars. (Consider that this was just two years after the initial announcement in New Haven and one year after Elizabeth left Toronto to begin a new and normal life.)

J. K. Lilly Sr. could not have been more proud of his sons. In one letter to Eli he wrote, "A glow of pride pervades my being as I contemplate the splendid manner in which you have steered the good ship Iletin to the harbor of success."

Each of the four members of the discovery team went on to make significant individual medical research contributions, with the possible exception of Banting. By March 1924 he was no longer engaged in the clinical investigation of insulin and had stopped advising patients. He devoted himself to the Banting Research Foundation, which was created to foster imaginative scientific research. He concentrated on trying to apply to other problems, primarily cancer, the model of sudden inspiration and insight that had led to the discovery of insulin. As he explained to an audience in Chicago in March 1925:

> *We do not know whence ideas come, but the importance of the idea in medical research cannot be overestimated. From the nature of things ideas do not come from prosperity, affluence and contentment, but rather from the blackness of despair, not in the bright light of day, nor the footlights' glare, but rather in the quiet, undisturbed hours of midnight, or early morning, when one can be alone to think. These are the grandest hours of all, when the progress of research, when the hewn stones of scientific fact are turned over and over, and fitted in so that the mosaic figure of truth, designed by Mother Nature long ago, be formed from the chaos.*

Many of the projects that the Banting Research Foundation pursued were related to military research. He was especially interested in biological and chemical warfare; at one point he suffered serious chemical burns after conducting an experiment in which he applied mustard gas to his own leg. The Banting Research Foundation played a major role in supporting the development of the first anti-gravity or G-suit, designed to prevent pilots from blacking out when subjected to extreme acceleration. These suits were used during World War II, and all G-suits worn by pilots, astronauts, and cosmonauts are based on this original design.

Banting married Marion Robertson on June 4, 1924. They had one son. Notwithstanding his dislike for public speaking, Banting joined the National Research Council of Canada in 1927 and became the country's leading spokesperson for medical research. Despite this distinction and although he would be knighted in 1934, he remained a man who looked and felt uncomfortable in a tuxedo. He once threatened that the next person who called him *sir* would "get his ass kicked."

Banting divorced Marion amid a well-publicized scandal in April 1932. Whatever favors the press had done him by launching his career and lionizing him in 1922, they withdrew ten years later by savaging his reputation as Canada's first-ever Nobel laureate. After the divorce, Banting struggled with depression. He married Henrietta Ball in 1937, but at Christmastime 1938, he was again beset with a dark mood. He wrote in his diary:

> God how I hate the whole fuss this so called festive season of the year. To me it is festering rather than festive. Cards. Presents. Gratuities. Sentiment. Good Lord how I hate the display of sentiment. Another word for sentiment is weakness. Christmas this year of 1938 symbolized futility . . . oh cruel time of year and assaying when one analyzes one soul to see if it is of any value.

And yet he would always have warm feelings for his early insulin patients. The same week he wrote to Teddy Ryder:

> I shall always follow your career with interest and you will forgive me if I add, a little pride, because I shall always remember the difficult times we had in the early days of insulin. The outstanding thing I remember was your strength and fortitude in observing your diet and the manly way in which you stood up to the punishment of hypodermic injections. I am sure that you will be a success in life if you maintain the same spirit in meeting the rebuffs of the world.

As Nazi Germany rose to power in Europe, Banting advocated the use of biological weapons in the event of a German invasion of England. When World War II began he applied to be sent to the front lines, but the Canadian government refused, holding that he would be of greater service in Canada. But Banting continued to worry about Canada's military vulnerabilities and in 1941 he embarked on a secret mission to England to test a G-suit developed at the Banting and Best Medical Research Institute.

On February 21, 1941, Banting boarded a Lockheed Hudson patrol bomber to go to England on a secret mission that was reportedly related to the use of chemical weapons or combat aviation problems. The plane crashed shortly after takeoff from Gander Airport in Newfoundland. Both the radio operator and the navigator were killed on impact. Banting and the pilot were badly injured. Banting was able to dress the pilot's wounds before he succumbed to his own injuries. The pilot survived to recount that in his final hours Banting, who was delirious, believed he was dictating a new scientific breakthrough to a stenographer. Banting was forty-nine years old at the time of his death and was survived by his second wife, Lady Henrietta Ball and his son by Marion, Bill. He spent his last night on earth in Montreal with Bert Collip, with whom he had become good friends.

John James Rickard Macleod continued to suffer the many indignities of Banting's hatred, and as the Ontario native's popularity increased so did acceptance of his view of Macleod. By 1928, Macleod's situation had become unbearable. He left Toronto to return to Scotland as the Regius Professor of Physiology at the University of Aberdeen. The University of Toronto hosted a lavish farewell dinner for him. Not only did Banting refuse to attend the dinner, he requested that an empty place be set at the table for him. Upon Macleod's return to Aberdeen, he was duly appreciated as a great physiologist, a brilliant scholar, and the author of eleven books and monographs. In 1930 he became a member of the Royal College of Physicians, London; and in 1932 he joined the Royal Society of Edinburgh. He never discussed his years in Toronto.

James Bertram Collip continued to work in endocrinological research. Always hoping to discover the next magic hormone, he undertook several collaborations with drug companies, including Eli Lilly. He significantly contributed to isolating the parathyroid hormone secreted by the parathyroid gland and adrenocorticotropic hormone (ACTH) secreted by the pituitary gland. In 1927 he declined an offer to join the Mayo Clinic. In 1928 he accepted a position as chair of biochemistry at McGill University in Montreal. Upon Banting's death, Collip succeeded him as senior administrator of medical research at the National Research Council Canada. After the war Collip moved to the University of Western Ontario, where Banting was working when he had had his inspiration.

While Collip and Banting had become friends, Best and Banting's relationship had cooled considerably. Charles Best never forgot the disappointment of not being officially recognized for his contribution to the discovery of insulin. In a letter dated 1945 to Dr. Elliott Joslin, Best wrote, "Dr. Ross was very friendly with me during the early stages of insulin but some years later he apparently decided that as I had not been born in Ontario little credit should be given me. I am told that he was largely responsible for the fact that the Dominion Government did not include me when they gave Banting his annuity. With Sir William Mulock, Dr. Ross apparently played a part in my complete exclusion from the tenth anniversary celebration of the discovery of insulin here in Toronto. It was on that occasion that Sir William announced that 'only the name of our Ontario bred boy will be mentioned.'" The 1972 official history of the Nobel Prize states that it was impossible to include Best in the 1923 prize because no one had nominated him.

From 1926 to 1928 Best did postgraduate research in the laboratory of Sir Henry Dale in London. This research led him to the discovery of histaminase, an antiallergic enzyme. He continued his research during his long and successful career at the University of Toronto. He had replaced Macleod there as professor of physiology. He was twenty-nine years old at the time of his appointment. In the 1930s, Best found that lecithin prevented depancreatized dogs from developing fatty livers. He and his colleagues isolated choline as the active nutritional component of lecithin, and studied the role of choline in metabolism. Also in the 1930s, Best became interested in the anticoagulant drug heparin, which had just been discovered, and worked to purify it for human use. In 1941, the year of Banting's death, Best was appointed director of the medical research unit of the Canadian navy.

Dr. John G. FitzGerald, Banting's good friend and director of the Connaught Laboratories, died shortly before Banting was killed. During the 1930s he had begun to suffer from mental illness and attempted suicide. He was sent to Connecticut for insulin shock treatments. After returning to Toronto and making another suicide attempt, he was admitted to Toronto General Hospital, where he managed to hide a knife after a meal. He opened an artery in his hip and bled to death.

Billy Ross, the Canadian patriot and Banting booster, suffered the loss of both of his sons, casualties of World War II.

Dr. Joseph Gilchrist, the self-described "human rabbit," died at Sunnybrook Hospital, suffering from poorly controlled diabetes and manic depressive psychosis.

J. K. Lilly Sr. had the privilege of making history when he signed the indenture with the University of Toronto in 1922. He took a personal interest in the lives of the early insulin patients and corresponded with many of them. A boy named Rodger MacQuigg wrote that he was sticking close to his diet and "feeling as frisky as ever." He promised Mr. Lilly, "After I get a little fatter, I will send you my picture and you can publish it in your paper [the company's internal newsletter, *Tile and Till*] and say, 'This is the result of taking Iletin!'" J. K. Lilly replied, "I hardly believe you can realize what a joy it is to me to have you and others benefit by the use of this new discovery. It is an everlasting joy day by day to get letters such as yours and to feel that good is being accomplished." Through regular correspondence, Elizabeth Mudge and J. K. Lilly developed a friendship. At her death the company had supplied her with insulin free of charge for twenty-five years. The elder Lilly turned the company over to his son Eli in 1932. In 1975 the company began providing sterling silver medals to men and women who had been kept alive by insulin injections for at least fifty years, and Eli Lilly (then in his ninetieth year) personally signed every one of the eighty-three letters that accompanied the medals during that year.

In 1947, Clowes was awarded the Banting Medal by the American Diabetes Association. It was the first time ever that an industrial corporation had been recognized for its contribution to medical research. Alec Clowes spent forty summers working at the laboratory at Woods Hole. At his home there in 1958 he died of a cerebral hemorrhage, two days before his eighty-first birthday. Three months later Eli Lilly and Company decided to discontinue operations at Woods Hole. A new generation of scientific research had begun. Collaboration between research universities and pharmaceutical companies was no longer uncommon, and extraordinary efforts to facilitate these alliances were no longer necessary.

George Walden remained an employee of Lilly for his entire career. He became vice president of biochemical manufacturing and a member of the board of directors. Reflecting later on his years at Lilly, Walden would say that the biggest thrill was being in on the romance of the development of insulin.

Eli Lilly Jr. shared his father's deep commitment to pharmaceutical research and development. He was president of Eli Lilly and Company from 1932 to 1948, subsequently becoming chairman of the board. Although he was never interested in politics, he became one of Indianapolis's most influential citizens through his major philanthropic efforts. His deep interest in local history led him to write two books and play a leading role in the Indiana Historical Society, the creation of the Glenn A. Black Laboratory of Archaeology at Indiana University in Bloomington, and the development of the Conner Prairie historic preservation and the prehistoric Angel Site. His significant personal financial contributions almost always came with the stipulation that they be anonymous.

J. K. Lilly Jr., who was known as "Joe," became president upon his brother's retirement in 1948. He was a man of many interests, from rare books and manuscripts to miniature soldiers to eighteenth-century paintings. His collection of rare books consists of 20,000 volumes and 17,000 manuscripts, including one of the 26 copies of the Dunlap broadside of the Declaration of Independence. It was considered among the finest general collections of books and manuscripts in the United States in the twentieth century. Lilly gave it to Indiana University in 1954, and it is housed today at the Lilly Library there. In the early 1950s, Mr. Lilly became a numismatist. His collection of gold coins quickly became one of the world's largest, eventually comprising 6,000 items. It now belongs to the Smithsonian Institution. The family's primary residence, Oldfields, now belongs to the Art Association of Indianapolis.

Together, J. K. Lilly Sr. and his sons established the Lilly Endowment in 1937. This private family foundation supports the causes of religion, education, and community development, with 60 to 70 percent of the grants paid each year going to charities in Indianapolis and Indiana. In 1968, the company established the Eli Lilly Foundation, a $7 billion organization that operates separately from the Endowment. The Foundation contributes almost $400 million annually to worthwhile charitable pursuits—50 percent of which has gone to universities, hospitals, and other nonprofit institutions in the state of Indiana. The Lilly family remains one of the largest benefactors to their home state.

Dr. Elliott Joslin devoted his life to diabetes treatment, education, and research and founded the Joslin Diabetes Center. Affiliated with Harvard Medical School, Joslin Diabetes Center is the world's largest diabetes research center, diabetes clinic, and provider of diabetes education. Joslin pioneered the idea of educating diabetics about their illness so that they could care for themselves. This approach, which is now widely accepted, is called DSME, for Diabetes Self-Management Education. Joslin maintained a diabetic registry for his entire career. In it he recorded each diabetic patient he treated, beginning with Mary Higgins in 1893, listing for each name, the address and age, as well as the dates of onset, diagnosis, and death. When he died at age ninety-two there were eighty volumes, representing some 58,784 names.

Dr. Joslin often described his experience witnessing the postinsulin resurrection of starved children in terms of what he called the "Banting Chapter" of the Bible (Ezekiel 37), which reads:

> *The hand of the Lord was upon me and set me in the middle of a valley; it was full of bones and He said to me, "Prophesy to these bones and say to them, 'Dry bones, hear the word of the Lord! I will make flesh come upon you and put breath in you, and you will come to life.' " So I prophesied as I was commanded and the bones came together but there was no breath in them. Then He said to me, "Prophesy to the breath; prophesy, son of man, and say to it, 'Come from the four winds, O breath, that they may live.' " So I prophesied as he commanded me, and breath entered them; they came to life and stood up on their feet.*

As Banting's star ascended, Allen's fell. The stock market crash of 1929 marked four crushing years of bankruptcy for Allen and the Physiatric Institute. Allen owed over $25,000 to Otto Kahn, who turned the matter over to an attorney. Allen tried to work out an arrangement with his creditors and committed his entire savings to ameliorating the situation, but it was not enough. Desperate for a second chance for his beloved institute, Allen returned to his initial investors, including Hughes, and begged for money. One by one the investors turned him down. Allen was incredulous. One of the founding ideals of the institute was that diabetics could find help there, regardless of their financial means. No worthy patient was ever refused help. Now Allen himself was being refused help. An eviction notice was nailed to a wooden stake and driven into the front lawn of the institute. Allen was given two weeks to vacate the premises. Later, the contents were auctioned off. Worst of all, he had buried his parents in a quiet corner of the grounds and hoped to be buried there himself. The bodies were now hurriedly exhumed and moved to a lot in a nearby town.

After the collapse of the Physiatric Institute, Dr. Allen and Belle Wishart Allen divorced. Allen persevered with his animal experiments in rented basements and outbuildings, drifting from one mediocre, ill-equipped facility to the next. Despite these impediments Allen continued to work on an idea that he had first experimented with while serving at the Army General Hospital in Lakewood in 1918—the relationship of dietary salt to high blood pressure. Now he introduced a low-salt diet for patients with hypertensive cardiovascular disease. Although this treatment was not as widely accepted as was his starvation diet for diabetics, the relationship of salt to high blood pressure was later proved.

Upon hearing of the collapse of the institute, a group of Allen's grateful patients scraped together a research fund of three hundred dollars a month for several years so that he could continue his work. It was an unprecedented amount of money for Allen, but, tragically, he had no laboratory facilities in which to continue his work at that time.

Allen was to remain an outsider for the rest of his career. In a letter to *The New York Times* dated May 14, 1937, Dr. Allen wrote:

> *Practically all medical discoveries have been made by individuals or small voluntary groups. The idea of an organized mass attack therefore lacks basis in past experience. . . . The great majority of medical investigators work on small salaries or none, and all their discoveries are given to humanity free. Secretiveness, selfish ambitions, and particularly the evil known as "politics" belong to institutional organizations rather than to the individual investigators, and they tend to increase, along with regimentation and barrenness, according to the size of the institution and its endowment.*

Otto Kahn's mansion was razed in 1939, and the ground was left vacant to reduce taxes. Although he lived another twenty-five years, Allen never returned to the property.

In 1949 Allen was awarded a Banting Medal by the American Diabetes Association. Accepting the award, Allen expressed "deep appreciation of your medal as a unique recognition of my mostly unsuccessful efforts" and said that his "ambition once was so high that I regarded both the diet and the extract as temporary steps toward a position where I could attack the real problem of cure." Frederick Allen is buried in Greenfield Cemetery on Long Island, New York. Not a single blood relative is buried with him. His is one of six plots purchased by his second wife, Anne. Allen's granite footstone bears the word "DOCTOR" in large capital letters, beneath which appear his name and the year of his death, 1964.

"The thing that has hurt me more than anything," Belle Wishart Allen wrote, decades later "was to see that very brilliant idealist, believing in the good in people, gradually becoming that bitter disillusioned old man."

Although Joslin always referred to the years of 1914 to 1922 as the "Allen era in diabetes," the contributions of Dr. Frederick M. Allen are now largely forgotten. His likeness is absent from the portraits of famous scientists displayed in the lobby of the Joslin center in Boston. The words of the eleventh century Persian poet, mathematician and astronomer Omar Khayyam, whose writing Allen especially favored, describe the brief, bright trajectory of the Physiatric Institute:

> *The Worldly Hope men set their Hearts upon*
> *Turns Ashes—or it prospers; and anon,*
> *Like Snow upon the Desert's dusty Face*
> *Lighting a little Hour or two—is gone.*

THIRTY-TWO

The Emergence of Elizabeth Gossett

Elizabeth returned to Washington, D.C., in 1922. There she commenced life as a normal teenager, finishing high school and applying to college. During these two and a half years she had one major setback. In August of 1924 she returned to Morristown to be treated by Dr. Allen. To her dismay, this visit was reported to the world.

MISS ELIZABETH HUGHES ILL
Secretary of State's
Daughter Suffers Diabetes Attack

MISS HUGHES IMPROVING
It Is Not Known How
Long She Will Remain in Sanitarium

In 1925 Elizabeth moved to her beloved New York City to attend Barnard College. From then until she graduated in 1929, Elizabeth pursued her dream of normalcy by living as any other Barnard student would—studying, dating, and enjoying the city. She even tempted fate with the occasional cocktail and cigarette. She told no one of her condition. In 1926 she weighed 150 pounds and took 38 units of insulin per day, which she administered herself, sharpening her own needle on a whetstone. Per special arrangement with Banting, her insulin—sometimes five thousand units at a time—was shipped directly from Connaught to "Miss E. E. Hughes, c/o State Department, Washington, D.C." She did not see a doctor once during these four years. She did not keep in touch with Banting or her Toronto cohort or Blanche. When her name did appear in print, it was unrelated to diabetes. She organized a club of Barnard undergraduates to support Hoover's presidential campaign and debated James Roosevelt, second son of Franklin Delano Roosevelt, on a bipartisan radio program. During the summers she often traveled with her parents to Europe, circulating among the most notable political and public figures of the day. She became a familiar face at The Hague, where her father served as a judge of the Permanent Court of International Justice from 1928 to 1930. The three of them continued to honor their agreement to forget the diabetic past, and soon the anguish of her life before Toronto seemed like a distant dream.

In 1928 Charles Evans Hughes hired a research assistant named William T. Gossett who was fresh out of law school. Like Hughes himself, Gossett worked his way through Columbia University Law School. In a further parallel to Hughes's life trajectory, Gossett became an associate at a law firm (Hughes, Rounds, Schurman and Dwight, now Hughes, Hubbard & Reed), and became engaged to his boss's daughter. Elizabeth did not tell Bill of her diabetes until a week after their engagement. Elizabeth and Bill were married in 1930, opting for a quiet ceremony at home, just as Antoinette and Charles had. Neither Banting nor Allen nor Blanche was invited to the wedding. Among the most beautiful of the wedding gifts was a pair of exquisitely wrought silver urns on pedestals given by President and Mrs. Herbert Hoover. Her willful amnesia about her illness was so complete that Elizabeth Gossett spent her honeymoon in Bermuda, where Elizabeth Hughes had suffered the very nadir of her four-year starvation.

In 1930, Charles Evans Hughes became chief justice of the United States after a two-week Senate debate on his suitability for the role, given his prolonged association with big business clients (e.g., Standard Oil). In eleven years as chief justice he administered the oath of office to President Franklin D. Roosevelt three times. It was to FDR that he submitted his letter of resignation in 1941. He was so concerned that his decision might be leaked to the press that he didn't tell his own children. They learned of his retirement by reading about it in the newspaper.

During the 1930s, Hughes became aware of the emerging trend among biographers, attributed largely to the British writer and critic Lytton Strachey, of irreverent portrayal in the guise of psychological insight and analysis. He may have been impressed also with Sir Frederick Banting's swift and decisive postdivorce humiliation in the popular press. To preempt the field and avoid becoming the target of an unflattering literary effort, the chief justice conceived the idea of composing an authoritative document that would set down the events of his life and career as he saw them and, more important, as he wanted them to be seen.

In 1933 Henry Beerits, a Princeton student majoring in politics, wrote his senior thesis about Charles Evans Hughes. His thesis advisor, Professor Edwin S. Corwin, an authority on constitutional law, proposed that the young man send a copy of the paper to Hughes himself. Just ten days later, Beerits received a reply from the chief justice. The letter thanked him for the paper and said that both he and Mrs. Hughes had read it and been impressed by it. Further, Hughes suggested that if Henry had no definite plans for the coming year, he might consider coming to Washington to work on a project with the chief justice. The project to which Hughes referred was the compilation of his autobiographical notes, which became known as the Beerits Memoranda.

Beerits arrived in Washington in September and would remain there, living at the Racquet Club and working on the memoranda until May. Hughes asked Beerits not to discuss the project with others. In an article published in 1992 entitled "Aftermath of a Senior Thesis" for the Princeton Class of '33 newsletter, Beerits described their process:

> Every Sunday afternoon I would go to his home, where he had a study on the ground floor, and he would reminisce about a stage of his career, referring me to various relevant books and articles. I would take careful notes and during the coming week, in my office at the Library of Congress, I would write a detailed account of his topic, with plenty of footnotes. On the next Sunday, at the beginning of our session, he would review this account and comment on it. It would be about 35 typewritten pages, and he would turn from one page to the next quickly with only a brief look, and I would think that my very careful presentation was not being appreciated. And then he would comment that a particular word

was a bit strong, and it was apparent that he was taking in everything on the page. He had this ability to fully absorb a whole page at a glance, and furthermore he had a photographic memory that would recall all that he read.

A highlight of the year was Beerits's being included in a very special dinner at the long stately table in the formal dining room with Elizabeth Gossett and her husband, Bill. Elizabeth was extremely interested in the young man and his project. After all, it had once been her fervent ambition to write her father's biography. Like her father, she knew that, victors and vanquished aside, history is written by the writers—and writers employ erasers as well as words.

In a final attempt to shape the record, Hughes composed "Autobiographical Notes" between November 1941 and the end of 1945, drawing heavily upon the Beerits Memoranda. Among the thousands of pages of these documents, there is no mention of diabetes or of Elizabeth's long struggle or of Banting. Having crossed the line, he was now redrawing it. He and Elizabeth were bound by blood and silence.

There were two things that Elizabeth was afraid of the public finding out: First, that Elizabeth Gossett, the dynamic, self-directed wife and mother was one and the same person as Elizabeth Hughes, the desperately ill diabetic girl; second, that her emancipation from the fatal destiny was, quite possibly, purchased at the expense of another child's life. She destroyed pictures of herself taken during the period of her declining health. Both to protect herself and to protect her father's reputation from any suggestion of impropriety she expunged all references to diabetes in her father's papers. In 1974 she founded the Supreme Court Historical Society with a friend on the Supreme Court, Chief Justice Warren Burger. For the rest of her life she guarded the reputation of Charles Evans Hughes. His image presided over the Gossett household in the form of a large portrait that hung above the mantle for as long as Elizabeth lived.

During Elizabeth's life, attitudes toward disease changed so dramatically that it is hard to imagine the stigma carried by the word "diabetes" in the first half of the twentieth century. Today it is common for those afflicted with a disease to use their personal experiences to educate, inspire, and assist fellow sufferers: Evelyn Lauder and Elizabeth Edwards did so for breast cancer; Ryan White and Magic Johnson did so for AIDS; Betty Ford and Kitty Dukakis did so for alcoholism; and Nancy Reagan did so on behalf of her husband for Alzheimer's.

Elizabeth Gossett did just the opposite. Throughout her desperate struggle to live, her family assiduously eschewed publicity about her condition. When the fact of her disease appeared in newspaper ink despite these efforts, she depended on the public's short attention span and insatiable appetite for news to allow her to slip into obscurity once she had endured her fifteen minutes of fame. She succeeded in fulfilling her dream of living a normal life. Insulin made that possible. For her to have received insulin and yet live as a diabetic would have betrayed Dr. Banting, her parents, and the anonymous child who may or may not have been denied the insulin that she received. It would be a dishonor to the miraculous transformation from invalid to normal girl that occurred in Toronto between August and November 1922. In living as she did, she was true to herself, if not to truth.

Just as Frederick Banting was born ordinary and lived an extraordinary life, Elizabeth Hughes was born extraordinary and lived an ordinary life. Elizabeth continued to protect the normalcy of her existence throughout her adult life, first in New York and then in Michigan. She volunteered for many community, educational, and professional organizations. She served as a trustee of Barnard College and Cranbrook Academy of Art. She was a founding trustee of Oakland University. She was founder and president of the Supreme Court Historical Society. The Hughes Gossett Award, named in her honor, is awarded annually by that society to the best student paper on the history of the court. In 1979 she received an honorary doctor of laws degree from New York Law School. When her name appeared in print, it was related to her philanthropic activities. As years went on, if people queried her about a childhood illness, she would often feign confusion and suggest that they must be thinking of her sister Helen. She never involved herself with any cause related to diabetes. Her will was devoid of any bequest to diabetic causes.

Other insulin takers in that era followed their own paths. As an adult, Myra Blaustein also devoted herself to nondiabetic-related charitable work. She coordinated volunteer activities at the only hospital for mentally ill people of color in Maryland. Her special project, which she introduced to the state of Maryland, was beauty-shop therapy. She never married.

Ruth Whitehill married John J. Leidy of Baltimore, cofounder and president of the Leidy Chemical Corporation. Both Myra and Ruth died in the Baltimore area at age forty-two, three years apart.

Jim Havens, the first American to receive insulin, had an unusual sensitivity to insulin produced from pork pancreas. He would have died, but Eli Lilly and Company supplied him with insulin produced solely from beef pancreas, which did not elicit a reaction. Jim married, fathered two children, and enjoyed a career as an artist. His prints and paintings are considered part of the color woodblock revival in America and may be found in the collections of the Library of Congress and the Metropolitan Museum of Art.

Teddy Ryder kept in touch with Banting until Banting's death in 1941. He spent his adult life working as a librarian in Hartford, Connecticut. He never married. On July 10, 1992, he celebrated a record seventy years of insulin injections, outlasting even Elizabeth Hughes. When he died in 1993 at age seventy-six, he was the last surviving member of the original group of patients treated by Banting. His scrapbook is now at the Thomas Fisher Rare Book Library at the University of Toronto.

Leonard Thompson, the first human trial case for injected insulin, died at Toronto General Hospital thirteen years and three months after his initial injection of "Macleod's serum." He was twenty-seven years old. Today, visitors to the anatomical museum at the Banting Institute at the University of Toronto may see Leonard Thompson's pancreas, which is displayed in a jar of formaldehyde as item 3030.

Blanche Burgess, the nurse and constant companion who played such an instrumental role in the life of Elizabeth Hughes, died of a urinary tract infection in 1967 at the age of seventy-seven. She died a widow, having never remarried. Her body was discovered by a neighbor. She is buried alone in a crypt in the "Corridor of Radiant Love" in the Great Mausoleum at the Forest Lawn Memorial Park Cemetery in Glendale, California.

After Antoinette died in 1945, one day after her fifty-seventh wedding anniversary, Charles grew increasingly close to Elizabeth. He died in

1948 in Osterville, Massachusetts, while summering with Elizabeth Gossett and her family. Truman ordered the nation's flags lowered to half-mast. He was buried next to Antoinette, Helen, and his parents in Woodlawn Cemetery.

Before his death, Hughes had named Merlo Pusey, the publisher of *The Washington Post,* as his authorized biographer. Elizabeth worked intensively with Pusey on the project. The Beerits Memoranda is frequently cited in the definitive, two-volume biography that was published in 1951. Among the eight hundred pages there is no mention of Elizabeth's diabetes. The biography won the Pulitzer Prize in 1952.

Elizabeth Hughes Gossett died unexpectedly of heart failure shortly after a good medical checkup in 1981. At the time of her death, she had received some 42,000 insulin injections over fifty-eight years. Had she lived to read her own obituary in the nation's leading newspapers, she would no doubt have been pleased to find not a single reference to diabetes or childhood illness. In the Hughes family plot at Woodlawn Cemetery in New York, the name Elizabeth Hughes is conspicuously absent from the gravestones commemorating her mother and father, sisters, brother, and grandparents. Even into death, Elizabeth abandoned the identity of Elizabeth Hughes. Elizabeth Gossett's final resting place is marked by a small brass plaque in the Memorial Garden at Christ Church Cranbrook in Bloomfield Hills, Michigan, where she and her husband raised their family. She was cremated, ensuring that no part of her would turn up in a jar.

Elizabeth Hughes Gossett had three children, none of them diabetic. In 1982, her grandson Dr. David Wemyss Denning broke the family silence by writing a letter to the editor of *The New England Journal of Medicine* in response to an article the *Journal* published earlier that year, "A Case of Diabetes Mellitus." The letter began, "It may interest your readers to hear about my grandmother, Elizabeth Gossett (née Hughes) who was Dr. Banting's and Dr. Best's third patient treated with insulin (by her own account). Her diabetes was a complete secret to all but her very close family. It is only since her death in April 1981 that it has become public knowledge."

POSTSCRIPT:
DIABETES AND INSULIN TODAY

THE STORY OF INSULIN HAS CONTINUED TO EVOLVE. IN LATE 1922 Dr. August Krogh returned to Denmark with the insulin formula, courtesy of Macleod. In the spring of 1923, Dr. Krogh and Professor H. C. Hagedorn founded the Nordisk Insulin Laboratorium, which began to manufacture the first Scandinavian insulin. Two years later, Novo Terapeutisk Laboratorium was founded and started producing insulin and a special syringe for injecting it. New, longer-acting insulin was introduced in 1935. The initial work that led to this new type of insulin took place in Denmark, where Dr. Hagedorn discovered that protamine, derived from fish sperm, when combined with insulin, slowed its action. The new protamine insulin allowed many diabetics to reduce their daily injections by half.

Connaught discovered that adding zinc to the protamine insulin slowed the action still further. In 1936 Toronto introduced protamine zinc insulin; it soon became the most widely used form of insulin in Canada. Despite manufacturing advances, two and a half tons of beef and pork pancreas were still required to produce eight ounces of purified insulin in 1948. Worldwide, that year, there were roughly three million insulin-dependent diabetics; one million of them lived in the United States. Under the pressure of this global demand, there were revivals of interest in fish insulin in 1941 and 1948, but while this source proved scientifically feasible, it was not economically practical.

Over time insulin resistance developed in patients after repeated injections of insulin derived from beef and pork pancreas. Some insulin-resistant diabetics died when their condition became uncontrollable. In the late 1950s and early 1960s a small research team at Connaught developed sulfated insulin, which was effective in patients with insulin resistance.

In 1978, Genentech, a small biotechnology startup, produced synthetic "human" insulin using recombinant DNA techniques, which it licensed to Eli Lilly for development and testing. It was approved by the United States Food and Drug Administration in 1982 and sold as Humulin in 1983.

Means of delivery have also advanced beyond the whetstone-sharpened steel needle that Elizabeth Hughes used in 1922. Today's diabetics may use disposable syringes, pens, or pumps. Other modes of delivery being researched include transdermal, oral, inhaled, and pancreatic transplant.

Eighty-five years after the discovery of insulin, diabetes care revenues represent over $3 billion in annual sales for Eli Lilly and Company, its second largest source of revenue. The company today has more than 40,000 employees worldwide—7,400 of whom are actively engaged in research and development of new medicines. Novo Nordisk—originally Nordisk Insulin Laboratorium—is also a world leader in diabetes care, with international production facilities in seven countries and more than 29,000 employees (as of December 2009).

The initial development of insulin took just under two years, whether you count from the first human trial in January 1922 to the official launch in October 1923 or from the first experiments on dogs in the spring of 1921 to the first successful large-scale production in the fall of 1922. Another way to look at it is that insulin became available for general distribution one year and four months after Lilly signed the indenture with Toronto. Today a new drug takes ten to fifteen years to wend its way through clinical development and regulatory review. Toronto's cost of developing insulin was $1,400 ($14,000 in today's dollars) and Eli Lilly's initial investment was $250,000 ($2.5 million in today's dollars). Today the cost of developing a new biotechnology product often exceeds $1 billion.

According to the American Diabetes Association, 23.6 million Americans, or 8 percent of the population, have diabetes. Of these, 5 to 10 percent have type 1 diabetes, which is defined by the body's failure to produce insulin. The remainder have type 2 diabetes, defined by the body's resistance to insulin or inability to produce sufficient insulin. A growing number of Americans—some 57 million—have a condition called prediabetes. This occurs when a person's blood glucose levels are higher than normal but not high enough to warrant a diagnosis of diabetes. The total prevalence of diabetes increased 13.5 percent from 2005 to 2007. The ADA estimates that about 24 percent of those with diabetes don't know they have it. In 2007, diabetes was the fifth leading killer of Americans, causing 73,000 deaths annually. The Centers for Disease Control predicts that if current trends continue, one in three Americans will develop diabetes at some point in their lifetime.

It is still not known what causes type 1 diabetes. Although insulin allows diabetics to live normal lives, there is no cure.

Should you wish to learn more about diabetes and insulin, contact the Juvenile Diabetes Research Foundation at www.jdrf.org or the American Diabetes Association at www.diabetes.org.

A portion of the proceeds from the sale of this book will be donated to the Juvenile Diabetes Research Foundation and the Life for a Child Program of the International Diabetes Federation.

NOTES AND SOURCES

The two geographic hubs of our research corresponded to the two primary locations of the development of insulin: Toronto, Canada, and Indianapolis, Indiana. We went to great lengths to physically place ourselves in the rooms and on the roads in which the primary characters lived, worked, and traveled nearly ninety years ago. In Toronto, we found a rich archive at the Thomas Fisher Rare Book Library at the University of Toronto. Here we were able to see and hold many primary documents and objects related to our story, including Elizabeth's daily dietary and insulin charts written in her own hand, Teddy Ryder's scrapbook, newspaper clippings from around the world, and Banting's desk diaries—not to mention the preserved pancreas of Leonard Thompson. Although Elizabeth destroyed many of the papers, photographs, and other materials that documented her illness, her letters to her mother during the pivotal years of 1921 to 1922 survive. They were essential to both the content and the mood of our narrative as far as she is concerned. We are grateful to the Hughes family for donating them to the Thomas Fisher Rare Book Library. In the University Archives, we found many documents relating to patent and royalty arrangements. We also visited the Banting House National Historic Site in London, Ontario—the house where Banting spent the sleepless night that ended in his scrawling twenty-five words in a bedside notebook.

At the Eli Lilly and Company corporate archive in Indianapolis, we found internal correspondence to and from Clowes and the Lilly family during the critical period in which he made so many trips to Toronto. The Lilly archive also yielded company newsletters, sales literature, and memoranda as well as pharmaceutical paraphernalia. Thanks to the prescience of the company leadership, which recognized the historical significance of the development of insulin even as it was happening, many important primary materials were magnificently catalogued and preserved for history. Moreover, the company celebrated significant anniversaries of the discovery and development of insulin, and the speeches made by Banting, Clowes, and others at these commemorative events provided excellent historical information and perspective.

A third likely geographic research hub would have been Morristown, New Jersey, but alas, the Physiatric Institute was demolished in 1937 and little evidence remains there of the great pioneering effort that Dr. Allen—"Dr. Diabetes"—so faithfully committed himself to carrying out. Information about the Physiatric Institute was drawn primarily from the Hughes papers at Columbia University, the superb collection at the New York Academy of Medicine, and the personal collection of Dr. Alfred Henderson. The property on which Otto Kahn's resplendent mansion stood and where so many desperately ill diabetics found help is now part of a corporate campus.

We read and reread *The Discovery of Insulin* and *Banting: A Biography*, both by Michael Bliss, professor of the history of medicine at the University of Toronto. These books were instrumental in navigating the chronological framework for our narrative. Also critical to our effort were *Charles Evans Hughes*, Merlo Pusey's comprehensive, two-volume biography; *The Autobiographical Notes of Charles Evans Hughes*, edited by David Danelski and Joseph Tulchin; *Sir Frederick Banting* by Dr. Lloyd Stevenson; *Starvation (Allen) Treatment of Diabetes* by Lewis Webb Hill, M.D., and Rena Eckman; *Elliott P. Joslin, M.D.: A Centennial Portrait* by Donald M. Barnett, M.D.; and the privately published commemorative volumes issued by Eli Lilly and Company on the occasion of the anniversary celebrations.

At the Library of Congress we found the Beerits memoranda, hundreds of newspaper articles, and letters and birthday cards written by Charles Evans Hughes to Antoinette Carter Hughes, often in verse, which provided insight into the nature of their relationship. At the Bentley Historical Library in Ann Arbor, Michigan, we discovered Dr. David Denning's letter to *The New England Journal of Medicine*, Elizabeth's obituaries, and biographical information about William Gossett.

We conducted meaningful research at and through the Lilly Library at Indiana University in Bloomington, Indiana; the Indiana Historical Society; the Indiana State Library; Mayo Clinic in Rochester, Minnesota; the New York State Library in Albany, New York; The American Philosophical Society in Philadelphia; the campus of The Silver Bay Association on Lake George, New York; Woodlawn Cemetery in the Bronx, New York; and Crown Hill Cemetery in Indianapolis.

Some of what we found is just plain curious, such as the fact that one of Banting's ancestors published a book about how to lose weight by avoiding fats, starch, and sugar and thus the word "banting" still appears in the Oxford English Dictionary as a synonym for dieting. Or the coincidence that, following the 1906 San Francisco earthquake, Eli Lilly and Company sent cases of much needed medicine to California, where the recently graduated Dr. Allen was helping with the recovery effort. Or the story that in 1925 Banting was in Washington and decided to stop by the house of Charles Evans Hughes on a whim. When he gave the driver the address, the cabbie looked skeptically at his passenger and informed him that he would never be admitted to the home of the secretary of state. Banting smirked and bet the cabbie: If Banting knocked on the door and was admitted, the cab ride would be free. If he was rebuffed, Banting would return to the taxi and pay double the fare. The cabbie lost the bet.

The character of Eddie at the Physiatric Institute is a composite of facts and anecdotes about several diabetics in different locations. The story of the birdseed is all too true. In their desperation diabetic children were driven to sneak food and to consume even nonfood items, including birdseed and toothpaste.

The phone call from Charles Evans Hughes to President Falconer at the University of Toronto is imagined, as is Antoinette's urging him to it. It is not known for certain exactly what prompted Frederick Banting to change his mind about accepting Elizabeth as a patient in August of 1922. However, we know that President Falconer and Charles Evans Hughes had been acquainted with each other for at least a decade; that Charles had never taken an extended trip such as the sail to Brazil without Antoinette since they were married; and that just ten days before the *Pan America* departed for Rio de Janeiro Antoinette delivered Elizabeth into Banting's care—and abruptly left her there.

Our depiction of Banting's burial and retrieval of the ring represents Banting's struggle to reach a final resolution about his engagement. We don't know how his struggle actually manifested itself. Likewise, we don't know that Antoinette took Elizabeth from the Physiatric Institute in the middle of the night. However, this is consistent with her dramatic efforts to save the lives of Elizabeth, Helen, and Charlie. Just as Elizabeth reinvented herself to stay true to herself, where we have invented components of our narrative we have done so to serve a greater understanding of the story and those involved.

One of the most interesting things about this story is that many of the characters who were most famous in 1922 are the most obscure now and vice versa. Charles Evans Hughes—a towering public figure in his time—is virtually unknown today. Likewise, Dr. Allen died poor and forgotten whereas the name of his colleague, Dr. Elliott Joslin, is emblazoned on diabetes centers around the world. Sadly, diabetes itself is still very much with us.

We sometimes learned as much through the pursuit of our research as we did through the research itself. For example, in our travels to Toronto we made it a habit to ask Canadians if they knew the name Frederick Banting. Most either did not recognize the name or had heard it but didn't know who he was. One man we asked knew quite a bit about Banting, but it turned out that he was an American physician. In Glens Falls, New York, the birthplace of Charles Evans Hughes, we discovered just how forgotten Hughes really is today. When we inquired about him at the information desk of the Crandall Public Library there, we were met with the reply, "How do you spell Hughes?"

Sometimes the experience of research was emotionally arresting, as when we found Elizabeth's name conspicuously absent among the graves of her siblings, parents, and grandparents in the Hughes family plot at Woodlawn Cemetery in the Bronx. Even in death Elizabeth abandoned the identity of Elizabeth Hughes. Elizabeth Gossett's final resting place is marked by a modest brass plaque in the columbarium at Christ Church Cranbrook in Bloomfield Hills, where she and her husband raised their family. Having lived in daily companionship with the character of Elizabeth for years, we intuited why she had chosen to be cremated—to avoid having her pancreas (or any other part of her body) suffer the ignominious fate of Leonard Thompson's.

Several questions remain frustratingly unanswered. One relates to Blanche Burgess and the mysterious Dr. McClintock, who, according to Elizabeth's letters, did not seem to need to work and spent much of his time courting Blanche in Toronto. It is our conjecture that McClintock might have been a Pinkerton agent hired by Hughes to ensure Elizabeth's safety shortly before Charles and Antoinette embarked on the *Pan America* to sail to Brazil. If it were to become public that Elizabeth had in effect "jumped the line" in order to secure insulin, her life might have been threatened.

The mystery that shapes the very fulcrum of the story is: How could Charles and Antoinette leave Elizabeth in Toronto when her condition was at its most precarious, and sail for Brazil? The trip was essentially a boondoggle, a trip with no critical political agenda. Wouldn't they want to be with Elizabeth at this decisive moment as they had been with Helen when she neared her end?

Finally, we are left to wonder at the choices Elizabeth made: How could she not keep in touch with Banting or her Toronto cohort or her devoted companion Blanche? How could she fail to dedicate herself in some way to diabetes research and to diabetics, to repay some of the luck and mercy that had spared her life? Could the answer lie in a dim awareness that at the heart of the glorious miracle through which she was saved lay the dark possibility that another child had died in her place?

This is a story punctuated with question marks. It is a story of lost diaries, censored manuscripts, and destroyed photographs. For Elizabeth, erasing was affirming; negation was preservation. This is the very kernel of Elizabeth's story, the calligraphic stroke of her life's work. The scant record of her four years of starvation is like the rippling rings of water that appear when something of substance has dropped beneath the water's surface. From a research perspective, the paucity of materials documenting the critical four years of Elizabeth's life is frustrating, but from a humanistic viewpoint it's hard not to feel just a little bit of an empathetic victory for her. This very lack of documentation is proof of the fulfillment of Elizabeth's impossible dream, one that so many of us take for granted: the chance to live a normal life. In our view, few people relished the extraordinary ordinariness of it as much as she did, and that makes the unanswered questions a little easier to accept.

ENDNOTES

Archival information for papers and collections is given in full in the listing of manuscripts in the bibliography. Shorts forms are used in the notes, as are some readily understandable abbreviations. Note that some papers are dispersed, as for Charles Evans Hughes, Elliott Joslin, and the Physiatric Institute Papers. For the depositories, see the list at the head of the bibliography.

Abbreviations

AH   Antoinette Hughes
EH   Elizabeth Hughes
CEH Charles Evans Hughes

Collections

Banting Papers
Beeman Papers
Best Papers
Best—Personal Collection
Collip Papers
Insulin Committee
Connaught Laboratories Papers
Feasby Papers
Gossett Papers

CEH Papers—LC
CEH Papers—BLCU
EH Papers
Joslin Papers, Marble Library
King Papers
Lilly Archives
Office of the President Papers, University of Toronto
Physiatric Institute Papers, Morristown Historical
   Society

Prologue

1 *Symptoms of diabetes:* Macfarlane, 3.
1 *It wouldn't be given its current name:* Ibid.
2 *urine of their diabetic patients tasted sweet:* Ibid., 4.
2 *In the eighteenth century:* Ibid., 5
2 *In 1856, Claude Bernard:* Ibid., 7.
2 *In 1889, Germany's:* Ibid., 7.
2 *In 1889, France's Edouard Laguesse:* Ibid., 7.
2 *Germany's Georg Zuelzer:* Bliss, *The Discovery of Insulin*, 29, 31.
3 *Allen era:* Joslin, "Diabetes for the Diabetics," (1956), 141.

1: Christ Church Cranbrook, Bloomfield Mills, Michigan, 1981

4 *"intellect, wisdom, quiet yet irresistible leadership"*: Eklund, "A Tribute to Elizabeth Hughes Gossett."

5 *"modesty, dignity, and grace"*: Ibid.

5 *"a champion of civil rights"*: Ibid.

5 *By the time of her death*: In 1982, Elizabeth's grandson, D. W. Denning, wrote Elizabeth took two injections of insulin daily for fifty-eight years. See D. W. Denning to *New England Journal of Medicine*, Mar. 8, 1982. Thomas Fisher Rare Book Library, University of Toronto, Toronto.

5 *And yet, at Elizabeth Gossett's own*: Ibid. Denning said only Elizabeth's close family knew she had diabetes. See also Elizabeth Hughes Gossett to Michael Bliss, ca. 1980, Thomas Fisher Rare Book Library.

6 *The last will*: Excerpt of Elizabeth's last will and testament found in the Polly Hoopes Beeman Collection at the Crandall Public Library, Glens Falls, N.Y.

2: Fifth Avenue, New York City, April 1919

7 *Known as "Dr. Diabetes"*: Barnett, 27.

7 *Born in Iowa*: Bliss, Transcribed unpublished biographical notes of Frederick M. Allen, Thomas Fisher Rare Book Library, 1.

7 *He attended the University of California*: Henderson, 41.

7 *He then volunteered at an animal lab*: Allen, Minutes of Banquet Session, *Proceedings of the American Diabetes Association* (1949), 33.

7 *After three years*: Ibid., 33–34.

8 *Shortly after the book was published*: Henderson, 42.

8 *He was let go*: Bliss, Transcribed unpublished biographical notes of Frederick M. Allen, 2–3.

8 *By this time the United States had entered*: Ibid., 3; Henderson, 43.

8 *One four-year-old boy*: Bliss, Transcribed unpublished biographical notes of Frederick M. Allen.

9 *Both experimented with a new model*: Allen preferred only to work with patients who "seriously co-operate toward their own improvement." See *The Physiatric Institute.*

3: The Breakfast Room of the Home of Charles Evans Hughes, New York City, April 1919

13 *"Work Done by Legal Aid"*: Jan. 27, 1919; *"Hughes Won't Act"*: Dec. 31, 1918; *"End War Policies Now"*: Dec. 1, 1918; *Hughes Points to Flaw"*: Mar. 27, 1919.

13 *"a bearded iceberg"*: Schoen, 68.

14 *Topping the list of blessings*: Pusey, 401; Beerits Memoranda, Biographical File: "1916–1921 Activities," CEH Papers–LC, 15a.

14 *On that morning*: Pusey, 226.

15 *She made a temporary home for them*: Pusey, 338–39.

15 *After politely disabusing them of the idea*: Pusey, 340.

16 *By 1917 he had resettled*: Beerits Memoranda, Biographical File: "1916–1921 Activities," CEH Papers–LC, 1.

16 *"fully one-third of [his] time"*: Danelski and Tulchin, 195.

16 *It was a formidable task*: Pusey, 370–71.

16 *It was called the Spanish flu*: Kolata, 10.

17 *The postwar movements*: Ibid., 247, 5.

17 *By the time it was over*: Ibid., 6–7.

17 *In one year, . . . life expectancy . . . dropped:* Ibid., 8.

17 *Unlike other outbreaks:* Ibid., 5.

17 *While the mortality rate:* Ibid., 7.

17 *Helen Hughes fell ill:* Beerits Memoranda, Biographical File: "1916–1921 Activities," CEH Papers—LC, 15a.

18 *Of the four Hughes children:* Danelski and Tulchin, 337; William T. Gossett to Myron E. Humphrey, Aug. 27, 1962, Gossett Papers.

18 *Further, the Hughes household:* Years later, an adult Elizabeth would recall sitting on Taft's lap during his visit to the Executive Mansion. "Oh! What a biggy man!" she exclaimed while running to her mother. See Elizabeth Hughes Gossett, "Charles Evans Hughes: My Father, the Chief Justice," 9. Hereafter "Charles Evans Hughes."

18 *while Elizabeth peered:* Pusey, 607. Antoinette Hughes used to tell her nosy daughter, "You'll come down with a crash some night."

19 *She had only just begun:* Pusey, 402; Beerits Memoranda, Biographical File: "1916–1921 Activities," CEH–LC, 15a; Worman, 57.

19 *to attend her fifth class reunion:* Beerits Memoranda, Biographical File: "1916–1921 Activities," CEH Papers–LC, 15a.

4: The Library of the Home of Charles Evans Hughes, New York City, April 1919

20 *"Without treatment, the life expectancy . . . less than a year":* Levinson.

21 *All of the patients listed:* Barnett, 20.

22 *She was known as a gracious hostess:* Pusey, 338.

23 *The sanitarium:* Charles Krouse, *Report: Preliminary to a Prospectus for the Establishment of an Institute for the Treatment and Investigation of Diabetes, Nephrites, High Blood Pressure, Etc.* Report commissioned by Charles E. Hughes, Jun. 19, 1920, CEH Papers: Frederick M. Allen file, Butler Library, Columbia University, 2–3.

23 *The nurses would be trained dieticians:* Ibid., 5.

25 *There was a contingent: JAMA* 77 no. 5 (July 1921).

25 *By 1920, the death rate from diabetes:* Lulu Hunt Peters, "Diet and Health: Diabetes," *Los Angeles Times,* Dec. 4, 1922: II9.

26 *The rise in diagnoses:* "The History of Diabetes and the Search for a Cure," fact sheet, Australian Juvenile Diabetes Research Foundation, 2004. Available digitally at: www.jdrf.org.au.

5: New York City, April 1919, Later That Afternoon

29 *"I believe in work":* www.thoughts.forbes.com.

29 *Hughes never stopped working:* Danelski and Tulchin, 191.

29 *He pursued law:* Pusey, 4, 5, 26, 111–12.

30 *The elder Hughes's letters:* Ibid., 30, 38. See Pusey, 28–42, for more correspondence between CEH and his parents during his college years.

30 *By the age of five:* Beerits Memoranda, Biographical File: "Ancestry and Early Life," CEH Papers–LC, 8.

30 *"The Charles E. Hughes Plan of Study":* "Charles E. Hughes: the Career and Public Services of the Republican Candidate for Governor," *New York,* Oct. 20, 1906: 2.

31 *By the age of eight:* Hughes, *Autobiographical Notes,* 15–16.

6: Toronto, Canada, and Cambrai, France, 1917–1918

32 *Great Britian and its empire:* Davis, 248.

33 *In 1917 the population of Toronto:* Careless, n.pag.

33 *By December 1916:* Banting, "The Story of the Discovery of Insulin" (1940), 23–24. Hereafter "Story of the Discovery."

33 *Banting was of Scottish and English descent:* Bliss, *Banting*, 16, 21.

33 *As each of the Banting sons:* Ibid., 23.

33 *Like the parents of Charles Evans Hughes:* Ibid., 26–28.

34 *he maintained the habit:* Bliss, *Banting*, 20, 24, 26, 28.

34 *He was interested in art:* Stevenson, 14, 15, 21.

34 *He was athletic:* Ibid., 15.

34 *According to one story:* Stevenson, 15–16.

34 *Edith Roach was part of Banting's plan:* Bliss, *Banting*, 44, 29, 36.

34 *Banting's ship crossed the Atlantic:* Stevenson, 40, 29.

34 *On the Western Front:* Ibid., 46.

34 *In the winter of 1917:* Ibid., 51.

35 *As a medical officer:* Ibid., 47.

35 *According to an oft-repeated . . . tale:* Ibid., 43.

35 *"Captain F. G. Banting, Medical Officer":* Ibid., 45.

35 *Dressing stations:* Ibid., 46, 48.

36 *At Lilac Farm:* Ibid., 48.

36 *While everyone at the front:* Ibid., 46.

36 *Occasionally Palmer would find Banting studying:* Ibid., 47.

36 *On September 28, 1918, Banting was operating:* Ibid., 48–49. For this day and its subsequent events, see Stevenson, 47–55.

7: War, Peace, and Politics, 1914–1918

40 *"He kept us out of war":* Pusey, 356.

40 *In Cleveland Macleod distinguished himself:* Michael J. Williams, "J. J. R. Macleod," 13, 27.

41 *In 1913 he published . . . Diabetes:* Ibid., 19. For more on Macleod's publications and studies during this time, see Williams, 15–21.

41 *Since moving to Ohio:* Ibid., 26.

41 *The son of a hardworking, popular reverend:* Ibid., 4.

41 *His brother Clement:* Ibid., 26.

41 *It was to be the bloodiest day:* Tucker, 506.

41 *He became increasingly critical of the university president:* Michael J. Williams, 27.

41 *His wife was unwell:* Ibid., 28.

42 *His brother Robert:* Ibid., 26.

42 *In June 1918:* Michael J. Williams, 29.

42 *Sir Robert Falconer:* Robert Falconer to Macleod, Dec. 16, 1916, Thomas Fisher Rare Book Library.

8: Glens Falls, New York, April 1920

43 *Charles Evans Hughes sat at his desk:* Hughes, *Autobiographical Notes,* 195.

43 *In the spring of 1919:* Beerits Memoranda, Biographical File: "1916–1921 Activities," CEH Papers–LC, 15a; Pusey, 402.

43 *Antoinette, Helen, Elizabeth, and Blanche moved:* Beerits Memoranda, Biographical File: "1916–1921 Activities," CEH Papers–LC, 15a.

44 *"Queen of Spas":* Sterngass, 12.

44 *All through the summer and fall:* Pusey, 402.

44 *He drove himself:* "Mrs. Hughes has been under a very severe strain all winter," Charles Evans Hughes wrote to John D. Rockefeller in April 1920, when he backed out of giv-

ing a speech at an upcoming Hippodrome meeting, "as she has been watching our daughter's decline." See CEH to John D. Rockefeller, Apr. 15, 1920, CEH Papers, Butler Library, Columbia University.

44 *Blanche was a . . . war widow:* Information on Blanche Burgess's background was gathered primarily through census records, vital records, and other archived material available through the New York Public Library's Ancestry database and California's Department of Public Health.

45 *She had taken to addressing letters:* It is likely that Elizabeth destroyed the letters she wrote to her mother from the sanitarium, as she had—by her own admission—done with other pieces of evidence related to this difficult time in her life. But for a vivid glimpse into her letter-writing style, see her surviving letters in the EH Collection at the Thomas Fisher Rare Book Library.

45 *"a ray of sunshine . . . just pure gold":* Pusey, 402.

45 *"a rare and joyous spirit":* Hughes, *Autobiographical Notes*, 196.

46 *Elizabeth, weighing in:* Banting et al., "Insulin in the Treatment of Diabetes Mellitus" (1922), 593.

46 *Elizabeth was consuming fewer than five hundred calories:* Ibid.

46 *Dr. Howk, Helen's doctor:* Pusey, 402.

47 *Catherine, the tallest and prettiest:* Not much is known about Catherine Hughes's personal life, except that which was drawn from the Pusey biography on Charles Evans Hughes and some general records obtained from Catherine's alma mater, Wellesley College. Pusey noted Catherine resisted her mother's restrictions as a teenager, bringing home groups of friends even when her father might be working at home (298). At Wellesley, she was a member of the debating club in 1918–1919 and Agora, a literacy club, in 1919–1920 (Wellesley College records).

47 *"Oh the pathos of it!":* Pusey, 402.

48 *She was buried:* Plot Folder: Lot. No. 12673: Lot Owner: Charles Evans Hughes and Antoinette Carter Hughes, Woodlawn Cemetery, N.Y.

48 *Woodlawn's necropolis:* Map of Woodlawn Cemetery, Bronx, N.Y.: Woodlawn Cemetery Office.

49 *To the end of his days:* Pusey, 403.

9: The Idea of the Physiatric Institute, May 1920

50 *Although some patients died of starvation:* Allen, "Diabetes Mellitus" (1920), 89.

50 *Elizabeth's health had improved:* Allen would later call Elizabeth a "remarkably intelligent and cooperative patient," a "model patient in all respects" who "has a thorough knowledge of all details of her diet." See Allen to Banting, Sept. 8, 1922, and Aug. 12, 1922, Banting Collection, Thomas Fisher Rare Book Library.

50 *He was to vacate the premises:* The exact date of Allen's eviction is unknown. Charles Evans Hughes notes in a letter that Allen must "go somewhere" else in July, and a report outlining Allen's acquisition of a private estate in Morristown, New Jersey, was rushed to Hughes on June 19, 1920. See CEH to J. H. Weaver, Esq., June 24, 1920: 4, CEH Papers: Frederick M. Allen file. Butler Library, Columbia University. See also Charles Krouse, *Report*.

51 *"the Baptist Pope":* Silas Hardy Strawn, "Chief Justice Hughes," *New York Herald*, Feb. 23, 1930: 70.

52 *Much to his amazement:* Krouse, *Report*, 6.

52 *The proposal described the purchase of the . . . estate:* Ibid., 6.

52 *The main building:* Ibid., 6.

52 *These would comfortably accommodate:* Ibid., 9.

52 *The other structures:* Ibid., 7.

53 *The estate had cost Kahn:* Henderson, 44.

53 *Mr. Kahn had employed:* Krouse, *Report*, 10.

53 *The medical purposes of the Physiatric Institute:* TK?

53 *Allen had worked out the operating costs:* Krouse, *Report*, 13.

53 *He was so committed:* Ibid., 9.

54 *Elizabeth was four feet eleven inches tall:* Banting et al., "Insulin in the Treatment of Diabetes Mellitus," 593; Bliss, *The Discovery of Insulin*, 43.

54 *Elizabeth herself had proved:* Allen would later praise Burgess as a nurse "especially qualified" in the treatment of diabetes, who had kept a "complete and accurate history" of Elizabeth's progress. See Allen to Banting, Aug. 12, 1922, Thomas Fisher Rare Book Library.

54 *After satisfying himself:* Hughes admitted his support of Allen's Institute rested solely on his daughter's affliction with diabetes and the hope Allen's work could be a great benefit in the treatment of the disease. See CEH to J. H. Weaver, Esq., June 24, 1920, CEH Papers: Frederick M. Allen file, Butler Library, Columbia University.

10: Banting's House in London, Ontario, October 30–31, 1920

56 *The next morning:* Banting, "Story of the Discovery" (1940), 45.

56 *Just a few weeks earlier:* Ibid., 38–39.

57 *He felt lost:* "It was the first time in my life," Banting would write in 1940, "that I have ever had time on my hands. I was lonesome [There were heavy expenses and I was not making any money] . . . I was deeply in debt—and became deeper as the months passed. I was very unhappy and worried." See Ibid., 35–37.

57 *Only four months before:* Stevenson, 61.

57 *The total purchase price:* Bliss, *Banting*, 48.

57 *He and Edith continued:* Ibid., 58.

58 *And the population continued to grow:* Careless, app., table V.

58 *While Banting had been in the trenches:* Bliss, *Banting*, 44, 45.

58 *Banting found temporary work:* Banting, "Story of the Discovery" (1940), 33–34.

58 *"Surgeons were very plentiful":* Ibid., 34.

58 *While in Toronto:* Stevenson, 60–61.

58 *He held fast to traditional:* Banting recounts with pride his creating a wooden foot and brace for a young patient. See Banting, "Story of the Discovery" (1940), 17–19.

59 *Bill Tew had also opened a practice:* Ibid., 36.

59 *Banting's income for his first month:* Banting, "The History of Insulin" (1929), 1; Banting, "Story of the Discovery" (1940), 35.

59 *In August his income rose:* Banting, Notebook Daily Accounts 1920–1921, MS Coll. 76 (Banting), Box 26, Thomas Fisher Rare Book Library.

59 *"Things fall apart":* The poem was first published in the American magazine *The Dial* in November 1920. Yeats later included it in a verse collection published in 1921. See Yeats, 19.

60 *"I've been thinking of joining up":* Banting, "Story of the Discovery" (1940), 48–50.

61 *At one o'clock:* For Banting's personal account of reading the article, see Banting, "Story of the Discovery" (1940), 45–48.

61 *Professor C. L. Starr:* C. L. Starr to Banting, Dec. 14, 1920, Thomas Fisher Rare Book Library.

61 *"Any reference to the pancreas":* Barron.

62 *"Diabetus [sic] Ligate pancreatic":* Banting, Notes, October 31, 1920, London, Ontario, Academy of Medicine Collection, 123 (Banting), Folder 1, Thomas Fisher Rare Book Library.

63 *It was not a new idea:* For more on Lydia DeWitt's findings, see DeWitt, 193–239.

63 *Ernest Lyman Scott:* See Scott, 306–10.

63 *Nicolas Paulesco . . . "pancreine":* Hazlett, 4. Paulesco's publication on this work appears in French. See Paulesco, 555–59.

63 *He would later say:* Genevieve Forbes, "Insulin Discoverer Says It Is Jealous Mistress," *Chicago Daily Tribune,* Mar. 7, 1924: 19.

11: Toronto or Bust, October 1920 to April 1921

64 *After the lecture, Banting met with Miller:* Banting, "Story of the Discovery" (1940), 56.

64 *Miller tried to sound encouraging:* Banting's recollection of Miller's reaction varies slightly. In his 1940 account, Miller liked his idea, but believed it had been attempted before. In Banting, "Account of the Discovery of Insulin," as requested by Col. Albert Gooderham in 1922, Banting writes that Miller didn't think it had been attempted before.

64 *In any case:* Bliss, *The Discovery of Insulin,* 48, 51.

65 *"And your timing couldn't be better":* Docket for Meeting of the Rockefeller Foundation, Feb. 23, 1921, "The Rockefeller Foundation, 1917–1921" file, CEH Papers, Butler Library, Columbia University, 24.

65 *Hadn't he claimed:* Isaacson, 387.

65 *"Lights All Askew":* "Lights All Askew in the Heavens," *New York Times,* Nov. 10, 1919.

65 *The* Times *of London carried the headline:* "Revolution in Science," *Times of London,* Nov. 15, 1919.

66 *Banting's first impression:* For Banting's account of his meeting with Macleod, see Banting, "Account of the Discovery of Insulin" (1922), 1–2; Banting, "Story of the Discovery" (1940), 61–63.

66 *There he had reunited with his parents:* Michael J. Williams, 30, 26.

66 *Banting was not at all:* Ibid., 38.

69 *Macleod had begun to make plans:* Ibid., 63; McCormick, "Insulin From Fish," 11.

69 *Macleod hoped to complete a paper:* For a summary of Macleod's findings at the Atlantic Biological Station in St. Andrews, see Macleod, "The Source of Insulin," 1–24.

70 *"if your offer":* Banting to Macleod, Mar. 8, 1921, app. 2 to Macleod, "History of the Researches Leading to the Discovery of Insulin," Sept. 20, 1922, Collip Collection. Hereafter "History of the Researches."

70 *Despite having written the letter:* Banting, "Story of the Discovery" (1940), 48–50.

70 *Three days later:* Macleod to Banting, Mar. 11, 1921, app. 4 to Macleod, "History of the Researches," Sept. 20, 1922, Collip Collection.

70 *When Macleod's letter reached Banting:* Banting, "Story of the Discovery" (1940), 50.

71 *On April 18, 1921, Banting accepted the offer:* Banting to Macleod, Apr. 18, 1921, app. 3 to Macleod, "History of the Researches," Sept. 20, 1922, Collip Collection.

12: Presidential Politics, 1916 and 1920

73 *Hughes, now fifty-eight:* Pusey, 401.

73 *Until now he had adhered to . . . Franklin's credo:* Elizabeth Hughes Gossett, "Charles Evans Hughes," 14.

73 *"a burden of incessant toil":* "Hughes Ignores Fusion Fight Here," *New York Times,* Oct. 19, 1907: 1.

73 *He was a very private, deeply thoughtful man:* Lesley Oelsner, "Supreme Court Society Seeks

to Expand," *New York Times,* July 24, 1975: 14; William T. Gossett, "The Human Side of Chief Justice Hughes," 1415–16; Pusey, 416.

74 *In 1920 Elizabeth was enthralled:* Ibid., 607.

74 *One of her earliest memories:* Elizabeth Hughes Gossett, "Charles Evans Hughes," 11.

74 *Hughes had seized the lead:* "California in Doubt; Majority for Wilson Turns to 1400 Lead for Hughes," *New York Times,* Nov. 8, 1916: 1; "Hughes Still 10 to 7 Among the Bettors," *New York Times,* Nov. 4, 1916: 4.

74 *There, huge celebratory bonfires:* "Election Lights to Be Signaled from Times Tower," *New York Times,* Nov. 6, 1916: 2; "100,000 Get Returns at Times Bulletins," *New York Times,* Nov. 8, 1916: 4; "Election Results by Times Building Flash," *New York Times,* Nov. 6, 1904: 3.

74 *At midnight, the signal flashed:* Elizabeth Hughes Gossett, "Charles Evans Hughes," 11.

75 *One such fire burned in Chicasha:* William T. Gossett to Myron E. Humphrey, Aug. 27, 1962, Gossett Papers, Bentley Library.

75 *The next morning the count was official:* Pusey, 362.

75 *"I have not desired the nomination":* Pusey, 332.

75 *So confident were Antoinette and Charles:* Pusey, 276.

76 *Antoinette . . . tooled around town:* Elizabeth Hughes Gossett, "Charles Evans Hughes," 8.

76 *There was an unspoken feeling:* Elizabeth Hughes Gossett, "Charles Evans Hughes," 8.

76 *Shortly before the Republican National Convention:* Pusey, 403.

76 *Hughes and Steinbrink met:* Pusey, 403.

77 *He predicted:* Ibid., 403.

77 *With these assets:* Pietrusza, 72–73.

77 *The Democratic presidential candidate:* "Roosevelt Makes 12 Speeches In Day," *New York Times* Oct. 30, 1920: 3.

78 *"America's present need":* Pietrusza, 86.

78 *"an army of pompous phrases":* Warren G. Harding biography, www.whitehouse.gov.

78 *To stabilize her metabolism:* Banting et al., "Insulin in the Treatment of Diabetes Mellitus," 593 (Chart).

78 *The Harding-Cox presidential election returns:* Pietrusza, 407.

79 *When her parents told Elizabeth the news:* Pusey, 607.

79 *She persuaded her parents:* Pusey, 606.

13: The Physiatric Institute, Morristown, New Jersey, 1921

80 *Physiatric Institute . . . opened with much fanfare:* "New Medical Institute; Jersey Institution for Diabetes and Metabolic Disorders Opens," *New York Times,* April 27, 1921: 8.

80 *A typical breakfast:* Elizabeth's typical diet is derived from her letters and the "Chart for Elizabeth Hughes," a meticulous food chart Elizabeth kept for herself in 1922. See the EH Papers and Banting Collection.

80 *The advanced kitchen:* Hill, Webb, and Eckman, 99, 103–106, 116–17.

81 *watchful gaze of the nurses:* Diabetes patients who were undergoing starvation therapy were known to eat a wide variety of things in desperation, including toothpaste. See Bunn.

81 *Teddy had been diagnosed:* Frank Jones, "Teddy Ryder: Banting's Living Miracle," *Toronto Star,* Feb. 20, 1983: A6.

81 *Nevertheless, on November 19, 1920, they committed Teddy:* Morton Ryder to Banting, June 25, 1922, Banting Collection.

81 *his caloric intake:* Jones, "Teddy Ryder," A6.

82 *When he went home:* Ibid.

82 *University of Mossouri and Cornell Medical College:* Krouse, *Report,* 5–6.

82 *Both Elizabeth and Eddie were fond of birds:* Elizabeth's adoration of birds can be seen in her letters to her mother, held in the Elizabeth Hughes Papers.

83 *The most famous war pigeon:* Home of Heroes Web site, www.homeofheroes.com.

14: The University of Toronto, Summer 1921

85 *On Saturday, May 14, 1921:* Banting, "Account of the Discovery of Insulin" (1922), 2.

85 *He had made plans:* Bliss, *Banting,* 61.

85 *Noble and Best decided to split the summer:* Banting, "Story of the Discovery" (1940), 66.

85 *It was hardly the gleaming vision:* Ibid., 66.

86 *Charley had grown up:* Charles Best, transcribed interview by Gene McCormick, Sept. 24, 1968, Lilly Archives.

86 *Banting's mother had been the first white child:* Bliss, *Banting,* 18, 19, 23, 24; Stevenson, 12.

87 *And so one of the greatest advances in medical science:* Ibid., 66–67.

87 *Their courtship sounded:* For a personal account of Best's relationship with Margaret, see *Margaret and Charley,* written by their son, Henry Best, in 2003.

87 *Banting learned:* Charles Best, transcribed interview by Gene McCormick, Sept. 24, 1968, Lilly Archives.

87 *Macleod had estimated:* Bliss, *Banting,* 63.

87 *On May 17 Macleod performed the first pancreatectomy:* Banting later recalls this surgery was the only time he ever saw Macleod in the operating room: Banting, "Account of the Discovery of Insulin" (1922), 2.

87 *Macleod demonstrated correct procedure:* Bliss, *Banting,* 62.

88 *Banting had performed his first operation:* Banting, "Story of the Discovery" (1940), 43–44.

88 *Banting and Best began:* Best, "Reminiscences . . .", 398.

88 *One of the most useful books:* "Minutes of Banquet Session," *Proceedings of the American Diabetes Association* 9 (1949), 33.

88 *When Charley wasn't in the lab:* Letters written by Charley to Margaret during this time are filled with professions of love and also how much he misses her—contrast to Banting's relationship with Edith, where no such letters were found (Best to Margaret Mahon, various dates, Best Personal Collection).

89 *The first dog:* Banting, Laboratory Notebook, May 18–19, 1921, Academy of Medicine, Banting Collection, 5, 7.

89 *By the time Macleod left:* Banting, "Account of the Discovery of Insulin" (1922), 2.

89 *The conditions in which they worked:* Ibid., 3.

89 *In May and June:* Bliss, *The Discovery of Insulin,* 74.

89 *At night, he often cooked:* Banting, "Story of the Discovery" (1940), 44–45.

89 *On Sundays, he frequented suppers:* Bliss, *The Discovery of Insulin,* 74.

89 *In mid-June, Best left for ten days:* Banting, "Story of the Discovery" (1940), 69–70.

89 *He was living in a boardinghouse:* Bliss, *The Discovery of Insulin,* 74.

90 *When Best returned in late June:* Banting, "Story of the Discovery" (1940), 70–73.

90 *When the time came:* Ibid., 69.

90 *Banting and Best depancreatized:* Bliss, *The Discovery of Insulin,* 67.

91 *After Banting and Best ran through the original allotment:* Bliss, *The Discovery of Insulin,* 61.

91 *Banting was quite fond of dogs:* Banting, "History of Insulin" (1929), 5.

91 *He said that one dog:* Banting, "Story of the Discovery" (1940), 22b–29b.

91 *On July 11:* Banting and Best, "The Internal Secretion of the Pancreas," 254. See also Bliss, *The Discovery of Insulin,* 67.

91 *Dog 410:* For some reason, Banting and Best only identified their canine subjects by physical descriptions and then assigned them apparently random numbers. They sometimes

numbered a new dog with the same number as a dog that had died, making notes they took that summer confusing. A series of Banting's original notebooks can be found at the Thomas Fisher Rare Book Library, MS Coll. 76 (Banting), and Academy of Medicine, 123 (Banting), Folders 1–11.

91 *On Saturday, July 30 they chloroformed donor Dog 391:* Banting, and Best, "Internal Secretion," 254; Bliss, *The Discovery of Insulin,* 67–68.

91 *At 10:15 in the morning they injected:* Banting, Notebook, Jan. 1921–Aug. 10, 1921, Banting Collection, 82–84. To read Banting's published account of the experiment with Dog 410, see Banting and Best, "Internal Secretion," 254–56.

92 *Despite this they left the lab:* Banting, Notebook, Jan. 1921–Aug. 10, 1921, Banting Collection, 84.

92 *In a paper . . . they speculated:* Banting and Best, "Internal Secretion," 255.

92 *On Monday, August 1 the collie . . . lay unconscious:* Banting. Notebook, Jan. 1921–Aug. 10, 1921, Banting Collection, 85; Banting, Chart for Dog 406, Jul. 31–Aug. 1, 1921, Banting Collection; Best to Macleod. Aug. 9, 1921, Banting Collection, 2.

92 *On Wednesday, August 3:* Banting and Best, "Internal Secretion," 259–61. See also Banting, Notebook, Jan. 1921–Aug. 10, 1921, Banting Collection, 86–88a, 40–49; Banting, Chart for Dog 408, Aug. 3–6, 1921, Banting Collection.

92 *"I have so much to tell you":* Banting to Macleod, Aug, 9, 1921, Banting Collection.

93 *"I am very anxious":* Ibid.

93 *The results of the comparative experiment:* For Best and Banting's notes on Dog 92 and Dog 409, see Banting, Notebook, Aug. 11–Sept. 16, 1921, Banting Collection, 54–83. Also see Banting, Chart for Dog 92 and 409, Aug 11–31, 1921, Banting Collection; Banting and Best, "Internal Secretion," 251–66.

94 *On August 19 . . . Banting conceived of a way:* Banting, Notebook, Aug. 11–Sept. 16, 1921, 67–69. Bliss, *The Discovery of Insulin,* 77.

94 *On the evening of August 20, Dog 92:* Ibid., 71–73.

94 *greatest experiences:* "I shall never forget the joy of opening the door of the cage and seeing this dog, which had been unable to walk, jump to the floor and run about the room in its normal fashion," (Banting, "The History of Insulin" [1929], 6).

94 *Over the next few days:* Banting, Notebook, Aug. 11–Sept. 16, 1921, Banting Collection, 74–83.

95 *She had lived . . . twenty days:* "I shall never forget that dog as long as I shall live," Banting wrote in 1940. "I have seen patients die and I have never shed a tear. But when that dog died I wanted to be alone for the tears would fall despite anything I could do. I was ashamed then. I hid my face from Best, but now I am not ashamed." See Banting, "Story of the Discovery" (1940), 30b.

95 *One of the people he persuaded:* Banting to Macleod, Aug. 9, 1921, Banting Collection.

95 *nickname of Vermin Henderson:* Bliss, *The Discovery of Insulin,* 81.

95 *Henderson agreed:* Velyien Henderson to Robert Falconer, Sept. 21, 1921, University of Toronto/Office of the President Collection, University of Toronto Archives.

15: Washington, D.C., and Bolton, New York, March to September 1921

97 *"Less government in business:* Harding first introduced the slogan in a signed article in *The World's Work*: "Harding Outlines Policies He Favors; Declares for Less Government in Business and More Business in Government," *New York Times,* Nov. 5, 1920: 7.

97 *Hughes had a perfect genius:* "Hughes Has Man's Job," *New York Times,* Mar. 27, 1921: XX3.

98 *She often hosted receptions:* Elizabeth Hughes Gossett, "Charles Evans Hughes," 11.

98 *Barely a month:* Pusey, 606–607.

98 *"CaCa":* Ibid., 219.

98 *Antoinette arranged for Elizabeth and Blanche:* Unless indicated otherwise, the descriptions of most of Elizabeth Hughes's day-to-day activities in Bolton, N.Y., were derived from her letters to her mother during her stay. They are held in the Elizabeth Hughes Papers.

99 *"There are 4 hydroairplanes [sic]":* EH to AH, Aug. 30, 1921, 3.

100 *"last night really was the night of all nights":* EH to AH, Aug. 24, 1921.

100 *"I want you to be very frank with me":* EH to AH, Sept. 2, 1921.

100 *"I don't know what's the matter":* EH to AH, Sept. 2, 1921.

101 *"If my St. Nicholas has come":* EH to AH, Sept. 5, 1921.

16: The Washington Conference, November 12, 1921, to February 6, 1922

102 *Occasionally he would emerge:* Danelski and Tulchin, xix.

103 *Antoinette led a procession:* Worman, 48.

103 *Despite this precaution:* Pusey, 464–65.

103 *In a proposal that was bold beyond all expectations:* "American Plan a Surprise; Long Applause by Great Audience Follows Presentation by Hughes," *New York Times,* Nov. 13, 1921.

104 *Tables were prepared:* Ibid.

104 *The admirals . . . were outraged:* Pusey, 477.

104 *Japan preferred a ratio of 10:7:* Ibid., 476, 479.

104 *"End of Conference Still Not in Sight":* New York Times, Jan. 27, 1922: 2.

17: The Physiatric Institute, Morristown, New Jersey, November 1921

108 *In November 1921 Elizabeth's weight:* Banting et al., "Insulin in the Treatment of Diabetes Mellitus," 593 (Chart).

110 *Despite his being a successful doctor:* Frederick Allen and Mary B. Wishart were married on October 22, 1921, at the Church of the Transfiguration in New York City. NYC Marriage License Records.

110 *Weren't they to stay:* Elizabeth wrote "Honeymoon Cottage" as the return address on all her letters home while she stayed in Bermuda.

18: The University of Toronto, September to December 1921

111 *During the first week:* Recounting the event over ten years later, Banting wrote "One mellows with the years but I still find it impossible to forget the awfulness the loneliness [sic] and the financial worries that were associated with London. Nor can I forget the feeling of defeat that came over me as I took my final leave on that foggy autumn morning . . ." Banting, "Story of the Discovery" (1940), 51–52.

111 *Banting could remain:* Macleod to Banting, Aug. 23, 1921, Banting Collection.

112 *"One result is no result":* Bliss, *The Discovery of Insulin,* 79.

112 *On September 5:* Banting, Notebook, Aug. 11–Sept. 16, 1921, Banting Collection, 84.

112 *While they waited:* Ibid., 84–94.

112 *On September 12:* Banting, Notebook 3, Sept. 12–16, 1921, Banting Collection, 12–16.

112 *On September 17:* Banting, Notebook 3A. Sept. 16–Dec. 22, 1921, Banting Collection, 1–5.

113 *In mid-September:* Velyien Henderson to Sir Robert Falconer, Sept. 21, 1921, University of Toronto Archives.

113 *"I told him":* Banting, "Account of the Discovery of Insulin" (1922), 4.

113 *Banting suggested:* A year later, Macleod would recount the meeting with Banting. He

recalls that he "pointed out that this being [Banting] and Best's research they should independently complete the work as outlined, and that then if the results continued satisfactory I would participate in the further investigations with my assistants." Banting does not mention this detail in his accounts. Macleod to Gooderham, "History of the Researches," Sept. 20, 1922, Collip Collection, 4.

113 *Then Banting suggested:* Banting, "Story of the Discovery" (1940), 3d. In W. R. Feasby, "The Discovery of Insulin," it is said that Best was at first "opposed" to bringing Collip into the group, as Best had "not been given the opportunity, with adequate help and testing facilities on diabetic dogs, to do more than a few experiments on the chemical properties of insulin." See Feasby, 68–84.

114 *Collip was a brilliant associate professor of biochemistry:* Barr, 238–40.

114 *Prior to Macleod's departure:* Banting, "Story of the Discovery" (1940), 3d.

114 *It seemed perfectly logical:* Macleod to Gooderham, "History of the Researches," Sept. 20, 1922, Collip Collection, 4.

114 *In October, Banting appeared on the payroll:* When Henderson propositioned Banting with the idea of a job, Banting recalls, "It was the only solution. . . . It would be a good experience. . . . [Henderson] was a man. He was honest, sincere, unselfish," (Banting, "Story of the Discovery" [1940]), 8b; Velyien Henderson to Sir Robert Falconer, Sept. 21, 1921, University of Toronto Archives.

114 *Macleod arranged:* Macleod to Robert Falconer, Sept. 30, 1921, University of Toronto Archives.

114 *Banting and Best visited a local abbatoir:* Banting and Best, "Pancreatic Extracts"; Bliss, *The Discovery of Insulin,* 92.

114 *For the first time Macleod seemed impressed:* When prominent diabetes doctor Elliott P. Joslin inquired if the research performed in Toronto could provide hope to his diabetic patients, Macleod wrote him on November 21, stating that while the work was inconclusive, "I may say privately that I believe we have something that may be of real value in the treatments of diabetics." Macleod to Joslin, Nov. 21, 1921, Best Collection.

114 *Macleod invited Banting and Best:* Macleod to Gooderham, "History of the Researches," Sept. 20, 1922, Collip Collection, 4–5.

115 *Banting would present:* See Banting, "Account of the Discovery of Insulin" (1922), 4–5.; Macleod to Gooderham, "History of the Researches," Sept. 20, 1922, Collip Collection, 4–5.

115 *according to Banting:* Banting, "Account of the Discovery of Insulin" (1922), 5. Macleod claims that he only found out Banting was angry with his introduction in January 1922. See Macleod to Gooderham, "History of the Researches," Sept. 20, 1922, Collip Collection, 4.

115 *"Half my life":* Banting Collection.

115 *The paper was published:* See Banting and Best, "Internal Secretion," 251–66. Banting and Best also expressed "our gratitude to Professor Macleod for helpful suggestions and laboratory facilities" (266).

115 *"At the meeting of the Southern Medical Association":* Joslin to Macleod, Nov. 19, 1921, Best Collection.

116 *"I have heard indirectly":* Leonard G. Rowntree to Macleod, Dec. 8, 1921.

116 *Dr. N. B. Taylor of the University of Toronto:* Macleod to Gooderham, "History of the Researches," Sept. 20, 1922, Collip Collection, 4–5.

116 *"terminologic horses [in the]":* McCormick, "History of Insulin," Lilly Archives, 124, *f. 141.*

116 *On November 23:* Banting, Laboratory Notebook 3A, Sept. 16–Dec. 22, 1921, Banting Collection, 43.

116 Sharpey-Schäfer, Edward. *An Introduction to the Study of Endocrine Glands and Internal Secretions: Lane Medical Lectures, 1913.* Palo Alto: Stanford University Press (1914): 84.

117 *Banting asked permission to add Macleod's name:* Macleod to Gooderham, "History of the Researches," Sept. 20, 1922, Collip Collection, 5.

19: The Crossroads of America, Indianapolis, Indiana, 1919–1921

118 *Alec Clowes was a dazzling tornado of a man:* As told by Linville A. Baker, hired by Clowes to work at Woods Hole in 1938, and Miss Lenora Clark, who became Clowes's secretary in 1940. Transcribed interview with Linville A. Baker Sept. 26, 1969, Lilly Archives; Leonora Clark,. "Biography of a Boss," Thomas Fisher Rare Book Library.

118 *"He lived more hours:* Madison, *Eli Lilly: A Life,* 55.

118 *At that time:* Clark, "Biography of a Boss." Lenora M. Clark was Clowes's longtime secretary at Eli Lilly and Company.

119 *Eli Lilly, grandson:* In October 1919, J. K. Lilly Sr. released a forty-page memorandum entitled "A Plan for Promoting the Affairs of Eli Lilly & Company During the Years 1920–21–22–23." Included in the memo was a plan to establish a "department of Experimental Medicine," Ibid., 46.

120 *He had been only fourteen years old:* Ibid. 4, 5.

120 *J. K. Sr. joined the company:* Ibid., 6, 14.

120 *Eli's careful analysis:* Ibid., 28.

120 *And taking a cue from Henry Ford:* Ibid., 46–51.

120 *The conservative argument:* Ibid., 41, 38.

121 *Clowes completed his medical studies:* George H. A. Clowes Jr., 199.

121 *When the war ended in 1918, Clowes:* Ibid., 204.

121 *Just then the Lillys:* Madison, *Eli Lilly: A Life,* 53.

121 *Built in 1852–53:* McDonald, 20.

121 *The huge numbers of workers:* McDonald, 33–34, 40; Tenuth, 110–11.

121 *In the year 1918 more than 7.5 million passengers:* Madison, *Indiana Through Tradition and Change,* 196.

122 *In 1920 the state's employment numbers:* Phillips, 273.

122 *The city competed:* Tenuth, 108–10; McDonald, 69–70.

123 *In 1898, empty . . . gelatin capsules:* McCormick, "McCormick History Redo 12.12.2007," CD-ROM, Lilly Archives, 119.

124 *In 1905, company sales:* "History in Chronological Order 1876 to 1950", Lilly Archives, CD-ROM, 48.

125 *One headline read:* "Conference Takes a Day Off At Last," Dec. 25, 1921, *New York Times:* 3.

125 *There stood L. S. Ayres:* Early description drawn from Tenuth, 59–60; McDonald, 45–46; an Ayres exhibit at the Indianapolis Historical Society seen by author.

126 *his fond nickname:* Transcribed interview with Allen Clowes, from a private collection provided by the Clowes family, Indiana Historical Society.

126 *Clowes would travel:* Anna Keltch Hickson, transcribed interview by Gene McCormick, Lilly Archives, 7.

20: The American Physiological Society Meeting, New Haven, Connecticut, December 28–30, 1921

128 *He assigned specific duties:* Macleod to Gooderham, "History of the Researches," Sept. 20, 1922. Collip Collection, 6, 9, 11–12; Bliss, *The Discovery of Insulin,* 108.

129 *Acutely aware of the enormous significance:* Barr, 242. R. L. Noble would describe this as the

"turning point" in Collip's career, when he would begin his specialization in endocrinology. See: Noble, R. L., 3.

129 *The two professors met:* Bliss, *The Discovery of Insulin,* 109.

129 *A diabetic Airedale:* Ibid., 102–103.

129 *With rabbits billed to the Department:* Bill for Toronto Dog and Cat Hospital to Prof. Macleod, Dept. of Physiology, June 1, 1921, Best Papers.

129 *It was Macleod:* E. Clark Noble, Mar. 12, 1977, unpublished account, Thomas Fisher Rare Book Library, 2.

129 *In addition to . . . assigned roles:* For notes on the experiments performed Dec. 6–16, see Banting, Laboratory Notebook 3A, Sept. 16, 1921–Dec. 22, 1921, Banting Papers, 53–66.

130 *On December 20, 1921:* Banting recorded this event on a single index card. See "Note card recording the first clinical use of extract," Banting Papers.

130 *Marjorie:* Dog 33 was depancreatized on November 18. See Banting, Laboratory Notebook 3A, Sept. 16–Dec. 22, 1921, Banting Papers, 36.

131 *The American Physiological Society:* Adolph, 12.

131 *The conference began:* For abstracts of all the lectures presented at the 1921 APS conference, see *Proceedings of the American Journal of Physiology, Thirty-Fourth Annual Meeting held in New Haven, December 28, 29, 30, 1921,* Baltimore: Feb. 1, 1922.

131 *He loathed public speaking:* E. Clark Noble would write Banting "was a notoriously poor speaker" when recounting the event fifty years later. Noble, unpublished account, October 1971, Thomas Fisher Rare Book Library, 4.

132 *As neither Banting nor Best was a member:* For their respective views of the meeting, see Banting, "Story of the Discovery" (1940), 7d; Macleod to Gooderham, "History of the Researches," Sept. 20, 1922, Collip Papers, 7. For a third-party account, see E. Clark Noble, October 1971, 4;, Thomas Fisher Rare Book Library, 3–4.

133 *Scott was among the first to reach him:* Macleod, "History of the Researches," Sept. 20, 1922, Collip Papers, 7. For more on Scott's findings, see Scott, 306–10.

133 *"Well done, Dr. Banting":* Clowes would later state, "It is true that Banting presented his material somewhat haltingly and certainly very modestly. However, anyone who was at all cognizant with the subject must have realized that a great discovery had been made and that provided the work could be brought to fruition there was every prospect that an important means of treating diabetes would be developed." See Clowes, "Banting Memorial Address" (1947), 53.

134 *Later, Clowes left a note:* See Macleod, "History of the Researches," Sept. 20, 1922, Collip Papers, 7. See also Michael J. Williams, 47.

134 *the brainchild of . . . professor John G. FitzGerald:* Rutty, "Couldn't Live Without It," 6.

134 *As far as he knew:* Macleod would write he only learned later that Banting was unhappy with his conduct and involvement in the experiments. See Macleod to Gooderham, "History of the Researches," Sept. 20, 1922, Collip Papers, 8.

134 *They had reserved a sleeping car:* Banting, "Story of the Discovery" (1940), 7d–8d.

135 *"They're all vultures and vipers":* Ibid.

21: Success and Failure, The University of Toronto, January 1922

137 *As the reality of a human trial:* Macleod to Gooderham, "History of the Researches," Sept. 20, 1922, Collip Papers, 8; Bliss, *The Discovery of Insulin,* 111–12.

137 *He had assumed he would be the one:* In 1954, Best claimed Banting said to him: "I think it would be much more appropriate, Charley, in view of our work together, if this first case should receive insulin made by your hands and tested by us on dogs and on ourselves" (Best to Sir Henry Dale, Feb. 22, 1954, Feasby Papers, 3).

137 *But Duncan Graham:* Banting, "Story of the Discovery" (1940), 18d.

138 *Although it galled him:* Macleod to Gooderham, "History of the Researches," Sept. 20, 1922, 8, Collip Papers. Macleod writes that after Banting's "repeated solicitations," he was able to "persuade" Graham to allow Banting's extract to be used clinically.

138 *Amid this high drama and posturing:* Patient Records for Leonard Thompson, Toronto, Dec. 1921–Jan. 1922, Banting Papers; and Banting et al., "Pancreatic Extracts in the Treatment of Diabetes Mellitus," 2–4; Bliss, *The Discovery of Insulin,* 112.

138 *He had lost most of his hair:* Banting et al., "Pancreatic Extracts," 4; Burrow, 341.

138 *On January 11:* See Patient Records for Leonard Thompson, Toronto, Dec. 1921–Jan. 1922, Banting Papers.

139 *The result was inconclusive:* Macleod to Gooderham, "History of the Researches," Sept. 20, 1922, Collip Papers, 8.

139 *Unwisely he confided his view to Duncan Graham:* Ibid.

140 *One of Ross's patients:* Bliss, *The Discovery of Insulin,* 125.

140 *Macleod was appalled:* Macleod to Gooderham, "History of the Researches," Sept. 20, 1922, Collip Papers, 9–10.

141 *Macleod painted a bright picture:* Macleod to Clowes, Apr. 3, 1922, Connaught Collection, Aventis Pasteur Limited Archives 95–025–01.

142 *"I experienced . . . the greatest thrill":* Bliss, *The Discovery of Insulin,* 117.

143 *His refusal . . . sent Banting into a rage:* Banting, "Story of the Discovery" (1940), 16d–17d. Also Best to Sir Henry Dale, Feb. 22, 1954, Feasby Papers.

143 *"Banting leaped on Collip":* "Medicine: Spark-Plug Man," *Time,* Mar 17, 1941.

143 *On January 21 Banting and Best discontinued . . . injections:* Banting and Best, "Pancreatic Extracts" (May 1922), 7.

143 *On Monday, January 23:* Banting et al., "Pancreatic Extracts in the Treatment of Diabetes Mellitus" (March 1922), 5; Patient Records for Leonard Thompson, Toronto, Dec. 1921–Jan. 1922, Banting Papers, 8; Bliss, *The Discovery of Insulin,* 120.

144 *By this time Marjorie could hardly . . . stand:* Banting and Best, "Pancreatic Extracts" (May 1922), 7.

144 *"Memorandum in Reference . . .":* "Memorandum," Jan. 25, 1922, Banting Papers, Scrapbook 2, 40.

145 *While Collip returned to the lab:* Banting et al., "Pancreatic Extracts in the Treatment of Diabetes Mellitus," 4–5.

146 *In order to dispel these doubts:* Banting and Best, "Pancreatic Extracts," 7.

146 *Later that day Banting was to learn:* Banting and Best, "Pancreatic Extracts," 8.

146 *Although he found no islets cells:* In 1940, Banting recalled that a closer inspection after the initial autopsy "revealed a microscopic group of cells so small that it was agreed that they could not be responsible for the survival of the dog." This contradicts Banting's acknowledgment in "Pancreatic Extracts," by Banting and Best, that the results were not conclusive. See Banting, "Story of the Discovery" (1940), 16b.

22: Failure and Success, The University of Toronto, February to April 1922

147 *At Toronto General Hospital:* Bliss, *The Discovery of Insulin,* 122, 130.

147 *In February, Banting began to drink heavily:* Banting, "Story of the Discovery" (1940), 19d.

148 *The pages of his diary suggest:* Bliss, *Banting,* 85.

148 *Reflecting on this time some years later:* Banting, "Story of the Discovery" (1940), 19d.

148 *Collip inexplicably lost his ability:* Ibid., 18d; Best, "A Report on the Discovery and Development" (Sept. 1922), 3–4.

148 *On the evening of March 31:* Banting recounts the event in 1940. See Banting, "Story of the Discovery" (1940), 20d–21d.

151 *The fact that he was not a practicing physician:* Ibid., 18d.

151 *It was decided that a diabetic clinic:* Banting, "Account of the Discovery of Insulin" (1922), 10; Banting, "History of Insulin" (1929), 9. For a report on the patients treated in the Soldiers' Civil Re-Establishment, see Gilchrist et al., "Observations With Insulin" (1923).

151 *By this time:* Decades later, Best would recall his disappointment with being assigned control of production, as he wanted to "get on with my M.A. thesis" in pursuit of his degree in 1922. Best interview by Gene E. McCormick, Sept. 24, 1968, Lilly Archives.

152 *"We have not as yet succeeded":* Macleod to Clowes, Apr. 3, 1922, Connaught Collection, Aventis Pasteur Limited Archives 95–025–01.

152 *composed a joint letter to Falconer:* Bliss, *The Discovery of Insulin*, 133.

152 *"So impressed with the feasibility":* "Toronto Doctor on Track of Diabetes Cure," Mar. 22, 1922, *Toronto Daily Star*, Banting Scrapbook, Thomas Fisher Rare Book Library.

153 *In 1922 a total of 161 patients:* Allen and Sherrill, "Clinical Observations," 804.

23: Honeymoon Cottage, Hamilton, Bermuda, January to July 1922

154 *They stayed in cabin number 18:* EH to AH, Jan. 13, 1922, Thomas Fisher Rare Book Library.

155 *Her letters to Mumsey:* Elizabeth's day-to-day activities during the stay in Bermuda are documented in letters held in the EH Papers.

155 *"I didn't come to Bermuda":* EH to AH, Jan. 8, 1922.

156 *Her diet:* EH to AH, Feb. 5, 1922.

157 *"A writer! Excellent!":* Gue, 256.

157 *Pauline Swalm:* Ibid., 257.

158 *Three times they reserved a cabin:* "Hughes Off for Bermuda; Secretary of State and Wife Taking Two Weeks' Vacation," *New York Times,* Feb. 16, 1922: 14.

158 *Despite a stinging sleet storm:* Ibid., 14.

158 *When the Hugheses arrived in Hamilton:* "Arrival of Mr. Hughes U.S. Secretary of State," *Royal Gazette* (Bermuda), Feb. 18, 1922: 1. Governor Willcocks let Elizabeth lead the way up the gangway to the ship so that she might be the first to greet her father.

159 *"Hughes Back From Trip": New York Times,* Mar. 7, 1922: 7.

159 *Unfortunately, Elizabeth:* Blanche Burgess to AH, May 26, 1922, EH Papers.

160 *By May Elizabeth's diet had been slashed:* Bliss, *The Discovery of Insulin*, 144.

160 *For the first time her weight . . . fell:* Banting et al., "Insulin in the Treatment of Diabetes Mellitus," 593.

160 *"I'm beginning to feel real hopeful":* EH to AH, Apr. 14, 1922.

160 *On Saturday, June 10, 1922:* "Miss Hughes First Bride of Cabinet; Secretary's Daughter Catherine Wed to Chauncey L. Waddell of New York by Bishop Harding," *New York Times,* Jun. 11, 1922: 17.

161 *The chapel's interior:* "Helen Hughes Memorial Dedicated in New York," *Indianapolis Star,* June 26, 1922: 10; author's visit to the chapel.

162 *At the top of the gangplank:* Elizabeth Hughes, transcribed interview by Michael Bliss, Nov. 22, 1980, Thomas Fisher Rare Book Library.

163 *"Because my daughter has Diabetes":* AH to Banting, July 3, 1922, Banting Papers.

24: Patents, Partnership, and Pancreases, Indianapolis and Toronto, April to August 1922

165 *In April 1922, in the middle of his workday:* Brown recounts his meeting with Mr. Lilly in his address at the 25 Year and Retired Employees Banquet, May 10, 1948. Copy is in the Lilly Archives. Also see M. C. McCormick, "History of Insulin," Lilly Archives, 136–37.

166 *Armed with Brown's affirmative reply:* Best would later estimate Clowes visited Toronto twenty-five times during 1922. Best, interview by Gene E. McCormick, Sept. 24, 1968, Lilly Archives,.

166 *While Clowes worked on Macleod:* M. C. McCormick, "History of Insulin," Lilly Archives, 136–37.

167 *Brown saw he would have to perform:* Ibid.

167 *Joslin would later say:* Joslin, "Pancreatic Extract," 654.

167 *At the last minute:* Macleod to Gooderham, Sept. 20, 1922, memorandum, "History of the Researches," Collip Papers, 5. When writing about the event years later, Banting didn't mention the reason for not attending the AAP meetings. He wrote simply that "Best and I stayed home and worked." He seems bitter, however, that Macleod presented the paper himself: "Macleod presented the work of the Toronto Group of workers. The usual time alloted [*sic*] is 10 minutes. He was given 20 minutes. At the end of his presentation, Eliot P. Joslyn [*sic*] rose and moved a standing vote of thanks to Macleod and his associates for their discovery of Insulin. Dr. G. H. A. Clowes of the Eli Lilly Co. of Indianapolis was present and his British sense of justice caused him to speak to Joslyn [*sic*] afterwards. Joslyn [*sic*] apparently did not know anything except from MacLeod. After the meeting Clowes wired me to come to Boston and bring reprints of the first two articles." (Banting, "Story of the Discovery" [1940], 26d–27d.)

167 *Within days of the conference:* Clowes to Macleod, May 11, 1922, Connaught Collection, Aventis Pasteur Limited Archives 95–025–01.

168 *Finally, in mid-May:* Macleod to Clowes, May 15, 1922.

168 *Working tirelessly at Connaught:* Banting would later write, "To Best must be given the greatest amount of credit for this phase of the [re]development [of insulin]. It was he more than anyone who bridged the gap between the test-tube and the beaker scale and later the large scale production." (Banting, "Story of the Discovery" (1940), 22d.)

168 *On May 15 Banting's friend Joe Gilchrist:* Banting, "History of Insulin" (1929), 15; Gilchrist et al., "Observations with Insulin," 7.

168 *With Best in charge:* Insulin Committee Minutes, Aug. 17, 1922–Sept. 29, 1925, University of Toronto/Board of Governors/Insulin Committee Collection, University of Toronto Archives, A1982–0001, Box 044.

168 *Williams had been promised insulin:* Woodbury, 54–57; John R. Williams, "Notes on Patient Jim Havens."

168 *In the fall of 1919:* Madeb et al., "The Discovery of Insulin: The Rochester, New York, Connection," 907. Hereafter, "The Discovery of Insulin."

168 *remained stable:* John R. Williams, "Notes on Patient Jim Havens"; idem., "A Clinical Study," 733–34. Case 1524.

168 *He was put on a diet:* Madeb et al., "The Discovery of Insulin," 907.

169 *By the spring of 1922:* John R. Williams, "A Clinical Study." 733–34. Case 1524.

169 *At first the miracle cure seemed ineffective:* Madeb et al., "The Discovery of Insulin," 909.

169 *On May 22, Clowes arrived in Toronto:* M. C. McCormick, "History of Insulin," 130–31, Lilly Archives; Madison, *Eli Lilly: A Life,* 56–57.

169 *Banting still refused:* Banting would later write that his "reason for abstaining from writing

my name to the Application in the first instance was because as a Physician and Physiologist, the idea of applying for a patent for any discovery or invention of mine was distasteful to me as a Medical Etiquette. Furthermore . . . I had taken the Hippocratic Oath." (Banting, "Declaration. In the Matter of British Patent Application No. 16360 of 1922," Thomas Fisher Rare Book Library.)

169 *These efforts were necessary:* Clowes to Macleod, May 11, 1922, Connaught Collection, Aventis Pasteur Limited Archives 95–025–01, University of Toronto.

170 *An advisory group was formed:* "Memorandum on the Course Pursued by the University of Toronto in the Development of the Manufacture of Insulin," Adapted From a Memorandum Prepared in January, 1924 for President Butler of Columbia University, University of Toronto Collection, University of Toronto Archives, A1967–0007, Box 86, Insulin Folder.

170 *Lilly agreed . . . to provide 28 percent:* Indenture between the Governors of the University of Toronto and the Eli Lilly Company, 30 May 1922, Collip Papers.

170 *Clowes estimated:* Clowes, telegram to Macleod, May 25, 1922, Thomas Fisher Rare Book Library.

171 *In an effort to avoid layoffs:* 1920 and 1921 Profits Summary, Lilly Archives.

171 *Eventually Mr. Lilly would choose:* Clowes to Macleod, Mar. 14, 1923, University of Toronto/Board of Governors/Insulin Committee Collection, University of Toronto Archives, A1982–0001, Box 12, Eli Lilly Folder.

171 *Within three days:* See Indenture between the Governors of the University of Toronto and the Eli Lilly Company, May 30, 1922, Collip Papers.

171 *George Walden was put in charge:* McCormick, "History of Insulin," Lilly Archives, 134–35.

171 *George Walden was a twenty-eight-year-old chemist:* Eli Lilly & Co. Application for Employment: George B. Walden, Sept. 25, 1917, Walden files, Lilly Archives.

172 *On June 2 and 3, he and Best went:* Bliss, *The Discovery of Insulin,* 140.

172 *Seventeen days later:* On June 22, Macleod wrote Clowes that "the delay has been due to the difficulty at this time of year of getting committees together, especially the Board of Governors." Macleod to Clowes, June 22, 1922, Connaught Collection, Aventis Pasteur Limited Archives 95–025–01.

172 *"Our chemists here have been working very intently":* Eli Lilly to Macleod, June 17, 1922, Lilly Archives.

172 *In Indianapolis, Billy Sylvester:* McCormick, "History of Insulin," Lilly Archives, 136, f. 158.

172 *Experimental runs were made almost daily:* Gene McCormick, "The Discovery and Manufacture of Insulin," Lilly Archives, 7.

172 *But it was not enough to supply clinicians:* Macleod to Dr. W. D. Sansum, June 21, 1922, University of Toronto/Board of Governors/Insulin Committee Collection, University of Toronto Archives; Macleod to Dr. Rollin T. Woodyatt, Jun. 21, 1922 University of Toronto/Board of Governors/Insulin Committee Collection, University of Toronto Archives.

172 *Macleod sent three copies of the indenture agreement:* Macleod to Clowes. Jun. 28, 1922, Connaught Collection, Aventis Pasteur Limited Archives 95–025–01, University of Toronto.

173 *Around this time Banting was approached:* Bliss, *Banting,* 95.

173 *With Doctors Campbell and Fletcher:* Banting, "Story of the Discovery" (1940), 36; "Memorandum on the Establishment of a Diabetic Clinic in the Toronto General Hospital"; "Memorandum on the Organization of the Diabetic Clinic" University of Toronto.

173 *Banting's friend from the Hospital for Sick Children:* Banting, "Story of the Discovery" 1940), 32.

173 *In mid-June Macleod left Toronto:* Bliss, *The Discovery of Insulin,* 141.

173 *The first factory-scale run was made . . . on June 26:* Gene McCormick, "The Discovery and Manufacture of Insulin," Lilly Archives, 7.

25: Fame and Famine, Summer 1922

175 *in July, the Toronto train stations teemed:* Banting, "Story of the Discovery" (1940), 26. TK

176 *"Is there any possible chance":* J. E. Paullin, telegram to Macleod, Jul. 1, 1922, Lilly Archives.

176 *"No insulin available":* Banting telegram to J. E. Paullin, Jul. 3, 1922, Lilly Archives.

176 *Dr. Morton Ryder:* Frank Jones, "Teddy Ryder: Banting's Living Miracle," *Toronto Star,* Feb. 20, 1983: A6.

176 *At Christie Street, several diabetics had suffered hypoglycemic shock:* Gilchrist et al., "Observations with Insulin" (1923).

176 *He finally accepted three new private patients:* Hamburger, 4, 5; Bliss, Historical Essay, 30.

176 *When Mildred Ryder:* Frank Jones, "Teddy Ryder: Banting's Living Miracle," *Toronto Star,* Feb. 20, 1983: A6.

177 *He came by Grenville Street:* Ibid.

177 *Several were living at the Athelma Apartments:* 78 Grosvenor Street was the return address on Elizabeth Hughes's letters to her mother.

177 *When he turned six:* Jones, "Teddy Ryder," *Toronto Star,* Feb. 20, 1983: A6.

178 *That summer Banting's old medical officer:* Notes on Charlotte Clarke; and Chart for Charlotte Clarke, Banting Papers. See also Banting, "Story of the Discovery" (1940), 45.

178 *During the journey he fell prey to his own paranoia:* "I have a hunch that Clowes is holding out on us," Banting wrote Best on July 21, just before making his trip to Indianapolis. See Bliss, *The Discovery of Insulin,* 147.

179 *He was met on the platform:* J. K. Lilly to Eli Lilly, July 26, 1922, Lilly Archives.

179 *It later came to light:* Clowes to Banting, July 18, 1922, Banting Papers.

179 *Eli Lilly and Company agreed to delay its own clinical work:* A diabetic clinic in the Methodist Hospital was created by Eli Lilly and Company during the early manufacturing phase of insulin in order to broaden "the Company's familiarity with clinical medicine and moreover, proved a valuable aid in gathering first-hand experience upon which to deal with the University of Toronto and investigators elsewhere" (McCormick, "McCormick History Re-Do", Dec. 12, 2007, Lilly CD-ROM, Lilly Archives, 366). Upon learning of the production problems in Toronto, Lilly delayed its investigational work. See Clowes to Banting, Aug. 11, 1922, Banting Papers, 2; Clowes to Macleod, Sept. 5, 1922, Lilly Archives, 3.

179 *Clowes pledged to do whatever he could:* Clowes's support for Banting to gain full credit for insulin is evident in letters written during the summer of 1922. He vows, among other things, to work with Allen to ensure Banting's papers get priority in publications; that Lilly will foot the bill to distribute Banting's papers across the country; to work toward Banting getting full credit for work; and that other researchers must hold the release of their publications until Banting is ready in exchange for material. See Clowes to Banting, Aug. 11, 1922 and Aug. 8, 1922, Banting Papers.

179 *Charlotte Clarke's wound:* Notes on Charlotte Clarke, Banting Papers.

179 *Banting went next:* Banting, "Story of the Discovery" (1940), 27–28; also Bliss, *The Discovery of Insulin,* 149.

180 *Next day he was in New York:* Banting, "Story of the Discovery" (1940), 29–30.

180 *Geyelin was appalled:* Banting, "The Story of Insulin" (1922), 19–20; Bliss, *Banting,* 100, 101.

180 *"We were sorry":* J. K. Lilly to Banting, July 26, 1922, Banting Papers.

181 *On July 29, Lilly sent 200 units:* A. L. Walters to Banting, July 31, 1922, Banting Papers.

181 *On August 8 they sent 500 units:* A. L. Walters to Banting, Aug. 8, 1922; J. K. Lilly to Clowes, Aug. 8, 1922, Lilly Archives; Clowes to Banting, Aug. 8, 1922, Lilly Archives.

181 *The question of who:* McCormick, "History of Insulin," Lilly Archives, 149

181 *Miss Elizabeth Mudge, a nurse:* Richard Dowling to Gene E. McCormick, April 24, 1969. Also Joslin, "Reminiscences. . . .", 67–68.

181 *Among the thousand or so names:* Joslin's Diabetic Registry.

182 *"I think I may have something for you":* Kienast, 14–15.

182 *By August, Walden and his team: FINAL DRAFT for Insulin Project,* CD-ROM, Lilly Archives, 45.

182 *Kingan . . . could not meet:* McCormick, "History of Insulin," Lilly Archives, 136, *f. 158.*

182 *The first shipment of frozen pancreas glands:* Ibid., 136.

182 *Now Indianapolis began to experience the problems:* Ibid., 139–40.

182 *In August 1922 Walden was near nervous collapse:* G. H. A. Clowes to Macleod, Sept. 23, 1922, Lilly Archives, 5.

182 *On August 8, he sent a telegram:* Clowes, telegram to Banting, Aug. 8, 1922, Banting Papers. Also J. K. Lilly to Clowes, Aug. 8, 1922, Lilly Archives.

183 *"Do anything you want with Frederick":* Bliss, *The Discovery of Insulin,* 160.

183 *The human trials at Banting's clinic:* Banting, "Story of the Discovery" (1940), 23d–25d; Gilchrist, et al, "Observations with Insulin."

183 *On August 10 Allen injected six patients:* Ibid., 151.

26: Four Trunks, Washington, D.C., August 1922

185 *"in the family way all the time":* Anthony, 36.

188 *"You started the Sunday school class":* Pusey, 133–34, 110.

189 *They had corresponded:* Robert Falconer, to CEH, Dec. 7, 1911; CEH to Falconer, Dec. 28, 1911, Thomas Fisher Rare Book Library.

189 *Hughes sat and stared:* Since we know that Banting denied Antoinette's initial request to help Elizabeth, it is likely that CEH stepped in on her behalf. While a phone call between Hughes and Falconer has never been documented, Falconer most likely would have been the person Hughes called. CEH's dedication to the integrity of his public position would have made him less apt to pull strings via other public officials, like Harding or Mackenzie King. We know that Falconer and Hughes knew each other since 1910 (see previous note), and in 1917 Falconer even wrote Hughes requesting a personal favor of his own when Hughes was chairman of the District Board of New York—that an American on the University of Toronto faculty be temporarily discharged from the military in order to teach medical students within the Department of Biochemistry. Hughes regretfully denied his request (Falconer to CEH, Nov. 13, 1917; CEH to Falconer, Nov. 15, 1917, Thomas Fisher Rare Book Library).

27: Escape from Morristown, August 1922

190 *One of Toronto's . . . accomplishments:* http://en.wikipedia.org/wiki/Gooderham Building; http://www. proudest architectural accomplishments.

190 *It had been Gooderham who donated the land:* Rutty, "Dr. Robert Davies Defries."

192 *Naval radio stations:* "War Radio Service for Hughes on Trip," *New York Times,* Aug. 23, 1922.

192 *She left a message:* Allen to Banting, Aug. 12, 1922.

28: The Transformation Begins, Toronto, August to November 1922

196 *"Height five feet"*: Banting, Frederick, Notes on First Examination of Elizabeth Hughes, Banting Papers, 3.

199 *"I take pleasure"*: Allen to Banting, Aug. 16, 1922, Banting Papers.

199 *After lunch, Robertson took Banting*: Banting, "Story of the Discovery" (1940), 42–43.

200 *On August 18, 1922*: "Daughter of U. S. Secretary of State Tries New Toronto Discovery," *Indianapolis News,* Aug. 17, 1922: 7.

200 *On August 22, 1922, Schley wrote*: George B. Schley to Clowes, Aug. 22, 1922, Banting Papers.

200 *At first, Banting dismissed the matter*: The Insulin Committee decided to withdraw the Best-Collip and Best patent applications to make way for an application for Banting, Best, and Collip. See patent papers located in the University of Toronto/ Board of Governors/Insulin Committee and Connaught papers at the Thomas Fisher Rare Book Library. See also Charles H. Riches to the Board of Governors, University of Toronto, Feb. 22, 1923, University of Toronto, Office of the President Papers.

200 *Through the summer and fall*: Rutty, 11; Clowes discovered the shortage problems in Toronto after a visit in July 1922. He immediately wired Indianapolis to send a supply to Toronto. Clowes Banting, July 18, 1922, Banting Papers. Correspondence during this period between Toronto and Indianapolis indicate Eli Lilly and Company were regularly sending batches of Iletin to Banting and his colleagues; this is further reflected in Clowes to Macleod, Oct. 20, 1922, Connaught Collection, Aventis Pasteur Limited Archives 95–025–01,1,5.

200 *The insulin directed to Banting's patients*: Rutty, 9. Banting would later recall stating at the time: "The indigent diabetic is our greatest problem. Every effort must be made to reduce the cost of insulin and remove the necessity of expensive diets so that they can look after themselves," (Banting, "Story of the Discovery" [1940], 22).

200 *Elizabeth took insulin twice daily*: Banting et al., "Insulin in the Treatment of Diabetes Mellitus," 592; also EH to AH, Aug. 22, 1922, Thomas Fisher Rare Book Library.

201 *Before 1922, hyperglycemic coma*: Joslin, "Diabetes for the Diabetics," 142.

201 *The first diabetic "resurrected"*: Bliss, *The Discovery of Insulin,* 161.

201 *Elizabeth called these . . . "the feels"*: EH to AH, Sept. 24, 1922, 2.

201 *In those early months of experimental insulin*: EH to AH, ibid..

202 *On August 21, Dr. Banting visited*: EH to AH, Aug. 22, 1922, 1.

203 *Banting was not nearly as cautious*: Banting et al., "Insulin in the Treatment of Diabetes Mellitus," 592.

203 *"unspeakably wonderful"*: EH to AH, Oct. 6, 1922, 2.

203 *"A week ago last Thursday*: James D. Havens to Banting, Dec. 11, 1922, Banting Papers.

203 *Banting encouraged Elizabeth*: EH to AH, Sept. 24, 1922, 3.

203 *"No body up here except Dr. Banting . . . knows"*: EH to AH, Sept. 29, 1922, 4

204 *"I could use up pages"*: EH to AH, Sept. 24, 1922, 3.

205 *"New Treatment Aids Miss Hughes"*: *New York American,* Oct. 15, 1922, Thomas Fisher Rare Book Library.

205 *"Permanently Cured by Insulin Treatment"*: *Toronto Daily Star,* Jan. 16, 1923, Thomas Fisher Rare Book Library.

206 *"New York Excited Over New Cure"*: *Toronto Daily Star,* Oct. 17, 1922, Thomas Fisher Rare Book Library.

206 *"Little Daughter of Hughes Seemingly Cured"*: *Fort Worth Star Telegram,* Dec. 16, 1922, Thomas Fisher Rare Book Library.

206 *"record case"*: EH to AH, Sept. 24, 1922, 2.

206 *"You'd think it was a fairy tale"*: EH to AH, Sept. 24, 1922, 1.

206 *"I hate to be written up like that"*: EH to AH, Oct. 21, 1922, 2.

206 *"With your letter this morning"*: EH to AH, Nov. 11, 1922, 2.

206 *"Yesterday morning"*: EH to AH, Oct. 8, 1922. **Omit salutation, begin:** Yesterday morning we were called . . .

29: Crossing the Line Aboard the SS *Pan America*, August to September 1922

208 *On Monday, August 21, 1922:* "Hughes Prepares for Trip; Arranges State Affairs for His Absence in Brazil," *New York Times,* Aug. 22, 1922: 4.

209 *"looks like God and talks like God"*: Danelski and Tulchin, xxviii.

209 *On Thursday, August 24:* "Hughes Sails Today; Admiral Vogelgesang Will Accompany Him to Brazil as Aide," *New York Times,* Aug. 24, 1922: 10.

209 *Ambassador Allencar of Brazil:* "Hughes Sails with Mission to Brazil; Secretary of State Carries Message of Good-will to Centennial Exposition," *New York Times*, Aug. 25, 1922: 7.

210 *After that the Pan America would proceed:* "War Radio Service for Hughes on Trip." *New York Times,* Aug. 23, 1922: 30.

210 *Hughes told reporters:* "Hughes Resting at Sea," *New York Times,* Aug. 26, 1922: 6.

210 *Secretary Hughes and his party:* "War Radio Service for Hughes on Trip," *New York Times,* Aug. 23, 1922: 30.

211 *"elaborate arrangements"*: Ibid.

212 *traditional ceremony:* "Try Secretary Hughes in Neptune's Court; Accused of Boisterous Conduct in Ceremonies When Pan America Crosses Equator," *New York Times,* Sept. 3, 1922: 13.

213 *Hughes and members of his delegation:* Ibid.

213 *"undermining the prestige of Neptune"*: Ibid.

213 *The secretary pleaded guilty:* Ibid.

213 *He participated in deck sports:* "Hughes in Deck Sports," *New York Times,* Aug. 28, 1922: 7.

213 *"One never can judge"*: "Hughes Pleads Guilty in Neptune's Court," n.p.: n.pub., n.d. . . . "one never can judge."

213 *"Every effort is being made"*: Allen's original letter resides in the Teddy Ryder Scrapbook at the Thomas Fisher Rare Book Library.

214 *Among the items Elizabeth inherited:* Elizabeth donated these artifacts to the Supreme Court Historical Society for an exhibit on her father. The medallions are described in detail in the "Hughes Exhibit Catalogue" by Gail Galloway and Susanne Owens in the 1981 Supreme Court Historical Society Yearbook. The Yearbooks are digitally available on the SCHS's Web site: http://www.supremecourthistory.org.

30: Fate, Fortune, and Forgetting, September to December 1922

215 *Sir William Bayliss:* See William Bayliss to *London Times,* Aug. 24, 1922.

215 *The University's patent attorney:* Gooderham to Banting, Sept. 16, 1922, Banting Papers.

216 *To exacerbate the matter:* See August Krogh to Macleod, Oct. 23, 1922, University of Toronto/Board of Governors/Insulin Committee Collection, University of Toronto Archives; Krogh to Macleod, Nov. 1922, Best Papers; Duncan Graham, to Macleod, Aug. 24, 1922, Best Papers; Banting to J. G. Fitzgerald, Oct. 5, 1922, Banting Papers.

216 *"I would then compare"*: Gooderham to Banting, Sept. 16, 1922, Banting Papers.

217 *Predictably, Banting's version reflected his view:* See Banting, "Account of the Discovery of Insulin" (1922).

217 *"complete credit . . . he could certainly":* Macleod to Gooderham, "History of the Researches," Sept. 20, 1922, Collip Papers, 2.

218 *"in many, if not most, laboratories":* Ibid., 3.

218 *"perfectly evident":* Ibid.

219 *In late November 1922 . . . August Krogh arrived: Novo Nordisk History,* 2.

219 *One of Dale's first . . . patients:* Bliss, *The Discovery of Insulin,* 167.

220 *"Now I know I am going to shock you":* EH to AH, Nov. 12, 1922.

221 *Charles Riches . . . appeal the rejection:* Charles H. Riches to Macleod, Nov. 1922, University of Toronto/Board of Governors/Insulin Committee Collection, University of Toronto Archives.

221 *Affidavits were requisitioned:* Macleod to Allen, Nov. 29, 1922, University of Toronto/Board of Governors/Insulin Committee Collection, University of Toronto Archives; Macleod to Clowes, Nov. 30, 1922, Connaught Collection, Aventis Pasteur Limited Archives 95–025–01.

221 *Banting asked . . . Hughes to help:* See Banting to CEH, Nov. 21, 1922, Banting Papers.

221 *"best possible attention:* CEH to Hon. Thomas F. Robertson, Commissioner of Patents, Nov. 24, 1922.

222 *In 1923, he helped to fund the Banting Research Foundation:* "Aid Banting Medical Fund," *Washington Post,* Nov. 2, 1923: 6; Edwin L. McCormick to Sir Robert Falconer, Nov. 2, 1923, University of Toronto/Office of the President Collection, University of Toronto Archives. For an overview of the Banting Foundation, see F. Lorne Hutchinson to *New York Times,* March 22, 1922; "The Banting Foundation: A Short Résumé of its Creation, Purposes and Organization." Written by the Banting Foundation, 1925, Banting Papers.

222 *"We've got to stay in all day":* EH to AH, Nov. 23, 1922.

222 *she and Blanche were sitting down to lunch:* See EH to AH, Nov. 28, 1922.

223 *Between August and January:* Banting et al., "Insulin in the Treatment of Diabetes Mellitus," 592–98.

223 *"Mrs. (rather) Lady van Hoofenbhouck Tulleken":* EH to AH, Nov. 23, 1922.

223 *In March of 1923:* George Ross to Mackenzie King, May 8, 1923, Banting Papers; See also Bliss, *The Discovery of Insulin,* 216–17.

223 *He wrote to . . . King:* CEH to Mackenzie King, Mar. 16, 1923, W. L. Mackenzie King Papers, vol. 93, Public Archives of Canada. See also the reply: King to CEH, Apr. 6, 1923.

223 *Banting was awarded:,* W.L. Mackenzie King to Banting, July 23, 1923, Banting Papers; Hector McKinnon, "Canada Rewards Banting's Service," *Toronto Daily Star,* June 28, 1923; "Plan Chair of Medicine to Honor Dr. Banting." n. pub., April–May 1923, Banting Papers.

223 *In June 1923:* "Rockefeller Gives Hospitals $150,000; Money to Be Extended in Promoting Use of Insulin for Diabetes," *Indianapolis Star,* Jun. 20, 1923: 2. The hospitals were: University Hospital in Ann Arbor; Johns-Hopkins Hospital in Baltimore; New England Deaconess Hospital in Boston; Presbyterian Hospital in Chicago; Lakeside Hospital in Cleveland; University Hospital in Iowa City; Royal Victoria Hospital in Montreal; Touro Infirmary in New Orleans, Presbyterian Hospital in New York City; Barnes Hospital in St. Louis; Lane Hospital in San Francisco; Hospital for Sick Children in Toronto; Toronto General Hospital in Toronto; the Banting-Best Fund at the University of Toronto; and the Physiatric Institute in Morristown.

224 *In the early insulin era:* White, 222.

224 *Only three . . . survived:* Bliss, *The Discovery of Insulin,* 160.

224   *Dr. Joslin also lost at least one early patient:* For results and case studies of these patients, see Joslin et al., "Insulin in Hospital and Home," 651; Woodyatt, 800; John R. Williams, 750.

224   *Paula Inge died:* Bliss, *The Discovery of Insulin,* 167.

31: The Nobel Prize and Beyond

225   *Throughout 1923, Nobel Prize nominations arrived:* Bliss, *The Discovery of Insulin,* 225–29.

225   *Banting reacted to the news:* Banting, "Story of the Discovery" (1940), 15e–16e.

225   *While Banting ultimately accepted the prize:* "Dr. Banting Shares Honors With Best," *Boston Globe,* Oct. 27, 1923: 11.

226   *This left Macleod with no choice:* "Macleod Awards Collip Half of His Nobel Prize," *Toronto Daily Star,* Nov. 7, 1923.

226   *The prize totaled $24,000:* "Four Men Will Share in the Nobel Prize; Prof. J. J. R. Macleod Divides His $20,000 With J. B. Collip," n.pub., Nov. 1923; "Macleod Awards Collip Half of His Nobel Prize; Total of $40,000 Has Now Been Divided Equally Among Four," *Toronto Daily Star,* Nov. 7, 1923; clippings appear in Banting Scrapbook and Collip Papers. Though reports at the time stated the total award money was $40,000, divided up among the four men at $10,000 apiece, Nobel records would indicate the real total was about $24,000 (Bliss, *The Discovery of Insulin,* 233).

226   *Privately, Macleod grumbled:* "Asks Time to Consider Award Disposal," *Toronto Daily Star,* Nov. 2, 1923.

226   *Neither Banting nor Macleod attended:* Banting would not go to Stockholm and deliver his Nobel Prize address until the following year. Banting, "Story of the Discovery" (1940), 18e.

226   *In November 1923 . . . a celebratory banquet:* "University Honours Professors Banting and Macleod as Winners of the Nobel Prize Award for Medicine in Board of Governors' Banquet Held at Hart House," *Toronto Globe,* Nov. 27, 1923. The only photo found of the event shows Sir Edmund Walker, chancellor, and Canon Cody, chairman of the board of governors, sitting between Banting and Macleod at the head table. See "Talented Workers in Research Field Paid High Honors," *Toronto Globe,* Nov. 28, 1923: 1.

226   *Georg Zuelzer and Nicholas Paulesco appealed:* Bliss, *The Discovery of Insulin,* 233.

226   *E. L. Scott published a claim:* Ibid., 238.

226   *Even Collip published a paper:* Collip, "Glucokinin: Second Paper," 77. For more on glucokinin, also see Collip's other two papers: "Glucokinin: A New Hormone Present," and "Glucokinin: An Apparent Synthesis."

227   *half of the insulin royalties:* "Agreement Between the Governors of the University of Toronto and James Bertram Collip," July 1, 1923, University of Toronto/Board of Governors/Insulin Committee Collection, University of Toronto Archives, 5.

227   *From 1923 to 1967:* Bliss, *The Discovery of Insulin,* 240.

227   *By separate arrangement with Lilly:* N. H. Noyes to Eli Lilly, Feb. 25, 1941; C. F. Eveleigh to Eli Lilly, Feb. 27, 1941; E. N. Beesley to F. B. Peck, Nov. 15, 1954, Lilly Archives.

227   *In October 1923 Iletin was released:* "McCormick History Re-Do 12–12–2007," CD-ROM. Lilly Archives: 307–308.

227   *The first-year sales:* 1923 Profit overview, Lilly Archives.

227   *By the end of 1923, Lilly had sold:* "McCormick History Re-Do 12–12–2007," CD-ROM. Lilly Archives: 307–308.

227   *"To give you some conception of the speed":* Clowes, "Insulin in Its Relation to Life Insurance," 2.

228 *"Many persons have the idea"*: "Indianapolis the Production and Distribution Center of Insulin," *Indianapolis News,* Oct. 27, 1923: 21.

228 *By the end of 1923 the cost of treatment:* Ibid., 3.

228 *"A glow of pride":* J. K. Lilly to Eli Lilly, ca. May 1923, Lilly Archives.

228 *He devoted himself to the Banting Research Foundation:* Best, "Frederick Grant Banting," 23–24.

229 *"We do not know whence ideas come":* Stevenson, 67.

229 *He was especially interested:* Stevenson, 398.

229 *The Banting Research Foundation played a major role:* Ibid., 401.

229 *"get his ass kicked":* Bliss, *The Discovery of Insulin,* 236.

230 *"God how I hate the whole fuss":* Banting diary, Thomas Fisher Rare Book Library.

230 *"I shall always follow your career":* Banting to Teddy Ryder, Dec. 27, 1938, Banting Papers.

230 *When World War II began:* Bliss, *Banting,* 254.

231 *John James Rickard Macleod:* Bliss, *The Discovery of Insulin,* 234.

231 *Upon Macleod's return to Aberdeen:* Michael J. Williams, 87.

231 *He significantly contributed:* Barr, 244–47.

231 *Upon Banting's death, Collip succeeded him:* Ibid., 249, 250.

231 *"Dr. Ross was very friendly with me":* Best to Joslin, June 28, 1945, Marble Library, Joslin Diabetes Center.

232 *From 1926 to 1928 Best did postgraduate work:* Charles Best biography, as part of PBS's "Red Gold: The Epic Story of Blood" Series. Available digitally at: http://www.pbs.org/wnet/redgold/.

232 *Dr. John G. FitzGerald:* Thomas Fisher Rare Book Library.

232 *Billy Ross:* Ibid.

232 *Dr. Joseph Gilchrist:* Ibid.

233 *"feeling as frisky as ever":* Roger McQuigg to J. K. Lilly Sr., Sept. 4, 1923, Lilly Archives.

233 *"After I get a little fatter":* Roger McQuigg to J. K. Lilly Sr., Sept. 12, 1923, Lilly Archives.

233 *"I hardly believe you can realize what a joy it is":* J. K. Lilly Sr. to Roger McQuigg, Sept. 18, 1923, Lilly Archives.

233 *Elizabeth Mudge and J. K. Lilly:* Ibid., 99.

233 *At her death:* Elizabeth Mudge to J. K. Lilly, April 22, 1941; Elizabeth Graham to Gene E. McCormick, Jun. 8, 1969, Lilly Archives.

233 *In 1975 the company began providing . . . medals:* Kahn, *All in a Century,* 101.

233 *In 1947, Clowes:* Kahn, 101; copy of Clowes's acceptance speech: Clowes, "Banting Memorial Address" (1947), 53.

233 *Alec Clowes spent forty summers:* Krahl, 335.

233 *At his home there . . . he died:* Krahl, 334; Miss Lenora Clark, interview by G. E. McCormick, Sept. 25, 1969, Lilly Archives, 2.

233 *Three months later:* T. P. Carney, memo to E. N. Beesley, Nov. 24, 1958. Lilly Archives.

233 *George Walden remained an employee:* Lilly News (press release), announcing retirement of George B. Walden, Feb. 24, 1960, Lilly Archives.

233 *His deep interest in local history:* Madison, *Eli Lilly: A History,* 166–68, 153–64, 149, 172–82, 142–51; Kahn, 70.

234 *He was a man of many interests:* Kahn, 78, 82; information on J. K. Lilly Jr. also available at the Indianapolis Museum of Art and the Lilly Library at Indiana University, Bloomington.

234 *In the early 1950s . . . gold coins:* Kahn, 80–81.

234 *Together, J. K. Lilly Sr. and his sons:* www.lilly.com.

235 *When he died:* Marble Library, Joslin Diabetes Center.

235 *postinsulin resurrection of skeletal children:* Joslin, "Address . . ." (1934), 39.
235 *Allen owed over $25,000:* Henderson, 47.
235 *Allen tried to work out an arrangement:* Ibid., 47.
235 *Desperate for a second chance:* See Allen to CEH, Jan. 4, 1929; CEH to Allen, Jan. 7, 1929, CEH Papers, Physiatric Institute file, Butler Library, Columbia University.
235 *An eviction notice:* Henderson, 48.
235 *Allen persevered with his animal experiments:* Henderson, 47; Bliss, *The Discovery of Insulin,* 239.
236 *Upon hearing of the collapse:* "Minutes of Banquet Session," *Proceedings of the American Diabetes Association* (1949): 35.
236 *It was an unprecedented amount:* American Diabetes Association of "Maurk of Banquet Session," (1949), 33–36.
236 *Otto Kahn's mansion was razed:* Henderson, 48.
236 *"deep appreciation of your medal":* American Diabetes Association, "Minutes of Banquet Session" (1949), 33–36.
237 *"The thing that has hurt me . . .":* Belle Wishart Allen in a letter to Dr. Alfred Henderson.
237 *The words of . . . Omar Khayyam:* Henderson, 48.

32: The Emergence of Elizabeth Gossett

238 *"Miss Elizabeth Hughes Ill":* New York Times, Aug. 8, 1924: 13.
238 *"Miss Hughes Improving":* New York Times, Aug. 10, 1924: 7.
238 *From then until she graduated:* Elizabeth Hughes, transcribed interview by Michael Bliss, Nov. 22, 1980, Thomas Fisher Rare Book Library.
238 *In 1926 she weighed 150 pounds:* EH to Banting, Nov. 2, 1926, Banting Papers.
239 *She did not see a doctor once:* See Elizabeth Hughes, transcribed interview by Michael Bliss, Nov. 22, 1980, Thomas Fisher Rare Book Library.
239 *She organized a club:* "Hoover Club Formed by Barnard Students; Miss Elizabeth Hughes Lines Up Girl Republicans—Smith Group to Organize Tomorrow," *New York Times,* Oct. 4, 1928: 5.
239 *debated James Roosevelt:* "Sons and Daughters," *Time* magazine, Nov. 5, 1928.
239 *During the summers:* Elizabeth Hughes Gossett, "Charles Evans Hughes," 11.
239 *their agreement to forget:* See Elizabeth Hughes Gossett, transcribed interview by Michael Bliss, Nov. 22, 1980, Thomas Fisher Rare Book Library.
239 *In 1928 Charles Evans Hughes hired . . . William T. Gossett:* William T. Gossett to Myron E. Humphrey, Aug. 27, 1962: 1; Gossett to Richard W. Hogue, Sept. 10, 1947: 1, 2, Bentley Library.
239 *Elizabeth did not tell Bill:* Elizabeth Hughes Gossett, transcribed interview by Michael Bliss, Nov. 22, 1980, Thomas Fisher Rare Book Library.
239 *Elizabeth and Bill were married in 1930:* "Elizabeth Hughes Weds W. T. Gossett," *New York Times,* Dec. 20, 1930: 14.
239 *In 1930, Charles Evans Hughes became chief justice:* Elizabeth Hughes Gossett, "Charles Evans Hughes," 12.
239 *In eleven years:* Ibid., 13.
239 *He was so concerned:* Ibid., 14.
240 *In 1933, Henry Beerits, a Princeton student:* Beerits, "Aftermath of a Senior Thesis," http://tigernet.princeton.edu/~cl1933/article.asp?year=1999&url=10henry-beertis.
240 *"Every Sunday afternoon":* Ibid.
241 *A highlight of the year:* Ibid.
241 *She destroyed pictures:* Elizabeth Hughes, transcribed interview by Michael Bliss, Nov. 22, 1980, Thomas Fisher Rare Book Library.

242 *She served as a trustee:* "History Ran in Elizabeth Gossett's Family," *Detroit Free Press,* April 26, 1981: 7C.

242 *As an adult, Myra:* "A Successful Volunteer Program Despite Handicaps," n.pub., Jacob Morganstern, *Ment. Hosp.,* 2: 2, June 1951, American Psychiatric Association. n.d.: 2.

243 *Ruth Whitehill married:* 1956 Baltimore City Directory.

243 *Both Myra and Ruth:* Myra Blaustein, Certificate of Death, Dec. 10, 1954; Mrs. Ruth Liedy, Certificate of Death, Feb. 19, 1957.

243 *Jim Havens:* Feudtner, 53.

243 *Jim married, fathered two children:* Biographical notes accompanying "Photograph of Jim Havens Holding One of His Children,.." Best Papers.

243 *He spent his adult life working as a librarian:* Nancy Papas, "Man Tells of Being a Medical First," *Hartford Courant,* Jan. 18, 1986: 1-A3; Katharine Martyn, "Teddy Ryder's Scrapbook," *Halcyon* no. 24 (Nov. 1999), Thomas Fisher Rare Book Library.

243 *On July 10, 1992:* Bliss, *The Discovery of Insulin,* 244.

243 *Leonard Thompson:* Digitized notes under "Formal Photograph of Leonard Thompson," Insulin Collection, Thomas Fisher Rare Book Library Online.

243 *After Antoinette died:* Pusey, 798–97, 803–805.

244 *At the time of her death:* See D. W. Denning to *New England Journal of Medicine,* Mar. 1982, Thomas Fisher Rare Book Library.

244 *Had she lived to read her own obituary:* The authors of this book have yet to see an obituary on Elizabeth Hughes that mentions her diabetic condition.

244 *"It may interest your readers":* Denning to *New England Journal of Medicine,* Mar. 8, 1982, Thomas Fisher Rare Book Library.

Postscript: Diabetes and Insulin Today

245 *In the spring of 1923:* Novo Nordisk History, Pamphlet, 6, 7. Available digitally at www.novonordisk.com.

245 *New, longer-acting insulin:* Rutty, "Couldn't Live Without It," 21–22.

245 *Connaught discovered that adding zinc:* Leibel and Wrenshall, 17.

245 *In 1936 Toronto introduced protomine zinc insulin:* Rutty, "Couldn't Live Without It," 22.

245 *Despite manufacturing advances:* Ibid., 26.

245 *Worldwide, that year:* Ibid., 26.

245 *Over time insulin resistance:* Ibid., 32.

246 *In 1978, Genentech:* Genentech, www.gene.com.

246 *It was approved:* Eli Lilly and Company, www.lilly.com.

246 *Eighty-five years after the discovery of insulin:* Eli Lilly and Company 2006 Annual Report, 12–13.

246 *The company today:* Eli Lilly and Company, www.lilly.com.

246 *Novo Nordisk:* www.novonordisk.com.

246 *Toronto's cost of developing insulin:* "Expenses Incurred in Initial Research on Insulin. June to December 1921, Thomas Fisher Rare Book Library; Kahn, 96.

246 *Today the average cost:* Neal Masia, "The Cost of Developing a New Drug." *Focus on Intellectual Property Rights,* Apr. 23, 2008. Also found at http://www.america.gov/st/econ-english/2008/April/20080429230904myleen0.5233981.html.

247 *In 2007, diabetes . . . fifth leading killer:* Amanda Schaffer, "In Diabetes, a Complex of Causes." *New York Times,* Oct. 16, 2007.

BIBLIOGRAPHY

Manuscripts

Frederick Banting Papers, Thomas Fisher Rare Book Library, University of Toronto
Polly Hoopes Beeman Papers, Crandall Public Library, Glens Falls
Charles Best Papers, Thomas Fisher Rare Book Library, University of Toronto
Charles Best Personal Collection, Thomas Fisher Rare Book Library, University of Toronto
Board of Governors, Insulin Committee, University of Toronto Archives
G. H. A. Clowes Papers, privately held
J. B. Collip Papers, Thomas Fisher Rare Book Library, University of Toronto
Connaught Laboratories Papers, Aventis Pasteur Limited, Toronto
Eli Lilly and Company Archives, Indianapolis
Sir Robert Falconer Papers, University of Toronto Archives
William R. Feasby Papers, Thomas Fisher Rare Book Library, University of Toronto
Simon Flexner Papers, American Philosophical Society, Philadelphia
William T. Gossett Papers, Bentley Library, University of Michigan
Charles Evans Hughes Papers, Butler Library, Columbia University
Charles Evans Hughes Papers, Library of Congress, Washington, D.C.
Charles Evans Hughes Papers, New York Public Library New York.
Elizabeth Hughes Papers, Thomas Fisher Rare Book Library, University of Toronto
Elliott P. Joslin Papers, Countway Library of Medicine, Harvard University
Elliott P. Joslin Papers, Marble Library, Joslin Center, Boston
W. L. Mackenzie King Papers, National Archives of Canada, Ottowa
J. J. R. Macleod Papers, Thomas Fisher Rare Book Library, University of Toronto
Office of the President Papers, Thomas Fisher Rare Book Library, University of Toronto
Physiatric Institute Papers, Morristown Historical Society, Morristown, New Jersey
Physiatric Institute Papers, Morristown Public Library, Morristown, New Jersey
Rockefeller Family Papers, Rockefeller Archive Center, Sleepy Hollow, New York
Rockefeller University Papers, Rockefeller Archive Center, Sleepy Hollow, New York

Books, Articles, Reports, Speeches

Adolph, Edward F. "Growing Up in the American Physiological Society." *Physiologist* 22, no. 5 (1979).

Allen, Frederick M. "Diabetes Mellitus." (1920), Reprinted from Nelson's Looseleaf, New York Academy of Medicine, New York.

———. "Present Results and Outlook of Diabetic Treatment." *Annals of Internal Medicine* 2, no. 2 (1928): 203–15.

———. *Glycosuria and Diabetes.* Cambridge: Harvard University Press, 1913.

———, and James W. Sherrill. "Clinical Observations With Insulin: 1. The Use of Insulin in Diabetic Treatment." *Journal of Metabolic Research* 2, no. 5–6 (1922): 803–985.

———, Edgar Stillman, and Reginald Fitz. *Total Dietary Regulation in the Treatment of Diabetes.* New York: Rockefeller Institute for Medical Research, 1919.

———. Unpublished Memoirs, private collection of Dr. Alfred Henderson.

American Diabetes Association. Minutes of Banquet Session. *The Proceedings of the American Diabetes Association* 9 (1949): 33–36.

American Journal of Physiology. *Proceedings of the American Journal of Physiology, Thirty-Fourth Annual Meeting held in New Haven, December 28, 29, 30, 1921,* Baltimore: Feb. 1, 1922.

Anthony, Carl Sferrazza. *Florence Harding: The First Lady, the Jazz Age, and the Death of America's Most Scandalous President.* New York: William Morrow and Company, 1998.

Banting, Frederick. "Account of the Discovery of Insulin." Sept. 1922. MS Coll. 76, Banting Papers, Thomas Fisher Rare Book Library, Toronto.

———. "Diabetes and Insulin: Nobel Lecture Delivered at Stockholm on Sept. 15, 1925." *Imprimerie Royale* (1925): 1–20.

———. "The History of Insulin." *Edinburgh Medical Journal* (Jan. 1929).

———. "Medical Research and the Discovery of Insulin." *Hygeia* (May 1924): 288–92.

———. Laboratory Notebook, May 18–19, 1921. Academy of Medicine, 123 (Banting), Folder 2, Thomas Fisher Rare Book Library.

———. Notebook, Jan. 1921–Aug. 10, 1921. MS Coll. 76, (Banting), Box 6A, Folder 3, Thomas Fisher Rare Book Library.

———. Notebook, Aug. 11–Sept. 16, 1921. MS Coll. 76 (Banting), Box 6A, Folder 7, Thomas Fisher Rare Book Library.

———. Notebook 3, Sep 12–16 1921. MS Coll. 76 (Banting), Box 6A, Folder 9, Thomas Fisher Rare Book Library.

———. Notebook 3A, Sept. 16–Dec. 22, 1921. MS Coll. 76 (Banting), Box 6A, Folder 11, Thomas Fisher Rare Book Library.

———. "Notes on First Examination of Elizabeth Hughes." Aug. 16, 1922. MS Coll. 76, Banting Papers, Thomas Fisher Rare Book Library, Toronto, Canada.

———. "Science and the Soviet Union." *Canadian Business* 9, no. 2 (Feb. 1936): 14+.

———. "The Story of the Discovery of Insulin" (1940). MS Coll. 76, Banting Papers, Thomas Fisher Rare Book Library, Toronto, Canada.

———, and C. H. Best. "The Internal Secretion of the Pancreas." *Journal of Laboratory and Clinical Medicine* 7, no. 5 (Feb. 1922): 251–66.

———, and C. H. Best. "Pancreatic Extracts." *Journal of Laboratory and Clinical Medicine* 7, no. 8 (May 1922).

———, C. H. Best, J. B. Collip, W. R. Campbell, J. J. R. Macleod, and E. C. Noble. "The Effect of Insulin on the Percentage Amounts of Fat and Glycogen in the Liver and Other Organs of Diabetic Animals." *Transactions of the Royal Society of Canada* 16, sec. V (1922): 13–16.

———, C. H. Best, J. B. Collip, W. R. Campbell, and A. A. Fletcher. "Pancreatic Extracts in the Treatment of Diabetes Mellitus." *Canadian Medical Association Journal* (March 1922).

———, C. H. Best, J. B. Collip, W. R. Campbell, and A. A. Fletcher. "Pancreatic Extracts in the Treatment of Diabetes Mellitus." *Canadian Medical Association Journal* (March 1922): 1–6.

———, C. H. Best, J. B. Collip, W. R. Campbell, A. A. Fletcher, J. J. R. Macleod, and E. C. Noble. "The Effect Produced on Diabetes by Extracts of Pancreas." *Transactions of the Association of American Physicians* (1922): 1–11.

———, C. H. Best, J. B. Collip, and J. J. R. Macleod. "The Preparation of Pancreatic Extracts Containing Insulin." *Transactions of the Royal Society of Canada* 16 Sec. V (1922).

———, C. H. Best, J. B. Collip, and J. J. R. Macleod. "The Effect of Insulin on the Excretion of Ketone Bodies by the Diabetic Dog." *Transactions of the Royal Society of Canada* 16, sec. V (1922): 17–18.

———, C. H. Best, J. B. Collip, J. J. R. Macleod, and E. C. Noble. "The Effects of Insulin on Experimental Hyperglycemia in Rabbits." *American Journal of Physiology* 62, no. 3 (1922): 559–80.

———, C. H. Best, J. B. Collip, J. J. R. Macleod, and E. C. Noble. "The Effect of Insulin on Normal Rabbits and on Rabbits Rendered Hyperglycaemia in Various Ways." *Transactions of the Royal Society of Canada* 16, sec. V (1922): 5–7.

———, W. R. Campbell, and A. A. Fletcher. "Insulin in the Treatment of Diabetes Mellitus." *Journal of Metabolic Research* 2, no. 5–6 (Nov.–Dec. 1922): 547–604.

———, and J. J. R. Macleod. *The Antidiabetic Functions of the Pancreas and the Successful Isolation of the Antidiabetic Hormone—Insulin.* Beaumont Foundation Annual Lecture Course II. St. Louis: C. V. Mosby Company, 1924.

"Banting the Artist." *Canadian Diabetic Association* 14 (First Quarter 1967): 8–13.

Barnett, Donald. *Elliott P. Joslin, M.D.: A Centennial Portrait.* Boston: Joslin Diabetes Center, 1998.

Barr, Murray Llewellyn. "James Bertram Collip, 1892–1965." *Biographical Memoirs of Fellows of the Royal Society* 19 (Dec. 1973). Bristol: John Wright and Sons Ltd., 1973: 235–67.

Barron, Moses. "Relation of the Islets of Langerhans to Diabetes With Special Reference to Cases of Pancreatic Lithiasis." *Surgery, Gynecology and Obstetrics* 31 (Nov. 1920): 437–48.

Batten, Jack. *The Annex: The Story of a Toronto Neighborhood.* Erin: Boston Mills Press, 2004.

Beerits, Henry. "Aftermath of a Senior Thesis." *Class of 1933 Newsletter,* 1992.

Bergman, Edward F. *Woodlawn Remembers: Cemetery of American History.* Utica, N.Y.: North Country Books, 1988.

Best, Charles. "Frederick Grant Banting, 1891–1941." *Obituary Notices of Fellows of the Royal Society* 4 (Nov. 1942): 21–26.

———. "Insulin and Diabetes—In Retrospect and in Prospect." *Canadian Medical Association Journal* 53 (1945): 204–12.

———. "Nineteen Hundred Twenty-One in Toronto." *Diabetes* 21, no. 2, suppl. (1972): 385–95.

———. "Reminiscences of the Researches Which Led to the Discovery of Insulin." *Canadian Medical Association Journal* 47 (Nov. 1942): 398–400.

———. "A Report of the Discovery and Development of the Knowledge of the Properties of Insulin." Sept. 1922. Unpublished. Feasby Collection, Thomas Fisher Rare Book Library.

Best, Henry B. M. *Margaret and Charley: The Personal Story of Dr. Charles Best, the Co-Discoverer of Insulin.* Toronto: Dundurn Group, 2003.

Bliss, Michael. *Banting: A Biography.* Toronto: University of Toronto Press, 1992.

———. *The Discovery of Insulin.* Chicago: University of Chicago Press, 1984.

———. "The Discovery of Insulin." *Textbook of Diabetes.* Vol. 1. London: Blackwell Scientific Publications, 1991.

———. "Historical Essay." *The Discovery of Insulin at the University of Toronto: An Exhibition*

Commemorating the 75th Anniversary. Ed. Katharine Martyn. Toronto: University of Toronto, 1996.

————. Transcribed unpublished biographical notes of Frederick M. Allen. Thomas Fisher Rare Book Library.

Bodenhamer, David J., and Robert G. Barrows, Eds. *The Encyclopedia of Indianapolis.* Bloomington: Indiana University Press, 1994.

Bridging the Years, Glens Falls, N.Y., 1763–1978. Glens Falls: Glens Falls Historical Association, 1978.

Brobeck, John R., Orr E. Reynolds, and Toby A. Appel, Eds. *History of the American Physiological Society: The First Century, 1887–1987.* Bethesda, Md.: American Physiological Society, 1987.

Brooks, Bradley C. *Oldfields.* Indianapolis: Indianapolis Museum of Art, 2004.

Bunn, Austin. "The Way We Live Now; 3-16-03; Body Check; The Bittersweet Science." *New York Times Magazine*, Mar. 16, 2003.

Burcar, Colleen. *You Know You're in Michigan When . . . 101 Quintessential Places, People, Events, Customs, Lingo, and Eats of the Great Lakes State.* Morris Book Publishing, 2005.

Burrow, Gerard N., et al. "A Case of Diabetes Mellitus." *New England Journal of Medicine* 306, no. 6 (Feb. 1982): 340–43.

Campbell, Walter R. "Dietetic Treatment in Diabetes Mellitus." *Canadian Medical Association Journal*: 13, no. 7 (July 1923): 487–92.

Campbell, Walter R. "Ketosis, Acidosis, and Coma Treated by Insulin." *Journal of Metabolic Research* 2, no. 5–6 (1922): 605–35.

Careless, J. M. S. *Toronto to 1918: An Illustrated History.* Toronto: James Lormer & Company, 1984.

Cavinder, Fred D. *The Indiana Book of Trivia.* Indianapolis: Indiana Historical Society Press, 2007.

Celebrating 75 Years Christ Church Cranbrook, 1928–2003. Christ Church Cranbrook, Published by University Lithoprinters, n.d.

"Charles E. Hughes: The Career and Public Services of the Republican Candidate for Governor." *New York*, Oct. 20, 1906.

Christ Church Cranbrook: A Visitor's Guide. Bloomfield Hills, Mich.: Christ Church Cranbrook, 1982.

Clark, Roscoe Collins. *Threescore Years and Ten: A Narrative of the First Seventy Years at Eli Lilly and Company, 1876–1946.* Chicago: Lakeside Press, 1946.

Clowes, G. H. A. "Banting Memorial Address." *Proceedings of the American Diabetes Association* 7 (1948): 49–60.

————. "Insulin in Its Relation to Life Insurance." Transcript of Address at the Seventeenth Annual Meeting of the Association of Life Insurance Presidents in New York, Dec. 7, 1923. Lilly Archives.

Clowes, George H. A., Jr. "George Henry Alexander Clowes: A Man of Science for All Seasons." *Journal of Surgical Oncology* 18 (1981): 197–217.

Collip, J. B. "Glucokinin: A New Hormone Present in Plant Tissue: Preliminary Paper." *Journal of Biological Chemistry* 56, no. 2 (June 1923): 513–43.

————. "Glucokinin: Second Paper." *Journal of Biological Chemistry* 57, no. 1 (Aug. 1923): 65–78.

————. "Glucokinin: An Apparent Synthesis in the Normal Animal of a Hypoglycemia— Producing Principle. Animal Passage of the Principle: Third Paper." *Journal of Biological Chemistry* 58, no. 1 (Nov. 1923): 163–208.

Cordery, Stacy A. *Alice Roosevelt Longworth, From White House Princess to Washington Power Broker.* New York: Viking, 2007.

Corner, George Washington A *History of the Rockefeller Institute: 1901–1953: Origins and Growth.* New York: Rockefeller Institute Press, 1964.

Cotter, Charis. *Toronto Between the Wars: Life in the City, 1919–1939.* Richmond Hill: Firefly Books, 2004.

Crosby, Alfred. *America's Forgotten Pandemic: The Influenza of 1918.* New York: Cambridge University Press, 2003.

Dale, Henry. "Fifty Years of Medical Research." *British Medical Journal* 2 (1963): 1287–1290.

Danelski, David J., and Joseph S. Tulchin, Eds. *The Autobiographical Notes of Charles Evans Hughes.* Cambridge, Mass.: Harvard University Press, 1973.

Davis, Kenneth C. *Don't Know Much About History: Everything You Need to Know About American History But Never Learned.* New York: Avon Books, 1990.

DeWitt, Lydia. "Morphology and Physiology of Areas of Langerhans in Some Vertebrates." *The Journal of Experimental Medicine* 8, no. 2 (March 1906): 193–239. *The Discovery of Insulin at the University of Toronto.* Thomas Fisher Rare Book Library, 1996.

Dominick, Angie. *Needles: A Memoir of Growing Up With Diabetes.* New York: Touchstone, 1998.

Duncan, Garfield G. "Frederick Madison Allen, 1879–1964." *Diabetes* 13, no. 3 (1964): 318–19.

Eckert, Kathryn Bishop. *Cranbrook.* New York: Princeton Architectural Press, 2001.

Eklund, Lowell. "A Tribute to Elizabeth Hughes Gossett." Christ Church Cranbrook, Bloomfield Hills, Mich. April 28, 1981.

Feasby, W. R. "The Discovery of Insulin." *Journal of the History of Medicine and Allied Sciences* 13, no. 1 (1958): 68–84.

Feudtner, Chris. *Bittersweet: Diabetes, Insulin and the Transformation of Illness.* Chapel Hill: University of North Carolina Press, 2003.

Filey, Mike. *A Toronto Album: Glimpses of the City That Was.* Toronto: Dundurn Press, 2001.

Fletcher, A. A., and W. R. Campbell. "The Blood Sugar Following Insulin Administration and The Symptom Complex—Hypoglycemia." *Journal of Metabolic Research* 2.5–6 (1922): 637–49.

Flexner, James Thomas. *An American Saga: The Story of Helen Thomas and Simon Flexner.* New York: Fordham University Press, 1993.

Freidel, Frank. *Presidents of the United States of America.* White House Historical Association, 1994.

Geyelin, Rawle H., et al. "The Use of Insulin in Juvenile Diabetes." *Journal of Metabolism Research* 2 (Nov. 1922): 767–91.

Gilchrist, Joseph, C. H. Best, and Frederick Banting. "Observations With Insulin on Department of Soldiers' Civil Re-Establishment Diabetics." *Canadian Medical Association Journal* (Aug. 1923).

Glad, Betty. *Charles Evans Hughes and the Illusions of Innocence.* Urbana: University of Illinois Press, 1966.

Goldstein, Erik. *The FirstWorld War Peace Settlements 1919–1925.* Essex: Pearson Education Limited, 2002.

———, and John Maurer, Eds. *The Washington Conference: 1921–22.* London: Frank Cass, 2002.

Gone but Not Forgotten—19th Century Mourning. Woodruff Fontaine House, APTA, Memphis Chapter. Memphis: 1989.

Gossett, Elizabeth Hughes. "Charles Evans Hughes: My Father the Chief Justice." *Supreme Court Historical Society Yearbook 1976.* Supreme Court Historical Society, 1976: 7–15.

Gossett, William T. "The Human Side of Chief Justice Hughes." *American Bar Association Journal* 59 (Dec. 1973), 1415–16.

———, Papers, Bentley Library, University of Michigan, Ann Arbor, Mich.

Gue, Benjamin F. *History of Iowa From the Earliest Times to the Beginning of the Twentieth Century.* Vol. 4, 1903.

Hamburger, Louis P. "Discussion of Dr. Banting's Paper on the Insulin Treatment of Diabetes Read Before the Baltimore City Medical Society." Dec. 14, 1922, Baltimore, Md. Unpublished. Banting Collection, Thomas Fisher Rare Book Library.

Hanlin, George. *Historic Photos of Indianapolis.* Nashville: Turner Publishing Company, 2006.

Harris, Captain E. S. *Lake George: All About It 1903.* Queensbury: Cambridge University Press, 2007.

Hazlett, Barbara E. "Historical Perspective: The Discovery of Insulin." *Clinical Diabetes Mellitus,* 3rd ed. Ed. Davidson, John K. New York, Thieme, 2000: 3–12.

Hendel, Samuel. *Charles Evans Hughes and the Supreme Court.* New York: King's Crown Press, 1951.

Henderson, Alfred R., "Frederick M. Allen, M.D., and the Psychiatric Institute at Morristown, N.J. (1920–1938)." *Academy of Medicine of New Jersey Bulletin* 16, no. 4 (1970).

Henretta, James A. "Charles Evans Hughes and the Strange Death of Liberal America." *Law and History Review* 24, no. 1 (2006).

Hill, Lewis Webb, and Rena S. Eckman. *The Starvation Treatment of Diabetes.* 3rd ed. Boston: W. M. Leonard, 1917.

Hughes, Charles Evans. *The Autobiographical Notes of Charles Evans Hughes.* Eds. David J. Danelski and Joseph S. Tulchin. Cambridge, Mass.: Harvard University Press, 1973.

Hutchinson, Woods. "Clearing the Skies for the Sugar-Poisoned." *Saturday Evening Post* 195, no. 50 (June 9, 1923).

Insulin Committee of the University of Toronto. "Insulin: Its Action, Its Therapeutic Value in Diabetes, and Its Manufacture." *Canadian Medical Association Journal* 13.7 (July 1923): 480–486.

Isaacson, Walter. *Einstein: His Life and Universe.* New York: Simon & Schuster, 2007.

Johnson, Steven. *The Ghost Map: The Story of London's Most Terrifying Epidemic and How it Changed Science, Cities, and the Modern World.* New York: RiverHead Books, 2006.

Joslin, Elliott P. "Address by Elliott P. Joslin." Dedication Exercises of the Lilly Research Laboratories, Oct. 11 and 12, 1934. *Lilly Research Laboratories Dedication.* Indianapolis: Eli Lilly and Company, 1934.

———. "Diabetes for the Diabetics: Ninth Banting Memorial Lecture of the British Diabetic Association." *Diabetes* 5, no. 2 (March–April 1956): 137–146.

———. *Diabetic Manual: Second Edition.* Philadelphia: Lea & Febiger, 1919.

———. "Pancreatic Extract in the Treatment of Diabetes." Letter to the Editor. *Boston Medical and Surgical Journal* 186, no. 19 (May 1922): 654. "Reminiscences of the Discovery of Insulin." *Diabetes* 5, no. 1 (Jan–Feb 1956): 67–68.

——— et al. "Insulin in Hospital and Home." *Journal of Metabolic Research* 2 (Nov.–Dec. 1922): 651–699.

Kahn, E.J., Jr. *All in a Century: The First 100 Years of Eli Lilly and Company.* Indianapolis: Eli Lilly and Co, 1976.

Kennedy, John F. *Profiles in Courage.* New York: Harper Collins, 2006.

Kettlewell, James K. *The Hyde Collection Catalogue.* Glens Falls, Hyde Collection, 1981.

Khalaf, Hala. *Young Voices: Life With Diabetes.* West Sussex, England: Novo Nordisk and John Wiley and Sons, 2005.

Kienast, Margate. "I Saw A Resurrection." *Saturday Evening* Post, July 2, 1938.

Knodel, Gerhardt. *Cranbrook Art Museum.* Bloomfield Hills: Cranbrook Art Museum, 2004.

Kolata, Gina. *Flu: The Story of the Great Influenza Pandemic of 1918 and the Search for the Virus That Caused It.* New York: Touchstone, 1999.

Krahl, M. E. "Obituary: George Henry Alexander Clowes, 1877–1958." *Cancer Research* 19, no. 3 (April 1959): 334–336.

Krouse, Charles. *Report: Preliminary to a Prospectus for the Establishment of an Institute for the Treatment and Investigation of Diabetes, Nephrites, High Blood Pressure, etc.* Report commissioned by Charles E. Hughes. June 19, 1920. Charles Evans Hughes Papers: Frederick M. Allen file. Butler Library, Columbia University, New York.

Leibel, B. S., and G. A. Wrenshall. *Insulin:* Toronto: Canadian Diabetic Association/University of Toronto Press, 1971.

Levinson, Paul D. "Eighty Years of Insulin Therapy: 1922–2002." *Medicine and Health Rhode Island* 86 (April 2003): 101–106.

Li, Alison, *J. B. Collip and the Development of Medical Research in Canada.* Quebec: McGill–Queens University Press, 2003.

Lilly Doll, The Children's Museum, Indianapolis.

The Lilly Library: The First Quarter Century 1960–1985. Bloomington: Indiana University Press, 1985.

Lilly Research Laboratories: Dedication. Indianapolis: Eli Lilly and Co, 1935.

Lowry, Edward G. *Washington Close-Ups: Intimate Views of Some Public Figures.* Boston: Houghton Mifflin Company, 1921.

Macfarlane, Ian A. "The Millenia Before Insulin." *Textbook of Diabetes.* Vol. 1. London: Blackwell Scientific Publications, 1991.

Macleod, J. J. R. "History of the Researches Leading to the Discovery of Insulin." *Bulletin of the History of Medicine* 52, no. 3 (1978): 295–312.

———. "Insulin." *Physiology Reviews* 4, no. 1 (Jan. 1924).

———. "The Physiology of Insulin and Its Source in the Animal Body: Nobel Lecture Delivered at Stockholm of May 26.1925." *Imprimerie Royale* (1925): 1–12.

———. "The Source of Insulin: A Study of the Effect Produced on Blood Sugar by Extracts of the Pancreas and Principal Islets of Fishes." *Journal of Metabolic Research* 2, no. 2 (Aug. 1922): 149–172.

———, and W. R. Campbell. *Insulin: Its Use in the Treatment of Diabetes.* Baltimore: William & Wilkins Company, 1925.

Madeb, Ralph, Leonidas G. Koniaris, and Seymour I. Schwartz, "The Discovery of Insulin: The Rochester, New York, Connection." *Annals of Internal Medicine*, vol. 143 no. 12 (Dec. 2005) 907–12.

Madison, James H. *Eli Lilly: A Life, 1885–1977.* Indianapolis: Indiana Historical Society Press, 2006.

———. *Indiana Through Tradition and Change: A History of the Hoosier State and Its People 1920–1945.* Indianapolis: Indianapolis Historical Society, 1982.

Mayer, Ann Margaret. *Sir Frederick Banting: Doctor Against Diabetes.* Mankato: Creative Education, 1974.

McAuliffe, Alicia. *Growing Up With Diabetes.* New York: John Wiley and Sons, 1998.

McCormick, Gene (former Eli Lilly and Company historian), unpublished notes, papers and interviews.

McCormick, N. A. "Insulin From Fish." *Bulletin of the Biological Board of Canada* (Dec. 1924).

McDonald, John P. *Images of America: Lost Indianapolis.* Charleston: Arcadia, 2002.

McMechan, Jervis Bell. *Christ Church Cranbrook: A History of the Parish to Commemorate the 50th Anniversary of the Consecration of the Church, 1928–1978.* Bloomfield Hills: Christ Church Cranbrook, 1979.

Messinger, Robert, and Laura Messinger. *Why Me? Why Did I Have to Get Diabetes?* Hiawatha: Little Mai Press, 2004.

Morganstern, Jacob. *Ment. Hosp.* 2: 2, June 1951, American Psychiatric Association.

The New York Society Library Annual Report. 2005–2006. Pamphlet.

Noble, E. Clark. Unpublished Account Outlining Discovery of Insulin. March 17, 1977. Thomas Fisher Rare Book Library, Toronto.

Noble, R. L. "Memories of James Bertram Collip." *The Canadian Medical Association Journal* 93 (Dec. 1965): 1356–64.

Palmer, Gwen, et al. *Images of America: Glens Falls.* Chicago: Arcadia Publishing, 2004.

Paulesco, Nicolas. "Action de l'extrait pancréatique injecté dans le sang, chez un animal diabétique." *Comptes Rendus Hebdomadaires des Séances et Mémoires de la Sociéte de Biologie* 85 (July 1921): 555–59.

Perkins, Dexter. *Charles Evans Hughes and American Democratic Statesmanship.* Boston: Little, Brown and Company: 1956.

Phillips, Clifton. *Indiana in Transition: 1880–1920.* Vol. 4. Indianapolis: Indiana Historical Bureau and Indiana Historical Society, 1968.

The Physiatric Institute. Morristown, N.J.: Physiatric Institute. Charles Evans Hughes Papers: Frederick M. Allen file. Butler Library, Columbia University.

Pickup, John, and Gareth Williams, Eds. *Textbook of Diabetes.* Vol. 1. London: Blackwell Scientific Publications, 1991.

Pietrusza, David. *1920: The Year of the Six Presidents.* New York: Carroll and Graf, 2007.

Price, Nelson. *Indianapolis: Then and Now.* San Diego: Thunder Bay Press, 2004.

Pusey, Merlo J. *Charles Evans Hughes.* New York: Macmillan, 1951.

Rinehart, Victoria E. *Portrait of Healing—Curing in the Woods.* Utica: North Country Books, 2002.

Rutty, Christopher J. "Couldn't Live Without It: Diabetes, the Cost of Innovation and the Price of Insulin in Canada, 1922–1984." *Canadian Bulletin of Medical History* 25, no. 2 (2008): 407–31.

———. "Robert Davies Defries (1889–1975): Canada's 'Mr. Public Health.'" *Doctors, Nurses and Practitioners.* Ed. Lois N. Magner. Westport: Greenwood Press, 1997: 62–69.

Sacks, Oliver. *Seeing Voices: A Journey Into the World of the Deaf.* New York: Harper Perennial Edition, 1990.

Schoen, Douglas. *On the Campaign Trail: The Long Road of Presidential Politics, 1860–2004.* New York: HarperCollins, 2004.

Scott, E. L. "On the Influence of Intravenous Injections of an Extract of the Pancreas on Experimental Pancreatic Diabetes. *American Journal of Physiology* 29, no. 3 (1912): 306–10.

Sharpey-Schäfer, Edward. *An Introduction to the Study of Endocrine Glands and Internal Secretions: Lane Medical Lectures, 1913.* Palo Alto: Stanford University Press (1914): 84.

Shaw, Margaret Mason. *He Conquered Death: The Story of Frederick Grant Banting.* Toronto: Macmillan, 1946.

The Scottish Society of the History of Medicine: Report of the Proceedings—Session 1996–97 and 1997–98.

Silver, Joel. *J. K. Lilly Jr., Bibliophile.* Bloomington: Lilly Library—Indiana University, 1993.

Silver Bay Association: Pictorial History 1900–1935. Silver Bay: Silver Bay Association, 1992.

Silver Bay YMCA of the Adirondacks.

Sinding, Christiane. "Making the Unit of Insulin: Standards, Clinical Work, and Industry, 1920–1925." *Bulletin of the History of Medicine* 76, no. 2 (2002) 231–70.

Smith, Kay. *Bloomfield Blossoms.* Bloomfield Hills: Bloomfield Township Bicentennial Commission, 1976.

Sterngass, Jon. *First Resorts: Pursuing Pleasure at Saratoga Springs, Newport, and Coney Island.* Baltimore: John Hopkins University Press, 2001.

Stevenson, Lloyd. *Sir Frederick Banting.* Toronto: Ryerson Press, 1946.

Striker, Cecil. *Famous Faces in Diabetes.* Boston: G. K. Hall and Co., 1961.

Tenuth, Jeffrey. *Indianapolis: A Circle City History.* Charleston: Arcadia Publishing, 2004.

Toobin, Jeffrey. *The Nine: Inside the Secret World of the Supreme Court.* New York: Doubleday, 2007.

Trachtman, Michael G. *The Supremes' Greatest Hits: The 34 Supreme Court Cases That Most Directly Affect Your Life.* New York: Sterling Publishing, 2006.

Tucker, Spencer, ed. *World War I; Encyclopedia.* Santa Barbara: ABC-CLIO, 2005.

U.S. Bureau of the Census. *Statistical Atlas of the United States, 1914.* Washington, D.C., 1914.

Waite, F. C. *Western Reserve University: Centennial History of the School of Medicine.* Cleveland: Western Reserve University Press, 1946.

Worman, E. Clark. *The Silver Bay Story.* Buffalo: Silver Bay Association, 1952.

White, Priscilla, M.D. "The Diabetic Child." *Pediatric Problems in Clinical Practice.* H. Michal-Smith, ed. New York: Grune and Stratton, 1954

Wilder, Russell M., Walter M. Boothby, Clifford J. Barborka, Hubert D. Kitchen, and Samuel F. Adams. "Clinical Observations on Insulin." *Journal of Metabolic Research* 2, no. 5–6 (Nov.–Dec. 1922): 703–728.

Williams, John R., "A Clinical Study of the Effects of Insulin in Severe Diabetes." *Journal of Metabolic Research* 2.5–6 (Nov.–Dec. 1922): 729–51.

Williams, Michael J. "J. J. R. Macleod: The Co-Discoverer of Insulin." *Proceeding of the Royal College of Physicians of Edinburgh* 23, no. 3 (July 1993): viii–125.

Woodbury, David Oakes. "Please Save My Son." *Reader's Digest* (Feb. 1963): 54–57. MS Coll. 241 (Best) Box 61, Folder 18, Thomas Fisher Rare Book Library, Toronto.

Woodyatt, R.T. "The Clinical Use of Insulin." *Journal of Metabolism Research* (Nov. 1922): 793–801.

World Health Organization. *World Health* (Feb.–March 1971).

Wrenshall, G.A., and G. Hetenyl. *The Story of Insulin: Forty Years of Success Against Diabetes.* Bloomington: Indiana University Press, 1964.

Yan, Kun. *The Story and Discovery of Insulin.* Bloomington: AuthorHouse, 2005.

Yapp, Nick. *1910s.* London: Könemann, 1998.

Yapp, Nick. *1920s.* London: Könemann, 1998.

ACKNOWLEDGMENTS

Many people gave generously of their time and attention in helping us tell this extraordinary story. We are very grateful to the Thomas Fisher Rare Book Library at the University of Toronto, especially Richard Landon, Director; Anne Dondertman, Assistant Director; Loryl MacDonald, Records Archivist; Garron Wells, University Archivist; and Jennifer Toews, Manuscript Collections; Lisa Bayne, Chief Archivist at Eli Lilly and Company; Morry Smulevitz, Scott MacGregor, Thane Wettig, Adam Fairfield, and Kelley Murphy of Eli Lilly and Company; Louise Mirrer, Jean Ashton, Stephen Edidin, Mary Kilbourn, Laura Washington, and Dale Gregory of the New-York Historical Society; and Rita Ormsby of the William and Anita Newman Library, Baruch College.

We thank Saundra Ketner at the Joslin Diabetes Center's Marble Library; Susan Sutton, Steve Haller, Paul Brockman, Dorothy Nicholson, and Betsy Caldwell of the Indiana Historical Society; Rebekah Marshall of the Indianapolis Museum of Art; Marcia Caudell and Rachael Adele Heger of the Indiana State Library; Breon Mitchell and Erika Dowell of the Lilly Library at Indiana University; Tara Craig, Janet Gertz, and Jane Siegel of Columbia University's Butler Library; Louisa Moy and Eric Neubacher of Baruch College; Karen Jania at the Bentley Historical Society; Jack Eckert of the Harvard Medical Library; Millie Seiler of the John R. Williams Health Science Library in Rochester, N.Y.; Professor James Madison of Indiana University; Daun Van Ee and the Manuscript Division at the Library of Congress; W. Bruce Fye, Hilary Lane, Robert A. Rizza, and Renee E. Ziemer of the

Mayo Clinic; Carie Levin of the Morris County Historical Society; Michael MacDonald of the National Archives of Canada; Winifred S. King at the New York Academy of Medicine; Charles Greifenstein and Valerie-Anne Lutz of the American Philosophical Society; Amy Fitch at the Rockefeller Archive Center; Paul G. Anderson and Pat Gunn of the Bernard Becker Medical Library at the Washington University School of Medicine; Christ Church Cranbrook in Bloomfield Hills, Michigan; the Bloomfield Hills Library and the Bloomfield Hills Historical Society; Janna Bennett at the Children's Museum in Indianapolis; Erica Burke at the Crandall Public Library in Glens Falls, New York; George Goodwin at the Bolton Historical Museum in Bolton Landing, New York; Grant Maltman at the Banting House Historical Site in London, Ontario; Hugh W. McNaught at Connaught Laboratories; Graeme McAlister of the Royal College of Physicians of Edinburgh, Scotland; Kathy Shurtleff at the Supreme Court Historical Society; Angela Klitzsch of the Clowes Fund; Marty Fink at the YMCA of the Adirondacks; Paul Mercer of the New York State Library; Kelli Crandall of the Crown Hill Funeral Home and Cemetery in Indianapolis; Woodlawn Cemetery in New York; Glens Falls Historical Society; Glens Falls Public Library; Wolfeboro Historical Society; and Cynthia L. Scott of the Wolfeboro Public Library.

We especially thank Jacqueline Anderson, wife of Maxwell Anderson, the director of the Indianapolis Museum of Art, for taking us on a tour of Westerly, G. H. A. Clowes's former residence. This house was donated by the Clowes family to the Indianapolis Museum of Art, and is now the residence of the museum's director. We also thank Bradley C. Brooks, who took us through Oldfields, the former home of J. K. Lilly Jr., which was donated to the Indianapolis Museum of Art.

A huge thank-you to our literary agent, Arthur Klebanoff, whose faith in the importance of our story helped transform it into the book you now hold in your hands. His hard work and effort are truly appreciated. We were inspired by the wisdom and encouragement of Michael Rudell, who during the past five years has reached out to a number of people to help shepherd this project.

At St. Martin's Press, we are grateful to our editor Phil Revzin and to president and publisher Sally Richarson for their early enthusiasm and oversight. Kenneth J. Silver and Kylah Goodfellow-McNeill steered our book along the final leg of its journey. Donald J. Davidson contributed thoughtful copyediting. John Murphy and his team helped with publicity. We thank you all.

We are also grateful to our administrative assistant, researcher, and friend Korenne Morelli, whose dedication and perseverance were invaluable to this project.

For their interest and support along the way, we thank Dr. Alfred Henderson and his daughters Mary Kaplan and Pat Lightfoot, without whom we would have a much poorer understanding of Dr. Allen's life. And for favors large and small we thank Sally Bock, Dr. Alexander Clowes, Maria Mercedes D'Antona, Dr. Susan Detweiler, Bruce and Mary Ann Gingles, Silissa Kenney, Mara and Stephen Kupperman, Christine Luu, Neil Rosini, Maxine Schweitzer, and Elizabeth Sugarman.

Finally, it would be hard to overstate how much we appreciate those few trusted and very carefully selected friends and family members who read and commented on early versions of the manuscript: Jessica and Joseph Ainsberg; Suzy and Richard Ainsberg; Marita Begley; Dale and Max Berger; Pam Bernstein; Robert Blinder; Dan and Jean Carmalt; Lynne Coll, Barbara Cooper, Jim Cooper, Harriette Delsener; Jeany Duncan; Linda and Richard Gesoff; Judy and Bob Golomb; Dr. Graham Ogle of the Life for a Child program; Paul Ridge, Craig Rochester, Mina Samuels and especially Michaela Murphy. Your time, thoughtful consideration, and encouragement buoyed our confidence and bettered our book.

INDEX

1. A few months after the initial batch of newspaper stories reporting her miraculous recovery, Elizabeth Hughes chose to disappear from the public eye and keep her diabetes and treatments a secret for the rest of her life, even from her own children until they were eighteen-years-old. Why do you think she made that decision? Does looking at the context of that era and her circumstances help explain it?

2. Elizabeth strives for "normalcy." How do you define normalcy? Is there such a thing?

3. When Charles Evans Hughes ponders whether he should call President Harding on Elizabeth's behalf, he wonders "[w]as his responsibility to the principles he had sworn to abide by greater than his responsibility to his daughter? One was broad, the other deep. Which was the greater good?" (p.186) What is your opinion?

4. When Banting attempts to secure research funding and a lab, he is rebuffed because his theories have been tested and failed before. His response is, "I'm not trying to be original. I'm trying to find something that works!" (p.67) What lessons can we learn from his ultimate success?

5. Discuss the nature of the rivalry between Banting and Macleod. Are such professional rivalries ultimately productive or counterproductive?

6. Consider these reflections about Charles Evans Hughes: "Living is by necessity a process of continuous loss. As we live we lose time, we lose innocence, we lose family and friends, we lose memories and the longer we live, the more we lose. Ultimately, we lose the process of losing itself, which is what living is to begin with." (p.212) Do you agree? How are we defined by our losses?

7. Banting once told an audience, "We do not know whence ideas come, but the importance of the idea in medical research cannot be overestimated. From the nature of things ideas do not come from prosperity, affluence and contentment, but rather from the blackness of despair, not in the

bright light of day … but rather in the quiet, undisturbed hours of midnight … when one can be alone to think.…" (p.229) Do you agree with Banting's view of the nature of ideas? If so, what does this mean for modern scientific breakthroughs?

8. Frederick Allen, like Banting, appeared to place financial compensation second to the goal of patient treatment. For example, when writing the budget for the Physiatric Institute, Allen did not include a personal salary in the budget. Allen often felt conflicted with his job as a doctor caring for patients, and raising the funds to keep the institute open. Are these roles necessarily at odds with one another? Do you think this conflict remains in modern medicine?

9. Throughout the book, Antoinette and Charles Evans Hughes are portrayed as sympathetic parents who dearly love their daughter. Yet, after bringing her to Toronto to be treated by Dr. Banting—with what was then an experimental treatment that could save her life or hasten her death—Charles and Antoinette sail for Brazil. It is with Dr. Banting and her nurse, Blanche, that Elizabeth spends the most crucial and precarious time of her young life. Were you surprised that her parents would leave her in Toronto? What does this say about the familial relationships of the time period, and how might that relationship have affected Elizabeth's perception of her disease? Why do you think she didn't stay in contact with Blanche or Dr. Banting after she recovered her health?

10. Ultimately the intervention of Eli Lilly enables the mass production of insulin as described in the book. Considered a radical idea at the time, Lilly believed the future of pharmaceutical manufacturing lay in fundamental biological research, saying, "Ideas don't cure people. Drugs cure people. … That's why we must bring the research scientists and the drug manufacturers together." Do you think this statement still holds true today? Would greater cooperation mean further advancements?

11. We get an extensive overview of the world in *Breakthrough*, including the political and social circumstances, and the myriad of conditions that led to, and at times hindered, the scientific advancement. What are some of the events that inadvertently affected this medical breakthrough? How precarious was the discovery? At what point can it be said that fate intervened?

12. How did reading this book affect, if at all, your view of what it's like to live with a chronic condition? Did it change your view of the research or pharmaceutical-production side of the equation?

A
Reading
Group
Guide

For more reading group suggestions, visit
www.readinggroupgold.com.

St. Martin's
Griffin